SPONTANEOUS BACTERIAL PERITONITIS

SPONTANEOUS BACTERIAL PERITONITIS

The Disease, Pathogenesis, and Treatment

Harold O. Conn

Yale University School of Medicine
New Haven, Connecticut, and
University of Miami School of Medicine
Miami, Florida

Juan Rodés
Miguel Navasa

Hospital Clínic i Provincial de Barcelona
University of Barcelona
Barcelona, Spain

with contributions by

Xavier Aldeguer, Vicente Arroyo, Pere Ginès,
Carlos Guarner, Josep Maria Llovet, Ramon Planas, Antoni Rimola,
Joan M. Salmerón, Germán Soriano, Pau Sort, Roser Vega

MARCEL DEKKER, INC.   NEW YORK · BASEL

ISBN: 0-8247-0355-3

This book is printed on acid-free paper.

Headquarters
Marcel Dekker, Inc.
270 Madison Avenue, New York, NY 10016
tel: 212-696-9000; fax: 212-685-4540

Eastern Hemisphere Distribution
Marcel Dekker AG
Hutgasse 4, Postfach 812, CH-4001 Basel, Switzerland
tel: 41-61-261-8482; fax: 41-61-261-8896

World Wide Web
http://www.dekker.com

The publisher offers discounts on this book when ordered in bulk quantities. For more
information, write to Special Sales/Professional Marketing at the headquarters address
above.

Current printing (last digit):
10 9 8 7 6 5 4 3 2 1

PRINTED IN THE UNITED STATES OF AMERICA

Preface

Although spontaneous bacterial peritonitis (SBP) is technically a new clinical syndrome that was reported for the first time in 1964, we suspect that it is really an old, overlooked disease that has existed as long as cirrhosis itself. Our suspicions are based on several lines of reasoning. First, we have identified 42 previously published case reports in the world's literature in which the key components of the SBP syndrome were described, but without recognition of the full syndrome per se. These features include cirrhosis, ascites, the sudden onset of abdominal pain, and evidence of intra-abdominal, enteric bacterial infection, in the absence of any obvious explanation such as the perforation of a hollow abdominal viscus or any possible exogenous source of contamination. Neither the name of the syndrome nor its probable pathogenesis as we understand it now was recognized in these early reports.

Second, there is nothing that is dramatically novel about any one component of the syndrome, such as the presence of a new infectious agent, that has characterized the recent discovery of other new syndromes such as the human immunodeficiency virus (HIV) in AIDS or a unique histological pattern such as the microvesicular fat deposition in the viscera as in Reye's syndrome. Rather, it appears to consist of the concurrence of common symptoms and signs arranged in a consistent pattern. Furthermore, there are no definitive histological lesions that, if found at autopsy, would unequivocally identify SBP.

Third, as is often the case, once SBP, or another new syndrome, is described it suddenly seems to be everywhere. SBP appears to be present in from 3% to 39% of recent retrospective and prospective series of cirrhotic patients (Chapter 4). These studies probably underestimate its prevalence, as suggested by new developments in the bacteriological diagnosis of SBP.

SBP has grown like Topsy and involves many variants of the basic syndrome—variations on a theme—each of which is described in detail and discussed from the clinical pathogenetic, diagnostic, and therapeutic points of view. Although we have attempted to make sure that none of these considerations is overlooked or omitted, there may be some repetition.

We have done several literature searches and estimate that approximately 4500 articles on this disorder have been cataloged under the term ''spontaneous bacterial peritonitis'' in the literature during the 35 years following the initial description of this syndrome. The sudden flood of publications on this subject is largely a ''me, too'' phenomenon. It baffles the authors of this volume how such a common, dramatic, frequently fatal disorder could have completely escaped detection for so long. Its acceptance as a bona fide disease has stimulated an enormous amount of interest and research about its diagnosis, pathogenesis, prognosis, treatment, and prevention. It has spawned a series of descriptions of variant syndromes and articles about new concepts of the pathobacteriology of the liver, the body's sequestration of bacteria within its anatomic compartments, and the ways in which bacteria traverse these boundaries. Bacterial translocation (BT), a new, pathogenetic concept that temporally parallels SBP, is an ideal example. All of these publications are creating a body of literature demonstrating that SBP is a well-defined and well-established disorder with far-reaching ramifications. Furthermore, we believe that we have seen only the tip of this iceberg.

The topic SBP has already generated many unanticipated findings. As indicated above, SBP has stimulated a new look at the process of bacterial translocation, the critical factor in the pathogenesis of SBP. The recently recognized association between SBP and gastrointestinal hemorrhage raises new and fascinating questions (J Goulis et al, Hepatology 27:1207, 1999). Similarly, the recognition of the concurrence of SBP and renal failure, although not completely elucidated, promises to improve our understanding and treatment of this disorder.

Our approach to organizing this book is relatively simple. We have divided the book into three parts: The Disease, Pathogenesis, and Treatment. The first two portions were written by Harold O. Conn, who was one of the first on the scene when SBP was recognized. He has presented the history of spontaneous bacterial peritonitis, including a chronological listing of major developments during the last 35 years, in Chapter 1. The clinical manifestations of these syndromes are described in Chapters 2 (typical) and 3 (atypical). Chapter 4, on the prevalence of SBP, follows. A concise description and discussion of tuberculous peritonitis (TBP) is then presented in Chapter 5.

Part II, on pathogenesis, begins with ''Clinical Pathogenesis of Sponta-

neous Bacterial Peritonitis'' (Chapter 6), which is based almost entirely on a
series of previously published descriptions of the pathogenesis of SBP that
defined this disorder. Chapters 7 and 8, which conclude the section on pathogenesis, emphasize the many disorders, procedures, and substances that may
induce or prevent the induction of bacterial translocation, which is the pathogenetic key to the puzzle of SBP.

We have specifically emphasized the plurality of the syndromes that
constitute SBP and related disorders. There are many variations on this theme.
Clinically silent SBP exists, and SBP may occur in the absence of any or all of
its laboratory abnormalities. There are parallel syndromes that follow similar
pathogenetic guidelines, such as *spontaneous pleuritis* (empyema), *spontaneous bacterial arthritis*, and *spontaneous bacterial meningitis*. Certainly, there
are specific pathogenetic differences from SBP in these related syndromes that
remain to be elucidated. Other related disorders may mimic SBP.

SBP may occur occasionally in patients without cirrhosis, including
those with chronic active or acute fulminant hepatitis. *Nonspontaneous bacterial peritonitis* may be one of the most difficult differential diagnoses in medicine. SBP may also occur in the absence of liver disease, such as in patients
with the nephrotic syndrome, rheumatoid arthritis, or disseminated lupus
erythematosus. Again, the reasons for the differences remain unclear. *Tuberculous peritonitis* (TBP), which is a spontaneous bacterial infection of the peritoneum, may occur precisely in the same way as SBP, except for the nature of the
infecting organism, but it carries its own stigmata and prognosis. The different
infectious agents give rise to different clinical and laboratory manifestations
and different host responses, as exemplified by the granulocytic leukocytosis
in SBP and the lymphocytosis of TBP. Usually the spread of the infection is
very different from the hematogenous dissemination of miliary tuberculosis,
which is more like that of SBP.

The third portion of the book was written by Dr. Juan Rodés and his
team of experts, led by Dr. Miguel Navasa, the third coauthor. They have
studied this disease extensively and have performed a large series of objective
investigations to assess the methods of making the diagnosis of SBP and of
treating it effectively over a period of many years. The chapters in this section,
which focus primarily on the prognosis, therapy, and prevention of SBP, were
prepared by Dr. Rodés and his team, who have performed innumerable randomized clinical trials to determine the most efficacious antibiotic agents in
the treatment and prophylaxis of SBP. They have compared antibiotic agents,
their routes of administration, their dosage, and the duration of therapy. Similarly, they have performed objective studies comparing large paracenteses with
diuretic therapy and portal decompressive procedures. Currently they are

studying renal impairment in SBP, the key prognostic complication of SBP. Finally, they have dealt with the effects and efficacy of liver transplantation in the management and elimination of ascites, and thereby of SBP, and present their opinions on diverse issues.

Harold O. Conn served as the Coordinating Editor of this volume. Each of the authors has devoted large portions of his professional life to SBP and related issues and hopes to transmit his interest, excitement, and knowledge about these disorders to the readers of this book.

Harold O. Conn
Juan Rodés
Miguel Navasa

ACKNOWLEDGMENTS

Two people who were absolutely essential to the creation of this volume, in addition to the contributors to its constituent chapters, especially my coauthors, Juan Rodés and Miguel Navasa, are Irene Cowern and Marilyn Barr Conn. Irene, who had been my last secretary at Yale, before I ''retired,'' eagerly returned to the fold at my request. Irene is a typist extraordinaire and a dedicated worker, who is willing to work in sickness and in health, and who has done so. In addition, she understands how a computer works and how to bypass its flaws when it doesn't do so properly, an invaluable expertise in these days of total dependence on cybernetics.

I am also grateful for the many thoughtful searches and great bibliographic assistance performed by Joan McGinnis, my long-time friend, colleague, and collaborator, and Chief Medical Librarian at the DVA Hospital, West Haven, Connecticut.

I also acknowledge the generous and invaluable assistance of Professor J. Wesley Alexander of the University of Cincinnati for providing the electron microscopic photomicrographs that illustrate Chapter 7, on the pathogenesis of SBP, and for reproviding them when they were lost during processing. I thank him for his generosity and his awesome display of faith.

I also acknowledge the contribution of many colleagues who contributed individual photomicrographs and tables to the greater glory of the volume.

Marilyn Barr Conn, who is a superb editor, typist, and office manager and my best friend and wife of too many years to enumerate, is my inspiration and my most valuable critic.

Harold O. Conn

Contents

Preface   *iii*

Contributors   *ix*

Part I   The Disease

1   History of Spontaneous Bacterial Peritonitis with an Appendix
    on the Chronology of the Disease   1
    Harold O. Conn

2   Clinical Patterns of Spontaneous Bacterial Peritonitis:
    Variations on a Theme   25
    Harold O. Conn

3   Unusual Presentations of Spontaneous Bacterial Peritonitis   47
    Harold O. Conn

4   Prevalence of Spontaneous Bacterial Peritonitis   75
    Harold O. Conn

5   Tuberculous Peritonitis   87
    Harold O. Conn

Part II: Pathogenesis

6   Clinical Pathogenesis of Spontaneous Bacterial Peritonitis   101
    Harold O. Conn

7   Bacterial Translocation: Studies of Mice and Men   113
    Harold O. Conn

8   Prevention of Bacterial Translocation   153
    Harold O. Conn

Part III: Treatment

9   Prognosis of Spontaneous Bacterial Peritonitis   187
    Xavier Aldeguer, Roser Vega, Josep Maria Llovet, and
    Ramon Planas

10 General Management of Patients with Spontaneous Bacterial
    Peritonitis   205
    Joan M. Salmerón, Miguel Navasa, and Juan Rodés

11 Antibiotic Therapy of Spontaneous Bacterial Peritonitis   219
    Miguel Navasa and Juan Rodés

12 Risk Factors for Spontaneous Bacterial Peritonitis in Cirrhosis:
    Efficacy of Norfloxacin in Preventing Recurrence of SBP   233
    Pere Ginès, Pau Sort, and Vicente Arroyo

13 Primary Prophylaxis of Spontaneous Bacterial Peritonitis   255
    Germán Soriano and Carlos Guarner

14 Liver Transplantation in Cirrhotic Patients with Spontaneous
    Bacterial Peritonitis   285
    Antoni Rimola

Index   297

Contributors

Xavier Aldeguer, M.D. Department of Gastroenterology, Hospital Universitari Germans Trias i Pujol, Badalona, Spain

Vicente Arroyo, M.D. Professor of Medicine, Liver Unit, Institut de Malalties Digestives, Hospital Clínic i Provincial de Barcelona, University of Barcelona, Barcelona, Spain

Harold O. Conn, M.S., M.D., F.R.C.P., F.A.C.P. Professor of Medicine, Emeritus, Department of Internal Medicine, Yale University School of Medicine, New Haven, Connecticut, and Clinical Professor of Surgery, Division of Liver and Bowel Transplantation, University of Miami School of Medicine, Miami, Florida

Pere Ginès, M.D. Liver Unit, Institut de Malalties Digestives, Hospital Clínic i Provincial de Barcelona, University of Barcelona, Barcelona, Spain

Carlos Guarner, M.D. Chief, Liver Section, Department of Gastroenterology, Hospital de la Santa Creu i Sant Pau, Universitat Autónoma de Barcelona, Barcelona, Spain

Josep Maria Llovet, M.D. Department of Gastroenterology, Hospital Universitari Germans Trias i Pujol, Badalona, Spain

Miguel Navasa, M.D.   Associate Professor of Medicine, Liver Unit, Hospital Clínic i Provincial de Barcelona, University of Barcelona, Barcelona, Spain

Ramon Planas, M.D.   Associate Professor and Head, Liver Section, Department of Gastroenterology, Hospital Universitari Germans Trias i Pujol, Badalona, Spain

Antoni Rimola, M.D.   Associate Professor of Medicine, Liver Unit, Hospital Clinic i Provincial de Barcelona, University of Barcelona, Barcelona, Spain

Juan Rodés, M.D., F.R.C.P.   Professor of Medicine and Head, Liver Unit, Hospital Clínic i Provincial de Barcelona, University of Barcelona, Barcelona, Spain

Joan M. Salmerón, M.D.   Senior Specialist, Liver Unit and Intensive Care Unit, Hospital Clínic i Provincial de Barcelona, University of Barcelona, Barcelona, Spain

Germán Soriano, M.D.   Liver Unit, Department of Gastroenterology, Hospital de la Santa Creu i Sant Pau, Universitat Autónoma de Barcelona, Barcelona, Spain

Pau Sort, M.D.   Liver Unit, Institut de Malalties Digestives, Hospital Clínic i Provincial de Barcelona, Barcelona, Spain

Roser Vega, M.D.   Department of Gastroenterology, Hospital Universitari Germans Trias i Pujol, Badalona, Spain

SPONTANEOUS BACTERIAL PERITONITIS

1

History of Spontaneous Bacterial Peritonitis with an Appendix on the Chronology of the Disease

Harold O. Conn
Yale University School of Medicine, New Haven, Connecticut, and University of Miami School of Medicine, Miami, Florida

You've come a long way, baby.

I. INTRODUCTION

The appearance of a random cluster of cases of spontaneous bacterial peritonitis (SBP) at the West Haven Veterans Administration Hospital (WHVAH) in Connecticut in the early 1960s was my first introduction to this syndrome, and a stroke of good fortune for me personally. As a faculty member of the Yale University School of Medicine assigned to the Liver Disease service at the WHVAH, I was in a position to serve as midwife at the birth of the SBP syndromes. Indeed, I use the plural—*SBP syndromes*—because SBP is a number of related disorders. Therefore, I shall present the history of SBP from a personal point of view.

I am convinced that SBP, which is now readily recognized, has existed as long as cirrhosis itself. Cirrhosis was first described in the 17th century (1) and Laënnec and others reported it formally in the early 19th century (2,3). Why had these syndromes not been discovered previously? It is my opinion that the first of half of the 20th century was the end of a long, dark, almost medieval period in medicine and the beginning of a renaissance of clinical curiosity and accomplishment. It was a time of rapid advancement in clinical

1

medicine, in increased research funds, and in the free expression of new clinical concepts. Our understanding of bacterial infections, of clinical bacteriology, and of new antibiotic agents was making rapid progress. One can appreciate this progress by reviewing the nature of medical articles published over a period of years in the *New England Journal of Medicine* (NEJM), the world's most respected and widely circulated medical journal for the past century.

In the 1950s, each issue of the NEJM contained five to seven clinical articles, of which almost half were case reports, i.e., observations of new symptoms, signs, or syndromes. Only a few were of true experimental nature, and clinical investigations—even uncontrolled studies—were extremely rare. This pattern has changed greatly over the past 50 years. In 1996, 40% of articles published in the NEJM were formal, prospective, clinical trials. In fact, the close collaboration between established medical schools and Veterans Administration (VA) hospitals, which was the brainchild of Dr. Paul Magnuson, the first Chief Medical Director of the VA (4), stimulated and funded a large amount of clinical investigation, especially dealing with chronic liver disease, one of the most common disorders among American war veterans.

After graduation from medical school, I had served an internship in Internal Medicine at The Johns Hopkins Hospital in Baltimore, a three-year residency that ended after my year as chief resident in 1956 at the Grace–New Haven Community Hospital at Yale University, and two years as a postdoctoral clinical research fellow in hepatic disorders under the preceptorship of Gerald Klatskin, who was a self-made hepatologist (i.e., a nongastroenterologist) and one of the first of that uncommon breed.

I was then assigned to the WHVAH, where William Hollingsworth was Chief of Service. I had been awarded a VA Clinical Investigatorship in Hepatology, which provided me with the freedom and support to roam the two 40-bed medical wards and to see in consultation all of the patients in the hospital referred with liver disease, which comprised almost one-third of the admissions to the medical service. Under such circumstances, only a blind physician could fail to accumulate extensive experience with patients with liver disease.

In early 1958 I saw a cirrhotic patient with what was for me a completely new disorder. It resulted in the initial description of the SBP syndrome (5). The patient, a 51-year-old chronic alcoholic man, had been admitted to the hospital with cirrhosis that was characterized by jaundice, ascites, diarrhea, and portal hypertension. His ascitic fluid was clear and sterile and contained only a few leukocytes. Several weeks after admission while undergoing diuresis he abruptly developed a fever of 104°F, chills, abdominal pain with generalized and rebound tenderness, and absent bowel sounds. He became hypotensive and exhibited early hepatic encephalopathy. His white-blood-cell (WBC) count was 15,000 per cubic millimeter. Paracentesis revealed cloudy fluid with numerous polymorphonuclear leukocytes, many of which contained Gram-negative rods. The ascitic fluid and blood cultures were positive for *Escherichia coli*. In the apparent absence of pancreatitis (serum amylase activity was <200 units per L) or other abdominal emergencies, the patient was treated with intraperitoneal neomycin and parenteral tetracycline and streptomycin. The fever and signs of peritonitis subsided within five days and the ascitic fluid became normal. One month later the same syndrome in every detail recurred and antibiotic therapy was restarted, but the patient died within a matter of hours. Autopsy showed an *Escherichia coli* bacterial peritonitis, without evidence of a perforation of any abdominal organ. It also showed a superficial acute jejunitis.

Careful review of textbooks of medicine and of liver disease did not turn up anything at all like this disorder. I discussed this case with Dr. Klatskin, but he, too, did not know what it was or how it came about. After I had seen a second, very similar patient, we again talked about it and made a more thorough search of the literature. Again we came up blank. I recall his saying, ''Harold, I think it's a fluke.''

''I know it's not a liver fluke,'' I replied.

When a third case was discovered we knew that it had to be a new syndrome.

The same syndrome was noted in four additional patients over the next four years. Two were caused by *Aeromonas liquifaciens*, a coliform, enteric species of bacteria, which is similar in many ways to *E. coli*. One was caused by *E. coli*, and another by enterococci. The same organisms were cultured from the blood of these patients at the same time. All died during their hospital admissions and no obvious cause for the bacterial peritonitis was discovered in any one of them. X-ray of the abdomen showed no free air in the peritoneal cavities of any of these patients, which ruled out gastrointestinal perforation. These six episodes in five patients were reported in April 1964 (5).

The reaction to this report was mixed. Some well-trained, experienced gastroenterologists thought that the report was in error because they had not seen patients with this disorder even though they had seen large numbers of decompensated cirrhotic patients. Others indicated that in searching for such cases retrospectively, they were able to confirm the frequent existence of this syndrome (F. Iber, personal communication).

Because the infecting organisms were all enteric in origin, we assumed that the infections had arisen in the gut from which the bacteria had escaped, inducing a bacteremia which had infected the ascitic fluid. Once the peritonitis had become established, we reasoned that the bacteria then escaped into the bloodstream, creating a secondary bacteremia. This second episode of bacteremia is the one that is seen at the time a diagnosis of SBP is made. The initial bacteremia we presumed was silent.

By 1971, Dr. J.M. Fessel and I had identified 28 patients at the WHVAH with this syndrome, which we termed "spontaneous bacterial peritonitis" (SBP) and which we reported (6). At that point we were seeing three or four new cases of SBP per year. It should be kept in mind that this large number of cases were seen on a relatively small medical service where the mean daily patient census was about 65 patients. More than one-half of these patients were men. Two-thirds of them had alcoholic cirrhosis, one-third had posthepatitic cirrhosis, and one patient had hemochromatosis. The mean age of these patients was 48 years. All had ascites, which was almost invariably cloudy. The WBC count in the ascitic fluid showed a great increase in the number of leukocytes, which ranged from 1,000 to 5,000 per cubic millimeter and which were predominantly polymorphonuclear in type. Almost all the patients exhibited jaundice, abdominal pain and tenderness, hypoactive or absent bowel sounds, and, usually, diarrhea. No free air was seen on roentgenograms of the abdomen in any of the 22 patients studied. About three-fourths of the patients had systemic hypotension and hepatic encephalopathy. Portal hypertension was established by the demonstration of esophageal varices or by abnormal ammonia tolerance tests (7). A single organism was cultured from the peritoneal fluid in a large majority of the patients. *E. coli* was the most common isolate (nine patients) and pneumococci the next most frequent (four patients). A variety of organisms, primarily enteric, made up the remainder, although streptococci of various types were common. Blood cultures were usually positive for the same organism. The infection was effectively treated with antibiotics in 60% of the patients. Nevertheless, only one of the 28 patients survived the admission, a mortality rate of 96%!

At the time of that report we had thoroughly reviewed the literature and had identified 46 previously published episodes of what we thought may have been SBP. It is intriguing that these patients had been reported predominantly from France, the first described in 1893 (8). Most of them were case reports describing one or two patients. All had overt ascites. Two patients had exhibited no signs or symptoms of SBP and were afebrile. Two others had had no abdominal pain. The WBC count was almost invariably elevated. Jaundice and decreased serum albumin concentrations were almost always present. *E. coli* had been isolated in 63%, pneumococci in 23%, streptococci in 12%, and *Candida* in 2%. Blood cultures were positive for the same species in about two-thirds of the patients. Ninety percent of the patients died.

These figures are startlingly close to those in our own series of 28 patients. No other series of any size was available at that time. In fact, the three largest collections of patients with similar or related disorders published in the literature consisted of 10 patients with coliform septicemia or peritonitis, reported by Caroli and Platteborse in 1958 (9); nine patients with enteric bacterial peritonitis described by Kerr et al. in 1964, which they attributed to prior paracenteses (10); and five patients with pneumococcal peritonitis in patients with posthepatitic, "postnecrotic" cirrhosis who were reported in 1968 (11). The last of these articles had been stimulated in part by our paper that was published in 1964. In none of these reports was the presence of an unexplained, enteric bacterial peritonitis and bacteremia recognized as a new clinical entity.

II. HISTORICAL VIGNETTE

It is of historical interest that Ludwig von Beethoven is probably the first patient known by name to have had SBP, especially since the clinical description of his case had been written 135 years before this syndrome was first described. Ever since I became aware of Beethoven's illness, it has seemed to me that SBP is the most likely explanation for his symptoms. It is even more astounding that this disease occurred in such an illustrious person. If he had not been so famous, his case history probably would not have been recorded at all. His diagnosis is based on a review of writings by Dr. Andreas Wawruch, Director of the Vienna Medical Clinic, who treated Beethoven during his final illness (12); by O.G. Sonneck, who translated his clinical description (13); and by Professor Anton Neumayr, a well-known and respected medical historian, physician, and concert pianist, who wrote a detailed medical biography of Beethoven in 1993 (14).

It has been unequivocally established that at the time of his death Beethoven had decompensated *alcoholic* cirrhosis. His enjoyment of alcoholic beverages, which started in his youth and continued throughout his life, is well known. He had drunk beer and wine freely for many years. It is not clear what his precise daily intake of alcohol was or, indeed, what mean daily consumption was required to cause cirrhosis (15). The postulated amount varies greatly among different individuals and different investigators. Nevertheless, the diagnosis of cirrhosis was established by its characteristic clinical course and by the findings at autopsy.

In May 1825 he had "abdominal dropsy" and epistaxis and had vomited blood, which may have come from esophageal varices. In addition, he had suffered an episode of jaundice of unknown etiology in 1821—presumably viral hepatitis—which probably did not contribute to his subsequent liver disease, although that possibility cannot be excluded. In December 1825, he had again vomited blood, was dyspneic and febrile and had severe abdominal pain.

At autopsy in March 1827, his liver was described as hard and shrunken to half normal size, and consisted of pea-sized nodules. In addition, his spleen was greatly enlarged. Four quarts of gray-brown fluid were present in his peritoneal cavity.

Dr. Wawruch's account of Beethoven's last illness was written in 1827 but was not published until 1842 in the *Allegemeine Wiener musikalishe Zeitung* (12). The following quotations are taken from Wawruch's description in O.G. Sonneck's book, *Beethoven: Impressions by his Contemporaries* (13), and Neumayr's book, *Music and Medicine* (14):

> On the eighth day, . . . at the morning visit, I found him stricken and suffering from jaundice over his entire body; the most dreadful vomiting and diarrhea had threatened to kill him the night before. . . . Shivering and shaking, he was doubled up with pains that raged in his liver and intestines, and his legs, which up to then were only moderately bloated, were terribly swollen. From now on, dropsy began to develop; the amount of urine voided was sparser, the liver showed clear signs of hard nodules, the jaundice increased. . . . By the third week, nightly attacks of suffocation appeared; the enormous amount of accumulated water required quick treatment, and I felt it necessary to recommend an abdominal incision, a tapping, to prevent the danger of sudden bursting.
>
> After a few moments of serious reflection, Beethoven gave his consent to the operation, all the more readily because Dr. Staudenheim, who had been asked to offer his medical advice, also strongly urged the same course as being absolutely mandatory. The chief surgeon of the General Hospital, Dr. Johann Seibert, made the tapping with his usual skill, so that Beethoven, happy to see the water pouring out, called out that the surgeon reminded him of Moses who struck the rock with his staff and brought forth the water. Relief came quickly. The amount of liquid weighed 25 pounds and the afterflow was surely five times as much. The rash act of loosening the tight bandage covering the incision in the night, presumably to bring about the rapid expulsion of remaining water, came close to spoiling Beethoven's pleasure in feeling better. A fierce, red, erysipelas-like inflammation appeared, displaying the first round patches on the skin, but careful drying of the incision's borders held the trouble in check.

The *"erysipelas-like" inflammation* was probably not caused by the Group A hemolytic streptococci, but rather by an infection of the abdominal wall caused by the organism responsible for the SBP, most probably *E. coli*, although other opportunistic organisms may have secondarily infected the edematous abdominal wall. We have seen "erysipelatic" lesions of the abdominal wall under similar circumstances in which leakage of the infected peritoneal fluid into the subcutaneous tissues resulted in infection with intense erythema and induration of the abdominal wall.

Four large *paracenteses* that drained from seven to more than 11 quarts of fluid each had been performed using glass cannulae at three- to four-week intervals during the winter of 1827, and large amounts of ascitic fluid continued to drain from the incisions, soaking the mattress and bedclothes, "which became infested with bed bugs." In view of Beethoven's hopeless situation, his physicians lifted their ban on alcoholic beverages and permitted him to drink rum punch, which refreshed him and led him to abuse this prescription. Following a series of intermittent episodes of encephalopathy, he died on March 26, 1828.

In my opinion, Beethoven's final illness was SBP, although with multiple draining wounds it was probably a peritonitis secondarily infected by multiple bacterial species, rather than the usual monomicrobial syndrome characteristic of SBP. Dr. Neumayr told me that he did not think that Beethoven had had SBP, but he did not suggest an alternative diagnosis. I agree with Neumayr that Beethoven probably did have Crohn's disease as well (14). I am unaware of any association between cirrhosis and Crohn's disease or between Crohn's disease and SBP. Of historical interest, Wawruch's innovative paracentesis therapy appears to represent the first use of massive paracenteses in the treatment of ascites, a technique which is currently in wide usage (16,17), especially when the paracenteses are associated with the administration of plasma or other volume-maintaining substances such as albumin, dextran, or hemaccel (16–19).

III. SUMMARY

Since its original description as a discrete syndrome, SBP has come a long way in a short period of time. As is typical of progress in science, the advances in our knowledge about SBP have come in fits and starts, but like the incoming tide it progressively advances along a broad front. A roughly chronological list of advances of significance in our knowledge of SBP are listed in the Appendix to this chapter. Each of these advances will be presented in much greater detail at the proper place later in this book.

APPENDIX: CHRONOLOGY OF SPONTANEOUS
BACTERIAL PERITONITIS

Table 1.1 lists in rough chronological order a number of the major developments that have occurred in the short life of spontaneous bacterial peritonitis (SBP). These observations cite first a description of Beethoven's final illness, which was probably an episode of SBP (Observation #1). We say "probably" because the diagnosis was completely clinical and because in the absence of mention of leukocyte counts in the ascitic fluid or of confirmatory cultures of the ascitic fluid it can only be a probable diagnosis. It is appropriate for clinicians to make clinical diagnoses especially since these features were not known to be important in the diagnosis of SBP until more than a century later.

There follows a citation to "primary peritonitis in children," which is also known as pediatric bacterial peritonitis (Observation #2). This preceded by a quarter of a century the recognition of SBP, the parent syndrome in adults. This citation is followed by the reference to a landmark investigation using state of the art methodology to study the transmural migration of *E. coli* through the bowel wall (Observation #3).

A series of other observations, which are cited roughly in the order in which they were recognized and reported, follow. Some of them are related to specific diseases and some to new concepts, but all of them are annotated and appropriate references from the literature are cited. (These references are presented in full in a separate list at the end of this chapter; see p. 19.) In this manner we have made a temporal map of the major steps in the cumulative growth of the SBP syndrome. Some significant steps have almost certainly been omitted and some minor steps have been included in this compilation. We welcome suggestions from readers.

This chronology is not rigid. All advances in knowledge are not created equal, nor do they appear on a regular, prearranged schedule. Furthermore, priority is sometimes established by the preliminary publication of an incomplete article or by a letter to the editor. When such articles are cited, one has the opportunity of using later, more definitive articles about that particular observation. SBP after endoscopic sclerotherapy (EST) (Observation #56) is a case in point. It took years to prove that EST does precipitate SBP. Other pertinent articles published before and since are cited as well. This is especially true when clusters of noteworthy observations are made at about the same time, as in the period from the mid-1970s until the mid-1980s, during which multiple articles are cited. In such an active period we have attempted to strike

(text continues on p. 18)

Table 1.1   Chronology of Major Developments in SBP

Dates	Observations
1825	1. *The first known clinical description of SBP*. Dr. Wawruch, Ludwig von Beethoven's personal physician, described Beethoven's final illness (1,2).
1940	2. *Primary peritonitis in children with the nephrotic syndrome*. The susceptibility to bacterial infection has been related to the hypogammaglobulinemia of nephrosis. The clinical pattern and bacterial spectrum, however, seem to be broadening (3).
1950	3. *Transmural migration of intestinal bacteria*. The use of radioactively labeled *E. coli* unequivocally identified the migrated bacteria in this superb application of basic clinical research (4).
1960	4. *Tuberculous peritonitis (TBP)*. This disease may be one facet of disseminated tuberculosis or it may be an example of spontaneous tuberculous infection of the peritoneum. TBP is a more serious disease in patients with underlying cirrhosis than in noncirrhotic patients (5).
1964	5. *The initial description of SBP syndrome in the modern era* (6).
1968	6. *SBP in posthepatitic, postnecrotic cirrhosis*. Curiously all five patients had pneumococcal SBP, and three of the five were children. This is an early report of SBP in *nonalcoholic cirrhosis* (7).
1971	7. *The pathogenesis of SBP*. The pathogenesis of SBP presented in this article is based on the clinical findings in 29 patients with bacteriologically proved SBP. This formulation remains the primary working hypothesis for the pathogenesis of SBP. The precise pathogenesis is not yet completely elucidated (8).
1971	8. *Original description of bacterascites*. The one patient with a positive ascitic fluid culture in the absence of symptoms or signs of SBP encountered in this study of 50 patients with cirrhosis and ascites was referred to as having ''asymptomatic'' bacterascites. This syndrome is assumed to represent the presence of bacteria in the ascitic fluid before or after an episode of SBP or simple contamination of the ascitic fluid (9).
1971	9. *Iatrogenic SBP*. A patient with pneumococcal SBP was retrospectively diagnosed as ''nonspontaneous'' because a splenoportogram had been performed one day after which massive bleeding into the ascitic fluid had occurred. A pre-existing pneumococcal bacteremia from a radiologically diagnosed pneumonia was presumed to have been the cause of the infection (10).
1986	10. *SBP in rheumatoid arthritis*. Only a single case of this concurrence has been reported in a patient with rheumatoid arthritis without cirrhosis. This phenomenon is unexplained except for the nonspecifically compromised immunity associated with collagen vascular disease (11).
1975	11. *SBP in disseminated lupus erythematosus (DLE)*. In DLE, SBP appears in patients without underlying cirrhosis. It is a relatively common syndrome

Table 1.1 Continued

Dates	Observations
	considering the fact the DLE is an uncommon disease. Susceptibility to bacteria may be the predisposition to infection of patients with collagen vascular disease or the immunoincompetence of patients receiving corticosteroid therapy (12).
1976	12. *Spontaneous bacterial empyema.* This syndrome represents the infection of fluid in a body cavity other than the peritoneal cavity. The pathogenesis is similar to that of SBP, but in addition diaphragmatic fenestrations may make the passage from the peritoneal to the pleural cavity more direct. A similar syndrome occurs in patients with chronic ambulatory peritoneal dialysis (CAPD) in which hydrothorax develops, rendering the CAPD ineffective. Repair of the diaphragmatic defect may permit reinitiation of CAPD (13,14).
1976	13. *Iatrogenic, vasopressin-associated SBP.* SBP of an atypical type was observed in several patients who were receiving intra-arterial vasopressin to constrict the splanchnic arteries for the treatment of hemorrhage from varices. These findings are similar to those in which atherosclerosis gives rise to ischemic gastroenteropathy (15).
1977	14. *Anaerobic bacteria in SBP.* It is unclear why anaerobic organisms only rarely cause SBP. Perhaps ascitic fluid has too high an oxygen concentration. Anaerobic organisms are seen in bacterial peritonitis after perforation of an abdominal viscus or in the vasopressin-induced variant of SBP (16).
1977	15. *The relationship of SBP and subacute bacterial endocarditis.* These two protean diseases have many thing in common, especially with regard to their pathogenesis (17).
1977	16. *SBP in neoplastic ascites.* There are two types of neoplastic ascites. One type, which simulates cirrhosis, exhibits an increased serum-ascites albumin gradient (SAAG) and supports bacterial growth. The other type has a low SAAG and is not a good medium for bacterial growth. As the ascitic albumin concentration increases, so do other proteins including complement (18).
1978	17. *Spontaneous meningococcal meningitis.* SBP frequently develops in patients with the same organism that is causing infection elsewhere in the body, such as *E. coli* in urinary tract infections or Salmonella in gastrointestinal salmonellosis. Is meningitis a complication of cirrhosis (19)?
1979	18. *Leukocytes in the ascitic fluid (AF).* Cloudy AF was recognized early as a reliable guide to the diagnosis of SBP. Based on 347 consecutive patients, the means and ranges were established for *normal AF* (e.g., 281–2600 WBC per cubic millimeter), AF in SBP (mean, 6084; range, 40–27,000 per cubic millimeter), and for pancreatitic and malignant AF. Later studies refined the numbers and showed that neutrophils are more useful than either the pH or lactate concentration (20).

Table 1.1 Continued

Dates	Observations
1979	19. *Perihepatitis as a form of SBP. Gonococcal perihepatitis*, which is also known as the Curtis-Fitz-Hugh syndrome, is a disease that represents the transfallopian passage of gonococci or other organisms from the pelvis to the peritoneal cavity. It may be caused by other organisms, of which chlamydia are the most common. However, the syndrome also occurs in men, which is a conundrum. Laparoscopy is effective both diagnostically and therapeutically (21–24).
1981	20. *Acute scrotal swelling in primary peritonitis.* This very rare syndrome is seen in patients with processus vaginalis, i.e., the persistence of the processus vaginalis peritonei, which traverses the vaginal canal and may give rise to a communication between the peritoneal cavity and the peritesticular tissues. It is similar in pathogenesis to postparacentesis scrotal edema (25).
1979	21. *Bacterial infection associated with prosthetic devices.* Such prostheses include ventriculoperitoneal shunts, peritoneovenous shunts, and intrauterine contraceptive devices (26–28).
1971	22. *Pediatric bacterial peritonitis.* This syndrome, which has rapidly decreased in prevalence and mortality over the last half century, is often seen in patients with the nephrotic syndrome and more commonly in girls than in boys. It is usually seen in the first seven years of life. These reductions and a marked change in etiology from gram-positive to gram-negative organisms may be related to the introduction of antibiotic drugs in the mid- 19th century. A variant of primary peritonitis has been reported from both the United States and India, which is almost always caused by gram-positive etiology (29–33).
1982	23. *Pediatric peritonitis in fulminant hepatic failure (FHF).* Six of these seven patients had bacterial peritonitis and one had no organisms recovered. These patients were characterized by defects in opsonization and by decreased concentrations of hemolytic C_3, C_4, and C_5. Opsonization was improved in these patients by infusions of fresh frozen plasma (34).
1980	24. *Hypothermia in SBP.* Hypothermia, like fever, represents a dysthermia, i.e., a resetting of the thermostat at a lower level, that is often seen in severe bacterial infections (35).
1980	25. *SBP in myelofibrosis with myeloid metaplasia.* The first reported case of SBP in a patient with myeloid metaplasia was observed in 1978. The metaplasia was secondary to myelofibrosis. The SBP was typical (36).
1980	26. *Increasing prevalence of SBP.* The prevalence of SBP appeared to be increasing at the Yale–New Haven Medical Center during the 15-year period following our initial report of SBP. To determine whether the prevalence was truly rising, we analyzed three consecutive seven-year periods (1958–1965, 1965–1972, and 1972–1979). The numbers of patients with SBP increased during these three periods from 6 to 25 to 53. The numbers of patients who had

Table 1.1 Continued

Dates	Observations
	autopsies and the percentage of patients with cirrhosis at autopsy increased from 3% to 8% to 15% in the three periods, respectively, a threefold increase, whereas the percentage of patients with cirrhosis at autopsy increased by less than half that rate (37).
1984	27. *pH of the ascitic fluid in the diagnosis of SBP.* A decrease in the pH of the ascitic fluid indicates the presence of bacterial infection, and the degree of the decrease in pH reflects the severity of infection in terms of the amount of carbohydrate metabolism stimulated by the infectious process. This metabolism may be a consequence of leukocyte metabolism, bacterial metabolism, or both. Neoplasic and other inflammatory lesions of the peritoneal cavity may also reduce pH (38).
1981	28. *Ascitic fluid lactate levels in SBP.* Lactate concentrations are not as accurate as pH in the diagnosis of SBP, and are certainly much less accurate than the polymorphonuclear leukocyte count. A comparison of these parameters was presented by Brook et al. (39) and Garcia-Tsao et al. (40).
1981	29. *Effects of diuresis on ascitic fluid composition.* Hoefs in 1981 reported the effects of diuresis on the concentrations of protein and the effects of white and red blood cells in serial measurements of the ascitic fluid of cirrhotic patients undergoing diuresis. The concentration of protein in the ascitic fluid doubled, as did the ascites to serum protein ratio over a period of two months as the ascites and edema fluid disappeared. The total WBC count, which consisted predominantly of long-lived lymphocytes, increased fourfold whereas the neutrophils, which have a very short half-life, showed only a small increase of about 50%. He reasoned that these findings, which could be predicted, resulted from the extraction of water (saline) from the ascitic fluid. In this seminal experiment the "dehydration" of the ascitic fluid resulted in an increase in the complement concentrations of the ascitic fluid, which suggested that diuresis can better protect cirrhotic patients from SBP than paracentesis (41–43).
1984	30. *The relationship between leukocytes in peripheral blood and in ascitic fluid in patients with and without SBP.* There is close positive correlation between the total concentrations of WBC and neutrophils in the ascitic fluid of patients with SBP, but not with mononuclear leukocytes. The increments in the neutrophil counts of ascitic fluid in SBP are so large and so variable that the correlations with the numbers and types of WBC in the peripheral blood are obscured. Thus, the changes in the number of neutrophils in the ascitic fluid are clinically useful in the management of patients with SBP whereas the changes in peripheral blood leukocytes are not (44).
1981	31. *Chronic ambulatory peritoneal dialysis (CAPD).* The bacterial spectrum of CAPD, which consists largely of *Staphylococcus albus* and other saprophytic bacteria such as rhodococci, suggests that the infections of the

Table 1.1 Continued

Dates	Observations
	dialysate fluid in the peritoneal cavity are derived from skin contamination. Yeasts, including *Candida albicans*, *Candida parapsilosis*, as well as *Aspergillus* and *Nocardial* species support a contaminatory pathogenesis (45–47).
1982	32. *Ecthyma gangrenosum and SBP*. Ecthyma granulosum is a necrotizing angiitis that occurs almost exclusively in patients with *Pseudomonas aeruginosa* infections and, occasionally, with other aerobic gram-negative enteric organisms such as *E. coli* or enterobacter species. It tends to occur in immunocompromised patients such as those with cirrhosis or with extensive burns. SBP caused by the same organism is not uncommon. The bacteria can be cultured from the skin lesions, the blood, and/or the ascitic fluid (48).
1982	33. *Large volume cultures of ascitic fluid* withdrawn at the bedside and inoculated directly into blood culture bottles enhance the diagnostic yield. Instead of the usual 5 ml inoculation used for blood cultures, volumes as large as 30 ml have been used, increasing the yield of positive culture threefold to sixfold (49).
1982	34. *Renal toxicity of aminoglycosides in patients with liver disease*. The use of aminoglycosides is often complicated by renal dysfunction. In patients with liver disease, this nephrotoxicity is greatly increased due to inhibition of prostaglandin synthesis (50,51).
1983	35. *SBP in nonalcoholic cirrhosis*. Although other instances of nonalcoholic cirrhosis in patients with SBP had been reported, the prospective demonstration of the frequency with which it occurs in this series establishes this point. Alcoholic cirrhosis is a less common etiologic factor in Italian cirrhosis than in American (52).
1983	36. *Chlamydial infections of ascitic fluid*. In addition to causing disease such as salpingitis or other genitourinary infections, *Chlamydia*, which are not easily detected, may be the explanation for peritonitis of unknown etiology (53).
1984	37. *SBP in hemochromatosis*. This syndrome appears to be simply the occurrence of SBP in a another type of cirrhosis, but in addition there appears to be a predisposition of iron storage disorders to infections with *Yersinial* organisms. The role of iron in the predisposition for such infections is purely circumstantial (54).
1984	38. *Culture-negative SBP (culture-negative neutrocytic ascites—CNNA)*. The explanations for the negative cultures are varied, but the absence of bacteria appears to carry a better prognosis than in confirmed SBP (55).
1984	39. *SBP in cardiac ascites*. Cardiac ascites, like neoplastic ascites, has a higher ascitic fluid protein concentration than that of cirrhotic peritoneal fluid. The presence of higher albumin and complement concentrations may inhibit the development of SBP (56).

Table 1.1 Continued

Dates	Observations
1984	40. *SBP vs. "perforation" bacterial peritonitis (PBP).* The differential diagnosis of PBP and SBP is important because failing to make the diagnosis of bacterial peritonitis after perforation of a hollow viscus greatly increases the mortality rate. Similarly, the erroneous, unnecessary performance of an exploratory laparotomy in patients with SBP doubles the morbidity and mortality rates. The most important clinical findings that are indicative of PBP are the presence of free gas, blood, or intestinal contents such as food particles or gastrointestinal enzymes in the ascitic fluid. Similarly, abdominal pain and/or tenderness are more severe in PBP than in SBP as are the laboratory abnormalities of SBP such as the neutrophil count, the number of bacteriological species cultured from the ascitic fluid, the presence of anaerobic species, and a putrid odor of the ascitic fluid (57–59).
1985	41. *Eosinophilic SBP.* A variant of this eosinophilic SBP occurs in patients with CAPD in whom the infusion of corticosteroids into the dialysate rapidly eliminates the eosinophilia (60,61).
1985	42. *SBP after bone marrow transplantation.* Bone marrow transplantation is a likely precipitant of SBP because the patients are usually immunocompromised by the preliminary antineoplastic chemotherapy and the use of corticosteroids (62).
1987	43. *SBP in Wilson's disease.* The association of Wilson's disease and SBP is rare. Could copper accumulation create an inhospitable environment for bacteria just as iron creates a hyperhospitable environment for Yersinial infections (63)?
1988	44. *Effect of diuresis on the ascitic fluid complement levels and opsonic activity and in preventing bacterial infection.* It has been established that cirrhotic patients with low ascitic fluid protein levels (<1 g per dl) also have decreased complement concentrations and deficient opsonic activity. Diuresis has been demonstrated to double the protein concentration of ascitic fluid and to increase opsonic activity 10-fold. Although not established by controlled clinical trials, it is likely that diuretic therapy decreases the risk of SBP and, certainly, is a more rational therapy of ascites in cirrhotic patients than paracentesis, which tends to decrease the protein-complement concentration. It has been suggested that ultrafiltration and reinfusion of the concentrated ascitic fluid can double the protein concentration of ascitic fluid and thus diminish susceptibility to SBP (64–66).
1986	45. *SBP after gastrointestinal hemorrhage.* Gastrointestinal bleeding is a very common precipitant for SBP and other bacterial infections. This susceptibility may well be a consequence of the overburdening of the reticuloendothelial system (RES) with the breakdown products of hemorrhage, hemolysis, and blood transfusions. Blockade of the RES can be caused by the administration of inert particles such as starch granules (67,68).

Table 1.1 Continued

Dates	Observations
1986	46. *Adenosine deaminase in the ascitic fluid of patients with tuberculous peritonitis.* Adenosine deaminase is the enzyme responsible for the deamination of adenosine to inosine, a reaction that stimulates T lymphocytes as part of the cell-mediated immune response. When increased in ascitic fluid, adenosine deaminase activity is an indication of TBP. It should be confirmed by laparoscopic, histologic, and bacteriologic methods (69).
1987	47. *Spontaneous cryptococcal bacterial peritonitis.* Spontaneous fungal peritonitis is a very uncommon disease. Four of the five hitherto reported cases had underlying hepatic disease and the fifth had disseminated lupus erythematosis, another disorder that predisposes patients to SBP. The patient cited here had alcoholic cirrhosis and the peritonitis was typical of SBP (70).
1987	48. *Encapsulating SBP.* This syndrome has been found primarily in patients with peritoneovenous shunts. It has also been observed in patients who were receiving β-adrenergic blockade with timolol and those who had CAPD (71–73).
1987	49. *Recurrent SBP.* Patients who survive the initial episode of SBP appear to be doomed to recurrences, often relentlessly until death (74).
1982	50. *SBP in acute viral hepatitis.* Although SBP in acute viral hepatitis is not common, a recent report from Taiwan indicates that one-fourth of patients with severe acute hepatitis with ascites develop SBP, a very high percentage. These patients tend to have portal hypertension, renal failure, coagulopathy, gastrointestinal bleeding, and a high fatality rate. This disorder is reminiscent of PSE in subacute hepatic failure (75–77).
1996	51. *Bacterial translocation in the pathogenesis of SBP.* Bacterial translocation is defined as the presence of bacteria in unusual extraenteric anatomic locations. The natural habitat of enteric bacteria is the gut; their presence in the peritoneal cavity is an undesirable, potentially lethal translocation. It represents either bacterial peritonitis or bacterascites. The translocation of enteric organisms, usually gram-negative bacteria to abdominal lymphoid tissue or blood is considered a step in the pathogenesis of SBP. It occurs in association with acute, severe liver injury or after hepatic resection. In experimental animals it can be induced by thermal injury or by galactosamine administration. It may be the result of the transmural migration of intestinal bacteria, although many other mechanisms may be involved (78–80).
1996	52. *Parvovirus infection in the pathogenesis of SBP.* The leukopenia associated with acute infection with *parvovirus B19* has been postulated to play a role in the pathogenesis of SBP. If this pathogenetic factor is established, other acute viral infections may similarly be implicated (81).
1996	53. *Differential diagnosis of tuberculous peritonitis (TBP) in patients with and without chronic liver disease.* The effect of the presence or absence of liver disease on the clinical picture and prognosis of TBP is extremely

Table 1.1 Continued

Dates	Observations
	detrimental. In Great Britain, TBP occurs eight times more frequently in Asians than in Caucasians (82,83).
1991	54. *Selective intestinal decontamination.* The process of suppressing enteric, anaerobic bacteria by the administration of oral, nontoxic antibiotic agents such as norfloxacin or oxacillin results in the prevention of SBP and other gram-negative infections in cirrhotic patients. This demonstration that merely reducing the population of potentially infectious bacteria in preventing SBP confirms our understanding of the pathogenesis of SBP (84).
1996	55. *Systemic antibiotic prophylaxis for patients at high risk of SBP.* In addition to oral decontamination of the gastrointestinal (GI) tract in cirrhotic patients at low risk of SBP antibiotic prophylaxis includes the treatment of patients at high risk of developing SBP. High risk patients for SBP include those (a) who have survived an episode of SBP, (b) who have Childs (Pugh) class C cirrhosis, or (c) who are about to undergo endoscopic sclerotherapy or ligation or other endoscopic procedures. Because in only about one-half of patients who develop SBP are the infections caused by gram-negative, aerobic organisms, systemic prophylaxis requires the use of antibiotic agents with sufficiently broad spectra to inhibit gram-positive bacteria and more potent antibiotic activity than norfloxacin or ofloxacin. Ciprofloxacin plus the combination of amoxillin and clavulanic acid appear at the time of writing to be effective, well-tolerated therapeutic combinations. In active bleeding these antibiotic agents can be administered intravenously initially and orally thereafter until three days after the bleeding has stopped (85).
1991	56. *Endoscopic sclerotherapy (EST) and SBP.* Bacteremia occurs after only invasive procedures, especially endoscopic therapies. Bacteremia is most common after EST, probably because of the multiple punctures and injections in a contaminated field. SBP, which may follow endoscopy, is therefor a common complication. This association is circumstantial but unquestioned. Because gastrointestinal bleeding itself is associated with SBP, it is not clear whether post-EST SBP is a consequence of the bleeding or of the SBP. Brain abscess, too, has followed EST (86–89).
1994	57. *Renal dysfunction in SBP.* Based on an analysis of almost 200 patients with SBP, it is clear that renal impairment typical of the hepatorenal syndrome occurs in one-third of patients with SBP, particularly in those who had exhibited evidence of azotemia prior to the onset of SBP. In almost half of them the renal impairment progresses thereafter. The occurrence of such renal failure is the single most important predictor of mortality in cirrhotic patients with SBP (90).
1996	58. *SBP in nephrogenic ascites.* Nephrogenic ascites is a controversial con-

Table 1.1 Continued

Dates	Observations
	cept that must be differentiated from cirrhotic, cardiac, pancreatitic, and other types of ascites. When associated with the nephrotic syndrome, end-stage renal disease, hemodialysis, or perhaps disseminated lupus erythomatosus SBP is an expected complication. When it is associated with peritoneal dialysis it does not represent true SBP because the peritoneal fluid is not true ascites. The case of SBP described by Horn et al. is acceptable as SBP, but it is unusual in that *Staphylococcus aureus* is normally an uncommon cause of SBP (91).
1990	59. *Effect of acute encephalopathy induced by sepsis on mortality.* The occurrence of an acutely altered mental state during sepsis is associated with a higher mortality (49%) than the presence of a pre-existing abnormal mental state (41%) or a normal mental state. Hypothermia, hypotension, thrombocytopenia, and the absence of shaking chills are all independent predictors of a fatal outcome (92).
1996	60. *Hospital acquired (nosocomial) SBP vs. community-acquired SBP in cirrhosis.* By definition SBP that precipitates admission to a hospital and/or that is present on admission to a hospital is considered community-acquired. Hospital-acquired SBP is usually defined as SBP that develops or becomes apparent 48 h or more after admission. In our early experience (Observations 5, 8, 13, 17, 18, and 26), SBP appears to be predominantly hospital-acquired. Ho et al. studied this problem by searching for the presence of other, pre-existing bacterial infections in the blood, urine, and elsewhere that may have predisposed patients to SBP. They studied retrospectively 176 cirrhotic patients with ascites who had been hospitalized over a five-year period. They compared 68 patients who had SBP on admission with 108 patients who did not. They found that blood cultures were positive in 57% of those with SBP versus 5% in those without SBP (p < 0.0001) and that urine cultures were positive for the same species of organisms (largely *E. coli*) in 61% of the patients with SBP versus 7% of those without (p < 0.0001). Furthermore, the same species of bacteria were recovered from the blood and urine. This association suggests but does not prove that a causal relationship exists between bacteriuria (or other infections) and SBP. In pregnancy asymptomatic bacteriuria has been found to be the cause of increased morbidity and mortality. On the other hand, antibiotic therapy of bacteriuria in nonpregnant women does not appear to be beneficial. Bacteriuria in primary biliary cirrhosis, which has been recognized for some years, is not apparently associated with SBP or other bacterial infections. The significance of bacteriuria in SBP is still not known, but circumstantial evidence suggests that it may be a critical factor in the pathogenesis of SBP (93–97).

a balance between the exact dates on which certain articles were published and their clinical, historical, or pathophysiological significance in relation to SBP. We hope that this chronology enhances the readers' understanding of SBP. Indeed, it has been a busy third of a century.

REFERENCES

1. Brown J. A remarkable account of a liver appearing glandulous to the eye. Phil Trans Roy Soc, 15:1266–1269, 1685.
2. Baillie M. The Morbid Anatomy of Some of the Most Important Parts of the Human Body, London: Bulmer, 1812, p. 101.
3. Laënnec RTH. Traité de l'auscultation médiate, Paris: Chaudé, 1826, II, p. 196.
4. Magnuson PB. Ring the Night Bell: The Autobiography of a Surgeon. Boston: Little Brown & Co., 1980, p. 376.
5. Conn HO. Spontaneous peritonitis and bacteremia in Laënnec's cirrhosis caused by enteric organisms. A relatively common but rarely recognized syndrome. Ann Intern Med, 60:568–580, 1964.
6. Conn HO, Fessel JM. Spontaneous bacterial peritonitis in cirrhosis. Variations on a theme. Medicine 50:161–197, 1971.
7. Conn HO. Ammonia tolerance as an index of portal-systemic collateral circulation in cirrhosis. Gastroenterology, 41:97–106, 1961.
8. Charrin, Veillon. Peritonite a pneumocoques sans pneumonie. Substitution apparente du bacterium coli an auneumocoque an moment de la mart. Comptes Rendus Soc Biol, 9S:1657–1670, 1893.
9. Caroli J, Platteborse R. Septicemie port-cave. Cirrhoses du foie et septicemie a colibacille. Sem Hop, 34:472–490, 1958.
10. Kerr DNS, Pearson DT, Read AE. Infection of ascitic fluid in patients with hepatic cirrhosis. Gut, 4:394–398, 1963.
11. Epstein M, Calia FM, Gabuzda GJ. Pneumococcal peritonitis in patients with postnecrotic cirrhosis. NEJM, 278:69–73, 1968.
12. Wawruch A. Ärzticher Rückblick auf L. van Beethoven's letzte Lebensepoche. Allgem. Wiener Musikzeitung II, 218–222, 1842.
13. Sonneck OG. Beethoven: Impressions by His Contemporaries. New York: Dover Publications, 1926.
14. Neumayr A. Music and Medicine. Bloomington, IL: Medi-Ed Press, 1994, p. 447.
15. Conn HO. Alcohol content of various beverages: all booze is created equal. Hepatology 12:1252–1254, 1990.
16. Gines P, Tito LL, Arroyo V. Randomized comparitive study of therapeutic paracentesis with and without intravenous albumen in cirrhosis. Gastroenterology 94:1493–1505, 1988.

17. Garcia-Compeán D, Villarreal JZ, Cuevas HB, et al. Total therapeutic paracente-
     sis (TTP) with and without intravenous albumin in the treatment of cirrhotic
     tense ascites: a randomized controlled trial. Liver 13:233–238, 1993.
18. Planas R, Gines P, Arroyo V, et al. Dextran-70 versus albumin as plasma expand-
     ers in cirrhotic patients with tense ascites treated with total paracentesis: results
     of a randomized study. Gastroenterology 99:1736–1744, 1990.
19. Salerno F, Badalamenti S, Lorenzano E, Moser P, Incerti P. Randomized compar-
     ative study of hemaccel vs. albumin infusion after total paracentesis in cirrhotic
     patients with refractory ascites. Hepatology 13:707–713, 1991.

REFERENCES FOR APPENDIX

1. Sonneck OG. Beethoven: Impressions by His Contemporaries. New York: Dover
    Publications, 1926.
2. Conn HO. Medical editor's notes in *Music and Medicine* by Anton Neumayr,
    Bloomington, IL: Medi-Ed Press, 1993, pp. 431–434.
3. Pahmer M: Pneumococcal peritonitis in nephrotic and non-nephrotic children. J
    Pediatr 17:90–106, 1940.
4. Schweinburg FB, Seligman AM, Fine J. Transmural migration of intestinal bac-
    teria. A study based on the use of radioactive *Escherichia coli*. NEJM 242:747–
    757, 1950.
5. Burack WR, Hollister RM. Tuberculous peritonitis. A study of forty-seven cases
    encountered by a general medical unit in twenty-five years, AJM 28:510–523,
    1960.
6. Conn HO. Spontaneous peritonitis and bacteremia in cirrhotic patients caused
    by enteric bacteria. Am J Med 60:568–580, 1964.
7. Epstein M, Calia FM, Gabuzda GJ. Pneumococcal peritonitis in patients with
    postnecrotic cirrhosis NEJM 278:59–73, 1968.
8. Conn HO, Fessel JM. Spontaneous bacterial peritonitis in cirrhosis. Variations
    on a theme. Medicine 50:161–197, 1971.
9. Ibid.
10. Ibid.
11. Skau T, Tegner Y. Spontaneous peritonitis and rheumatoid arthritis: A case re-
    port. Acta Chir Scand 152:317–318, 1986.
12. Lipsky PE, Hardin JA, Schour L, et al. Spontaneous peritonitis and systemic
    lupus erythematosus: importance of accurate diagnosis of gram-positive abacte-
    rial infections. JAMA 232:929–931, 1975.
13. Flaum MA. Spontaneous bacterial empyema in cirrhosis. Gastroenterology 70:
    416–417, 1976.
14. Kawaguchi AL, Dunn JCY, Fonkalsrud RE. Management of peritoneal dialysis-
    induced hydrothorax in children. Am Surgeon 62:820–824, 1996.

15. Bar Meir S, Conn HO. Spontaneous bacterial peritonitis induced by intra-arterial vasopressin therapy. Gastroenterology 70:418–421, 1976.

16. Targan SR, Chow AW, Guze LB. Role of anaerobic bacteria in spontaneous peritonitis of cirrhosis. AJM 62:387–403, 1977.

17. Snyder N, Atterbury CE, Correia JP, Conn HO. Increased concurrence of cirrhosis and bacterial endocarditis: a clinical and postmortem study. Gastroenterology 73:1107–1113, 1977.

18. Isner J, MacDonald JS, Schein PS. Spontaneous streptococcus pneumonia peritonitis in a patient with metastatic gastric cancer: a case report and etiologic consideration. Cancer 39:2306–2309, 1977.

19. Bar Meir S, Chojkier M, Groszmann RJ, Conn HO. Spontaneous meningococcal peritonitis: A report of two cases. Am J Dig Dis 23:119–122, 1978.

20. Bar-Meir S, Lerner E, Conn HO. Analysis of ascitic fluid in cirrhosis. Dig Dis Sci 24:136–144, 1979.

21. Husebö OS, Bjerkeseth T, Kalager T. Acute perihepatitis. Acta Chir Scand 145:483–485, 1979.

22. Wang S-P, Eschenbach DA, Holmes KK, Wager G, Grayston, JT. *Chlamydia trachomatis* infection in Fitz-Hugh-Curtis syndrome. Am J Obstet Gynecol 138:1034–1038, 1980.

23. Cano A, Fernandez C, Scapa M, Boixeda D, Plaza G. Gonococcal perihepatitis: Diagnostic and therapeutic value of laparoscopy. Am J Gastroenterol 79:280–282, 1984.

24. Brinson RR, Kolts BE, Monif GRG. ''Spontaneous'' bacterial peritonitis: transfallopian route of infection confirmed. Gastroenterology 89:1214–1216, 1985.

25. Udall DA, Drake DJ, Jr. Rosenberg RS. Acute scrotal swelling: A physical sign of primary peritonitis. J Urol 125:750–751, 1981.

26. Hubschmann OR, Countee RW. Gram-positive peritonitis in patients with infected ventriculoperitoneal shunts. Surg Gynecol Obstet 149:69–71, 1979.

27. Wormser P, Hubbard RC. Peritonitis in cirrhotic patients with LeVeen shunts. Am J Med 71:358–362, 1981.

28. Brinson RR, Kolts BE, Monif GRG. Spontaneous bacterial peritonitis associated with an intrauterine device. J Clin Gastroenterol 8:82–84, 1986.

29. Fowler R. Primary peritonitis: Changing aspects 1956–1970. Aust Pediat J 7:73–83, 1971.

30. Harken AH, Shochat SJ. Gram-positive peritonitis in children. Am J Surg 125:769–772, 1973.

31. Speck WT, Dresdale SS, McMillan RW. Primary peritonitis and the nephrotic syndrome. Am J Surg 127:267–274, 1976.

32. Sen S, Lalitha MK, Fenn AS, Mammen KE. Primary peritonitis in children. Ann Trop Paed 3:53–56, 1983.

33. Clark JH, Fitzgerald JF, Kleiman MB. Spontaneous bacterial peritonitis. J Ped 104:495–500, 1984.

34. Larcher VF, Wyke RJ, Mowat AP, Williams R. Bacterial and fungal infection

in children with fulminant hepatic failure: Possible role of opsonisation and complement deficiency. Gut 23:1037–1043, 1982.

35. LeCarrer M, Poupon R-Y, Ballet F, Darnis F. Les infections du liquide d'ascite chez le cirrhotique: Etude clinique et biologique de 36 episodes observes au cours d'une annee. Gastroenterol Clin Biol 4:640–645, 1980.

36. Conn HO, Goldfarb J. Spontaneous bacterial peritonitis: an endemic epidemic. In: *Hepatic, Biliary and Pancreatic Surgery*, Cohen JH, ed. Symposia Specialists. Miami, 1980, pp. 441–452.

37. Ibid.

38. Gitlin N, Stauffer JI, Silvestri RC. The pH of ascitic fluid in the diagnosis of spontaneous bacterial peritonits in alcoholic cirrhosis. Hepatology 1:511, 1981.

39. Brook I, Altman RS, Loebman WW, Seeff LB. Measurement of lactate in ascitic fluid. An aid in the diagnosis of peritonitis with particular relevance to spontaneous bacterial peritonitis of the cirrhotic. Dig Dis Sci 26:1089–1094, 1981.

40. Garcia-Tsao G, Conn HO, Lerner E. The diagnosis of bacterial peritonitis: Comparison of pH, lactate concentration and leukocyte count. Hepatology 5:91–96, 1985.

41. Hoefs JC. Increase in ascites white blood cell and protein concentrations during diuresis in patients with chronic liver disease. Hepatology 1:249–254, 1981.

42. Kato A, Ohtake T, Furuya R, et al. Spontaneous bacterial peritonitis in an adult patient with nephrotic syndrome. Intern Med 12:719–721, 1993.

43. Runyon BA, Van Epps DE. Diuresis of cirrhotic ascites increases its opsonic activity and may help prevent spontaneous bacterial peritonitis. Hepatology 6: 396–399, 1986.

44. Vinel JP, Conn HO, Lerner E, Goldfarb J. Studies of spontaneous bacterial peritonitis: the relationship of leukocytes in ascitic fluid and in peripheral blood. Neth J Med 27:253–257, 1984.

45. Arfania D, Everett ED, Nolph KD, Rubin J. Uncommon causes of peritonitis in patients undergoing peritoneal dialysis. Arch Intern Med 141:61–64, 1981.

46. Fenton SS, Wu G, Cattran D, et al. Clinical aspects of peritonitis in patients on chronic ambulatory peritoneal dialysis. Peritoneal Dialysis Bull 1:S1–S58, 1981.

47. Tang S, Lo CY, Lo WK, Ho M, Cheng IK. Rhodococcus peritonitis in continuous ambulatory peritoneal dialysis. Neph, Dial, Transplant 11:201–202, 1996.

48. Rajan RK. Spontaneous bacterial peritonitis with ecthyma gangrenosum due to *Escherichia coli*. J Clin Gastroenterol 4:145–148, 1982.

49. Kammerer J, Dupeyron C, Vuillemin H, Leluan G, Fouet P. Apport des exams cytologiques et bactériologiques du liquide d'ascite cirrhotique au diagnostic de péritonite bactérienne. Med Chir Dig 11:243–251, 1982.

50. Cabrera J, Arroyo V, Ballesta AM, et al. Increased risk of renal dysfunction due to interaction of liver disease and aminoglycosides. Gastroenterology 82:49–105, 1981.

51. Moore RD, Smith CR, Lietman PS. Increased risk of renal dysfunction due to

interaction of liver disease and aminoglycosides. Am J Med 80:1093–1097, 1986.

52. Pinzello G, Simonetti RG, Craxi A, Di Piazza S, Spano C, Pagliaro L. Spontaneous bacterial peritonitis: a prospective investigation in predominantly nonalcoholic cirrhotic patients. Hepatology 3:545–549, 1983.

53. Shabot JM, Road GD, Truant AL. *Chlamydia trachomatis* in the ascitic fluid of patients with chronic liver disease. Am J Gastroenterol 78:291–294, 1983.

54. Capron JP, Capron-Chivrac D, Tossou H, Delamarre J, Eb F. Spontaneous *Yersinia enterocolitica* peritonitis in idiopathic hemochromatosis. Gastroenterology 87:1371–1375, 1984.

55. Runyon BA, Hoefs JC. Culture-negative neutrocytic ascites: A variant of spontaneous bacterial peritonitis. Hepatology 4:1209–1211, 1984.

56. Runyon BA. Spontaneous bacterial peritonitis associated with cardiac ascites. Am J Gastroenterol 79:796–803, 1984.

57. Caralis PV, Sprung CL, Schiff ER. Secondary bacterial peritonitis in cirrhotic patients with ascites. South Med J 77:579–583, 1984.

58. Conn HO. The differential diagnosis of spontaneous versus ''perforation'' bacterial peritonitis in cirrhotic patients with ascites. Ergeb Gastroenterol 24:292–298, 1989.

59. Akriviadis EA, Runyon BA. Utility of an algorithm in differentiating spontaneous from secondary bacterial peritonitis. Gastroenterology 98:127–133, 1990.

60. Leung ACT, Orange G, Henderson IS. Intraperitoneal hydrocortisone in eosinophilic peritonitis associated with continuous ambulatory peritoneal dialysis. Br M J 286:766–769, 1983.

61. Rowland M, Brown RB, Geldman M. Eosinophilic peritonitis: an unusual manifestation of spontaneous bacterial peritonitis. J Clin Gastroenterol 7:369–371, 1985.

62. Julia A, Acebedo G, Jornet J, Zuazu J. Spontaneous pneumococcal peritonitis: late infection after bone marrow transplantation. N Engl J Med 312:587, 1985.

63. Person JL, Anderson DS, Brower RA. Spontaneous bacterial peritonitis in Wilson's disease. Am J Gasteroenterol 82:66–68, 1987.

64. Stabellini N, De Paoli Vitali E, Fiocchi O, et al. Extracorporeal ascitic ultrafiltration with intraperitoneal reinfusion of the concentrate ascites. In: *Artificial Support and Hemodetoxification in Severe Organ Failure*. Rome, Italy: Acta Medical Ed. Congressi Srl, 1985, pp. 137–140.

65. Runyon BA. Patients with deficient ascitic fluid opsonic activity and predisposed to spontaneous bacterial peritonitis. Hepatology 8:632–635, 1988.

66. Runyon BA, Antillon MR, Mc Hutchison JG. Diuresis increases ascitic fluid opsonic activity in patients who survive spontaneous bacterial peritonitis. J Hepat 14:249–252, 1992.

67. Bleichner G, Boulanger R, Squara P, Sollet JP, Parent A. Frequency of infections in cirrhotic patients presenting with acute gastrointestinal hemorrhage. Br J Surg 73:724–726, 1986.

68.   Goulis J, Armonis A, Patch D, Sabin C, Greensdale L, Burroughs AK. Bacterial infection is independently associated with failure to control bleeding in cirrhotic patients with gastrointestinal hemorrhage. Hepatology 27:1207–1212, 1998.

69.   Martinez-Vasquez JM, Ocaña I, Ribera E, Segura RM, Pascual C. Adenosine deaminase activity in the diagnosis of tuberculous peritonitis. Gut 27:1049–1053, 1986.

70.   Poblete RB, Kirby BD. Cryptococcal peritonitis: Report of a case and review of the literature. Am J Med 82:665–667, 1987.

71.   Brown P, Baddeley H, Read AE, Davies JD, McGarry J. Sclerosing peritonitis in patients on timolol. Lancet 2:1477–1481, 1974.

72.   Leport J, du Mayne JFD, Hay JM, Cerf M. Chylous ascites and encapsulating peritonitis: Unusual complications of spontaneous bacterial peritonitis. Am J Gastroenterol 82:463–466, 1987.

73.   Stanley MM, Reyes CV, Greenlee HB, Nemchausky B, Reinhardt GF. Peritoneal fibrosis in cirrhotics treated with peritoneovenous shunting for ascites. An autopsy study with clinical correlations. Dig Dis Sci 41:571–577, 1996.

74.   Tito L, Rimola A, Gines P, Llach J, Arroyo V, Radés J. Recurrence of spontaneous bacterial peritonitis in cirrhosis: Frequency and predictive factors. Hepatology 8:27–32, 1987.

75.   Thomas FB, Fromkes JJ. Spontaneous bacterial peritonitis associated with acute viral hepatitis. J Clin Gastroenterol 4:259–262, 1982.

76.   Rolando N, Harvey F, Brahm J. Prospective study of bacterial infection in acute liver failure: An analysis of fifty patients. Hepatology 11:49–53, 1990.

77.   Chu C-M, Chiu D-W, Liaw Y-F. The prevalence and prognostic significance of spontaneous bacterial peritonitis in severe acute hepatitis with ascites. Hepatology 15:799–803, 1992.

78.   Runyon BA, Sunano S, Kanei G, et al. A rodent model of cirrhosis, ascites and bacterial peritonitis. Gastroenterology 100:489–493, 1991.

79.   Herndon DN, Zeigler ST. Bacterial translocation after thermal injury. Critical Care Med 21:S50–S54, 1993.

80.   Kasravi FB, Wang L, Wang X-D, et al. Bacterial translocation in acute liver injury induced by D-galactosamine. Hepatology 23:97–103, 1996.

81.   Yamamoto T, Ise K, Nunoue T, et al. Parvovirus B19 as a trigger for spontaneous bacterial peritonitis in a patient with cirrhotic ascites. Am J Gastroenterol 91: 1857–1859, 1996.

82.   Wolfe JH, Behr AR, Jackson BT. Tuberculous peritonitis and role of diagnostic laparoscopy. Lancet 1:852–853, 1979.

83.   Shakil AO, Korula J, Kanel GC, Murray NGB, Reynolds TB. Diagnostic features of tuberculous peritonitis in the absence and presence of chronic liver disease: a case control study. Am J Med 100:179–185, 1996.

84.   Rimola A. Infections in liver disease. In: *Oxford Textbook of Clinical Hepatology*, McIntyre N, Benhamou J-P, Bircher, J, Rizetto M, Rodes J, eds., New York: Oxford University Press, 1991.

85.   Pauwels A, Mostefa-Kara N, Debenes B, et al. Systemic antibiotic prophylaxis

after gastrointestinal hemorrhage in cirrhotic patients with a high risk of infection. Hepatology 24:802–806, 1996.

86. Cohen FL, Koerner RS, Taub SJ. Solitary brain abscess following endoscopic injection sclerosis of esophageal varices. Gastrointest Endosc 31:331–333, 1985.

87. Tam F, Chow H, Prindiville T, Cornish D, Haulk CD, Trudeau W, Hoeprich P. Bacterial peritonitis following esophageal injection sclerotherapy for variceal hemorrhage. Gastrointest Endosc 36:131–133, 1990.

88. Schembre D, Bjorkman DJ. Post-sclerotherapy bacterial peritonitis. Am J Gastroenterol 86:481–486, 1991.

89. Bac DJ, De Marie S, Van Blankenstein M. Spontaneous bacterial peritonitis complicating malignancy-related ascites. Dig Dis Sc 41:131–132, 1996.

90. Follo A, Llovet JM, Navasa M, et al. Renal impairment after spontaneous bacterial peritonitis in cirrhosis: incidence, clinical course, predictive factors and prognosis. Hepatology 20:1495–1501, 1994.

91. Horn S, Holtzer H, Horina JH. Spontaneous bacterial peritonitis in a patient with nephrogenic ascites during an episode of acute renal transplant rejection. Am J Kid Dis 27:442–443, 1996.

92. Sprung CL, Peduzzi PH, Shatney CH, Wilson MF, Sheagren JN. Impact of encephalopathy on mortality in the sepsis syndrome. The Veterans Administration Systemic Sepsis Cooperative Study Group. Crit Care Med 18:801–806, 1990.

93. Burroughs AK, Rosenstein IJ, Epstein O, Hamilton-Miller JM, Brumfitt W, Sherlock S. Bacteriuria and primary biliary cirrhosis. Gut 25:133–137, 1984.

94. Boscia JA, Abrutyn E, Kaye D. Asymptomatic bacteriuria in elderly persons. Treat or not treat? Ann Intern Ed 106:764–766, 1987.

95. Patterson TF, Andriole VT. Bacteriuria in pregnancy. Infect Dis Clin North Am 1:807–822, 1987.

96. Probst T, Probst A, Schauer G, Judmaier G, Braunsteiner H, Vogel W. Is spontaneous bacterial peritonitis a complication of hospitalization? J Hepatol 19:184–189, 1993.

97. Ho H, Zuckerman MJ, Ho TK, et al. Prevalence of associated infections in community-acquired spontaneous bacterial peritonitis. Am J Gastroenterol 91:735–742, 1996.

2

Clinical Patterns of Spontaneous Bacterial Peritonitis: Variations on a Theme

Harold O. Conn
*Yale University School of Medicine, New Haven, Connecticut, and
University of Miami School of Medicine, Miami, Florida*

I. INTRODUCTION

The first article published on spontaneous bacterial peritonitis (SBP), which consisted of a description of six episodes of SBP in five patients and a hypothesis about the pathogenesis of the syndrome, emphasized the homogeneity of the clinical picture (1):

> In each instance it started abruptly with sudden fever and shaking chills, accompanied by nausea, vomiting, and progressive abdominal discomfort. Hypotension, which was present in each patient, was usually severe. In each patient diffuse abdominal tenderness, nonlocalizing rebound tenderness, and, usually, hypoactive bowel sounds were present. There was rapid deterioration in mental state characterized by confusion, disorientation, delirium, and asterixis. Although blood ammonia levels tended to be increased, there was no consistent elevation. Leukocytosis of the peripheral blood was found in all of the patients. Upright and lateral decubitus roentgenograms of the abdomen showed no free air in the peritoneal cavity. Peritonitis was proven by paracentesis. The ascitic fluid in each instance was turbid and showed an increase in polymorphonuclear leukocytes. The specific gravity ranged from 1.012 to 1.018. Gram stains of the centrifuged sediment showed many polymorphonuclear leukocytes, and in three instances gram-negative rods were identified. Cultures of ascitic fluid grew *Escherichia coli* in three instances, *Aeromonas liquefa-*

ciens in one and *Streptococcus faecalis* in one. In each patient blood cultures were positive for the same organism. Although these bacteria were not classified further, the organisms obtained from the blood and ascitic fluid were culturally identical and showed the same antibiotic sensitivities.

Therapy with tetracycline and streptomycin gave rapid and dramatic results. Fever, abdominal pain, and hypotension disappeared, and the blood and ascitic fluid became sterile. Despite prompt control of the coliform peritonitis and bacteremia there followed in each of the patients a profound worsening of hepatic function characterized by an increase in serum bilirubin and glutamic-oxalacetic transaminase levels. These changes were attributed to the hypotension and transient renal decompensation associated with gram-negative bacteremia. All of these patients died of decompensated cirrhosis or its complications within three months.

By the time our second paper on SBP had been published, seven years after the first (2), we had observed 33 episodes of SBP in 29 patients at the VA Hospital in West Haven, Connecticut, and its affiliated hospitals.

Based on these products the sine qua non of SBP was the triad of cirrhosis, portal hypertension with ascites, and an extensive portosystemic collateral circulation. Almost immediately the pattern started to broaden—not with major changes, but rather with variations on the theme.

Among the 24 additional patients a number of subtle variations, which were described in the two articles, had been noted. Some represented the absence of a clinical sign or symptom that was usually seen in SBP (patients 13 and 28). When all of the signs and symptoms were missing it was referred to as "silent SBP."

Another patient (patient 15), had a pleural effusion infected with the same organisms as those found in the ascitic fluid, which is termed *spontaneous bacterial empyema* (SBEmp).

A bizarre variant of SBP was encountered in another patient (patient 23), who had bled from esophageal varices and who had been treated with intraarterial vasopressin. In this patient the clinical pattern was complete and typical of SBP, except that many bacterial organisms, including two species of Bacteroides, *E. coli, Proteus morgani*, and anaerobic and gram-positive rods were all recovered from the ascitic fluid. We postulated that "vasopressin-induced SBP" represented the effects of the arterial vasoconstrictor on the integrity of the intestinal mucosa barrier to bacteria. In similar syndromes of inadequate celiac arterial blood flow, enteric bacteria may escape through the bowel-blood or bowel-lymphatic barrier giving rise to SBP. This iatrogenic syndrome appears to permit the peritoneal fluid to be infected by multiple intestinal bacteria, especially anaerobic species, which are otherwise only rarely responsible for SBP (3).

One of the patients in this series (patient 19) survived the infection and thus represented our first case of *nonfatal SBP*.

We also noted two patients who responded promptly to antibiotic therapy, but who shortly thereafter developed *recurrent SBP* caused either by the same bacterial species (patient 10) or another organism.

In addition, other variants of the prototypical pattern were observed. One occurred in a noncirrhotic patient with ascites induced by a reticulum cell sarcoma rather than by cirrhosis, a syndrome which has been termed *malignant* or *neoplastic* SBP (patient 1). Actually, there are two different types of neoplastic ascites. One type results from intrahepatic metastases, which induce postsinusoidal portal hypertension characterized by a low ascitic fluid protein concentration, a large serum-ascites albumin gradient (SAAG), and reduced opsonic and bacteriocidal activity (4). The other type results from peritoneal metastases in which the tumor exudes neoplastic fluid into the peritoneal cavity. This type of ascites is characterized by high ascitic fluid protein and complement concentrations, a low serum-ascites albumin ratio, and increased opsonic and bacteriocidal activity (5). Recurrent bacteremia will be discussed in detail in Chapter 14.

In the period from July 1974 through December 1979 we reported an additional 35 new patients with SBP as well as four other previously unreported patients with proven SBP who had been observed at our hospital between 1964 and 1970. Of these 39 patients, 36 had alcoholic cirrhosis, one had primary biliary cirrhosis, and two did not have cirrhosis. In one the ascites was a manifestation of a metastatic hepatic malignancy and in the other it represented myelofibrosis and myeloid metaplasia (6).

One unique patient (patient 29), who had the typical SBP syndrome, had a single colony of *Mycobacterium tuberculosis* cultured from the ascitic fluid in addition to *enterococci*. This patient may represent the first patient that was discovered with *spontaneous tuberculous peritonitis*, or, perhaps, represents a case of secondary contamination from a previously infected peritoneal tuberculous focus.

Another patient (#12) provided insight into how iatrogenic bacterial peritonitis may occasionally develop. This patient had portal hypertension during the investigation of which a splenoportogram had been performed. After the procedure the patient experienced severe intra-abdominal bleeding, and 24 hours later he developed overt Type III pneumococcal SBP. It was postulated that the patient, who was shown at that time to have a lobar pneumonia by X-ray, had had a pneumococcal bacteremia at the time of the splenoportogram. At autopsy an intrasplenic hemorrhage was found.

Furthermore, a variety of bacteria other than the anticipated aerobic, gram-negative bacilli have been isolated. These bacteria included various types of streptococci (patients 12, 19, and 21). The only other previously unidentified organisms we encountered during the period was *Neisseria perflava*, propionibacteria, and citrobacter species.

II. DIFFERENT TYPES OF CIRRHOSIS WITH SBP

This pattern of "variations on a theme" has continued, virtually every possible variable has been documented, and thus the syndrome has been broadened considerably. All of the first 29 patients, for example, had micronodular *alcoholic cirrhosis*. It was not difficult to predict that other types of cirrhosis would also be associated with SBP. These variations, some of which were observed in our series, but most of which have been reported by other investigators elsewhere, will be documented here.

Initially the patients all seemed to have alcoholic cirrhosis, which was known then as Laennec's cirrhosis (1,2). That pattern changed quickly. Epstein reported SBP in *posthepatitic cirrhosis*, exclusively caused by pneumococci (7). The association of pneumococcal SBP that occurred only in patients with posthepatitic cirrhosis infection was short lived. Indeed, in most large series the pneumococcus is the second or third most frequent bacterial agent responsible (2) after *E. coli* and *Klebsiella pneumoniae*. Other types of cirrhosis quickly followed, e.g., *hemochromatosis* and other iron-storage disorders (8), which has developed a curious relationship with the Yersinial species (9–11), which in turn seems to be dependent on abundant amounts of iron for its well being (12,13). In young children with α_1-*antitrypsin-deficiency-associated* cirrhosis appears to be the cirrhosis of choice for the development of SBP (15). SBP has been reported in both cardiac (16) and neoplastic (17) ascites, especially the type associated with intrahepatic metastases as opposed to the type characterized by peritoneal metastases (18).

A. SBP in Wilson's Disease

Person et al. have reported two patients with Wilson's disease who developed SBP (14). Both were 20-year-old men who had cirrhosis without any known reason for developing chronic liver disease. Both patients had decreased ceruloplasmin levels and increased urinary copper excretion, and one (patient 2) had Kayser-Fleischer rings. The first patient (patient 1) had a classic presentation of SBP, i.e., abdominal pain, ascites, fever, and a large increase in the number of ascitic fluid leukocytes (6400 per cubic millimeter), 98% of which were polymorphonuclear. His ascitic fluid and blood both grew *Klebsiella pneumoniae*. The infection was fatal. The second patient (patient 2) developed abnormal liver function tests, fever (100.6°F), and diffuse abdominal pain. The ascitic fluid contained 14,800 WBCs per cubic millimeter, of which 85% were polymorphonuclear. No bacteria were cultured from the ascitic fluid or blood, i.e., he had culture-negative SBP (CNSBP, CNNA). The patient responded promptly to broad spectrum antibiotic therapy. One other case of SBP in Wilson's disease has been reported (19). One additional case of probable SBP in Wilson's disease has been described, but the results of the ascitic fluid examination were not reported (20). No explanation for the rarity of this association has been established. Perhaps, it is related in some unknown way to the needs of these bacteria for increased copper concentrations.

Biliary cirrhosis and SBP have been associated, but only rarely (14a,b). Similarly, schistosomiasis and portal vein thrombosis, both of which are presinusoidal types of portal hypertension that are not prone to develop ascites, have not yet been reported in patients with SBP.

B. Species of Bacteria Causing SBP

The SBP syndrome was originally recognized as being caused by aerobic, gram-negative enteric species, and this pattern has persisted. *E. coli* are by far the most common organisms responsible and *Klebsiella* species are second. Almost all of the other gram-negative organisms known have been reported, but pneumococci and *Klebsiella* species appear to be tied for third place.

The list of bacterial organisms that have been cultured from the peritoneal fluid of patients with SBP has grown enormously (see Table 3.4).

It is of interest that SBP in adults was first reported in 1964 (1), whereas primary peritonitis, the similar syndrome seen in children with the nephrotic syndrome, had been recognized and described at least 25 years earlier (21) and, conceivably, several centuries earlier (22). Perhaps pediatricians are more perceptive than internists. Since pediatric SBP was described before the adult syndrome we shall discuss it first.

C. Pediatric SBP Syndromes

Primary peritonitis is the term that has been most commonly used to describe bacterial peritonitis in children (21,23). It was well recognized 25 years before

SBP was described. This serious infection is usually caused by pneumococci, beta-hemolytic streptococci, or *Haemophilus influenzae*. It has been postulated that these patients were often hypogammaglobulinemic secondary to the nephrosis, and that this antibody deficiency predisposed them to develop pneumococcal and streptococcal infections. By comparison, SBP is a similar infection that occurs primarily in adult patients with cirrhosis, usually of alcoholic origin. Recent reports have suggested that the profile of the infecting organisms in primary peritonitis appears to be changing so that it is becoming more enteric in nature, similar to that seen in adult SBP (24,25).

Primary peritonitis should be differentiated from the pediatric SBP syndrome reported by Larcher et al. (26), which is virtually identical to that seen in adult SBP. Ten of the 11 children in their series, who averaged 5.5 years of age, had cirrhosis and ascites prior to the development of SBP. The etiology of the cirrhosis, however, differed in the two groups. In the children the SBP was associated with pediatric types of chronic liver disease such as α_1-antitrypsin-deficiency-associated cirrhosis, cryptogenic hepatitis of infancy, and biliary atresia, among others. Eleven of the 79 patients with chronic liver disease developed SBP (14%), a percentage similar to that seen in adult SBP (2,19). The clinical syndrome in the children closely mimics that seen in adults. It consists of abdominal pain, rebound tenderness, fever, and often diarrhea or vomiting. The WBC counts in the ascitic fluid averaged 2500 per cubic millimeter, which is similar to that observed in adults. The bacteria isolated were quite different, however. They consisted predominantly of *Streptococcus pneumoniae* (73%), *Klebsiella pneumoniae* (18%), and *Haemophilus influenzae* (9%). In adults the bacteria are usually gram-negative, enteric bacilli (67%), primarily *E. coli* and *K. pneumoniae*, whereas pneumococci were found in about 15%. In 82% of the pediatric patients the same species was isolated from the ascitic fluid and from the blood at the time of diagnosis.

Larcher et al. demonstrated that their patients frequently exhibited reduced opsonizing capacity for pneumococci prior to their subsequent development of pneumococcal SBP (27). All of these patients had reduced complement levels. Thus, both the classical antibody-dependent pathway and the alternate complement pathways appear to be deficient in those patients destined to develop SBP. Similar deficiencies in complement and opsonizing capacities have been shown for adult SBP (28–30), suggesting that the ultimate defect in both types of SBP may be related to complement deficiency and impaired clearance of bacteria. This same group of investigators had previously shown that children with fulminant hepatic failure had shown enhanced susceptibility to bacterial and fungal infections that were associated with decreased concentrations of complement concentration in vivo (31) and diminished opsonization in vitro.

In their quite different series of primary peritonitis in Indian children, Kumaravel and Ramakrishnan reported 48 children with SBP, 75% of whom were female (32), and differentiated them from 102 children with "perforative" peritonitis who were predominantly male (62%) and in whom perforation of a hollow viscus was found at laparotomy. Their "primary peritonitis" was defined as patients who had an acute abdomen with purulent material in the peritoneal cavity, but in whom no perforation was found at laparotomy. In both subgroups abdominal pain, fever, and vomiting were common. Bacteriologic cultures of peritoneal fluid showed no growth in 75%. Many of these patients had received antibiotic therapy, however. Thus, several different types of Indian pediatric SBP apparently exist.

Sen et al. reported a rather common syndrome in Indian girls (33). They described 31 children from a single hospital, only one of whom had underlying nephrosis. Although these girls were otherwise normal, the disease was highly lethal. I propose that it be called *Indian childhood SBP*. Incidentally, the term *primary*, as in *primary peritonitis*, means "essential" or idiopathic. By comparison, *spontaneous* in spontaneous bacterial peritonitis is a conscious misnomer that means "without apparent cause" and not "spontaneous" as in *spontaneous combustion*.

D. Fever vs. Hypothermia in SBP

Hippocrates recognized fever to be a beneficial sign of infection and this concept has persisted for two millennia. Galen stated that "Fever is Nature's engine, which she brings into the field to remove her enemy" (34). Fever is caused by the release of androgenous pyrogens, including pyrogenic cytokines such as interleukin-1, interleukin-6, etc., which raise the thermoregulatory set point in the anterior thalamus (34,35). Presumably hypothermia, which is induced by a variety of endogenous antipyretic substances known as cryogens such as α-melanin-stimulating hormone and glucocorticosteroids that reduce the thermoregulatory set point, may therefore be considered an enemy of Nature. Indeed, experiments in animals tend to show that hypothermia is harmful to the hosts. Presumably, the occurrence of hypothermia in serious bacterial infections such as bacteremia, pyogenic infections, and SBP has negative prognostic implications.

One of the few significant additions to the original clinical syndrome of SBP was the recognition that *hypothermia*, like fever, may be a primary component of SBP. It is not clear who made the first observation that hypothermia is common in SBP. The earliest report of which I am aware is in an article by Le Carrer et al. in 1980 that hypothermia, i.e., temperatures >38°C or <36°C, as well as fever, were common in SBP (36). Our group at the WHVAMC has been aware of this association for many years. We had noted years ago that hypothermia, even in the absence of other signs of SBP, was useful in suggesting the diagnosis of silent or at least "very quiet" SBP. We have been suspicious of temperatures of 96°F or less in ascitic cirrhotic patients. We taught that the occurrence of even a single, confirmed episode of hypothermia demanded prompt paracentesis and examination of the ascitic fluid. We were able to make the diagnosis of SBP in several patients on the basis of that observation alone (2). Of course, hypothermia has long been known to be associated with bacterial infection, especially bacteremia.

Hypothermia may occur in a variety of circumstances: exposure to low temperatures, usually extrinsic, but sometimes intrinsic exposures such as the intravenous infusions of cold solutions or gastric lavage, or peritoneal dialysis with cold fluids. The administration of hypnotic or tranquilizing substances such as barbiturates or phenothiazines and the presence of metabolic disorders such as myxedema, hypopituitarism, uremia, diabetes with ketoacidosis, or sepsis are often associated with hypothermia (37).

In sepsis, hypothermia is usually seen in patients with bacterial infections, especially those of gram-negative origin, although fever is a much more common sign (38–40). Hypothermia is frequently seen in elderly patients and often occurs in association with hypotension and bacterial peritonitis is a common cause (41,42). The mechanism of hypothermia is not known, but it is postulated to be the result of a reduced hypothalamic temperature set point, and decreased levels of tri-iodothyronine probably play a role (42,43). Hypothermia probably occurs in virtually every cirrhotic patient with renal failure in the terminal stages (44).

E. Variations in the Clinical Syndrome

SBP is not a static syndrome. Several new, previously unreported physical signs have been added to the clinical picture, each of which has broadened the scope of this syndrome. One such new sign is *erythema gangrenosum*, bullous dermatologic lesions that are seen almost exclusively in patients with *Pseudomonas aeruginosa* infections. Occasionally it is seen with *E. coli* infections (45). Another new sign is *acute scrotal edema* as an early manifestation of SBP in children (46). This sign may well be associated with the sudden scrotal edema syndrome that results from a communication between the peritoneal and the subcutaneous tissues of the abdominal wall as has been reported following paracentesis (47). *Cutaneous pigmentation of the abdominal wall* has been described as a manifestation of chronic SBP (48). The occurrence of hemorrhagic *vesicles and bullae* of the skin of a patient with SBP from whom *Vibrio vulnificus* had been cultured from both the peritoneal cavity and the vesicular fluid has also been reported (49).

III. LABORATORY VARIATIONS IN SBP

A. Culture-Negative SBP (CNSBP) and Culture-Negative Neutrocytic Ascites (CNNA)

CNSBP is defined as the presence of the clinical picture of SBP, ascites that contains more than 250 polymorphonuclear leukocytes (PMNs) per cubic millimeter, a sterile ascitic fluid culture, and no explanation for the abdominal finding (50). In the most simple sense it represents culture-negative SBP. How can such a syndrome develop? What does it signify? First, it may represent SBP at an early phase in its course, prior to the peritoneal infection becoming fully developed. Second, it may represent SBP at a late stage in its course, after the body's defenses have defeated the invading organisms, when the bacteria are too inhibited or too few in number to show a positive culture. Third, organisms may be too fastidious to grow on the culture media employed or on a culture medium that is for any reason not as hospitable to bacteria as it usually is. Conceivably, the patient may have received an antibiotic substance that is too small to eradicate the infection, but is large enough to suppress the growth of the organism in vitro. Fourth, the number of bacteria may be so small that the inoculum contains "no" bacteria. If, for example, the number of organisms in the ascitic fluid were less than 1 per ml, inocula of 1 ml of ascitic fluid would sometimes be free of bacteria and would consequently show no growth. (See Table 2.1.)

In an attempt to assess the situation, Pelletier et al. compared 38 cirrhotic patients with SBP and 15 with CNSBP selected especially by virtue of their

Table 2.1 Clinical Variants of the Spontaneous Bacterial Peritonitis Syndrome

1. Spontaneous bacterial peritonitis (culture-positive SBP)
2. Culture-negative SBP (false-negative SBP or "probable SBP")
3. Asymptomatic bacterascites (ABA)
4. Symptomatic bacterascites (SBA)

not having received any antibiotic agents for at least one month, and, of course, of not having any intra-abdominal source of infection (51). Most of the patients had alcoholic cirrhosis. The majority of their patients with SBP were infected with *E. coli.* The two groups were similar in clinical and laboratory features. The only statistically significant differences were a higher mean serum creatinine concentration (1.6 vs. 1.3 mg%; $p < 0.03$), a higher mean serum bilirubin concentration, and a higher percentage of positive blood cultures (39 vs. 13%; $p < 0.05$) in those with SBP (see Table 3.3). In addition, the mean leukocyte and PMN counts in the ascitic fluid were lower in the CNSBP group than in the SBP group (3177 vs. 8064 per cubic millimeter; and 2367 vs. 6663, respectively; $p < 0.02$). Recovery rates were higher and 30 day mortality rates were lower in the CNSBP than in the SBP group (87 vs. 69%; $p < 0.05$ and 20 vs. 50%; $p < 0.05$, respectively). Although the exact explanation is not known, it is reasonable to accept the original hypothesis that CNSBP is a more serious variant of SBP than ABA, which may equally well be called culture-positive, neutrocytic ascites (CPNA). The cirrhosis was less severe in CNSBP than in CPNA according to Pugh's criteria (52).

Tam and associates published an almost identical paper (53) in which the patients with CNSBP responded to antibiotic therapy in terms of a decrease in the numbers of WBCs and PMNs in the ascitic fluid. They, too, believe that CNSBP is a less severe type of SBP, and one that requires antibiotic therapy.

A very similar quandary exists for culture-negative bacterial endocarditis (54), which, like CNSBP, occurs in about 20% of patients with bacterial endocarditis (55).

B. Other Variants of SBP

Another syndrome that appears to be related pathogenetically to acute scrotal edema, which occasionally occurs after paracentesis (47), is unilateral abdominal or chest wall edema that follows laparotomy or thoracotomy in ascitic cirrhotic patients (56). In principle, such patients suffer from fistulae between the peritoneal cavity and the subcutaneous tissues of the body wall. The ascitic fluid dissects into the subcutaneous spaces where its distribution is determined by the site of incision and by gravity. Because subcutaneous fluids do not cross the midline freely, the fluid is usually localized to the side of the incision. When the incision crosses the midline, the fluid may be distributed bilaterally. Occasionally, such collections of edema may dissect into the subcutaneous tissue of the lower extremity if the attachments of Scarpa's fascia to the fascia lata are incomplete, and may give rise to edema of the lower extremity and/or the scrotum and penis. When the ascitic fluid is infected by bacteria in SBP, either spontaneously or secondarily, one may see the ''erysipelas'' described in Beethoven after his paracentesis (see Chap. 1) (57) because the infected ascitic fluid may induce a severe, erysipelas-like erythemia.

Secondary ''complications'' of unilateral trunkal edema, such as *unilateral jaundice*, may occur when the accumulated fluid is ascitic in origin (56). This phenomenon occurs because ascitic fluid is high in albumin concentration and because bilirubin binds to albumin. Subcutaneous dissections of ascitic fluid in which the albumin concentrations is high, tend to be brightly jaundiced if the serum bilirubin concentrations are elevated whereas collections of edema fluid in patients with heart disease or nephrosis, in which the albumin concentrations are low, do not. Edema associated with burns or allergic reactions have a high albumin concentration and appear jaundiced. Indeed, this is the basis of the histamine wheal test for jaundice, in which wheals induced by subcutaneous injections of histamine appear jaundiced whereas the surrounding tissue does not.

C. Spontaneous Eosinophilic Bacterial Peritonitis

This rare syndrome is of little clinical importance. *Eosinophilic ascites*, i.e., ascitic fluid with a high concentration of eosinophilic leukocytes, has been reported in patients with eosinophilic gastroenteritis or the hypereosinophilic syndrome (58), and may occur in patients with progressive cardiac failure. The mechanism of the eosinophilia is unknown. It is assumed that allergy may be responsible, but the cause has never been elucidated. Eosinophilic SBP appears to be typical SBP in which the polymorphonuclear response to the infection is primarily eosinophilic for unknown reasons. Apparently, these eosinophilic polymorphonuclear leukocytes function well. Rowland described an alcoholic cirrhotic patient who developed the classical syndrome of SBP except that 80% of the 12,400 leukocytes per cubic millimeter of ascitic fluid were eosinophilic (59). Surprisingly, there were no eosinophilic leukocytes among the 7000 WBC per cubic millimeter in the patient's blood. The patients responded promptly to conventional antibiotic therapy with the disappearance of the peritoneal leukocytosis and the peritoneoeosinophilocytosis.

Eosinophilic peritonitis of unknown cause may be associated with chronic ambulatory peritoneal dialysis (60), and may be rapidly corrected by the administration of intraperitoneal hydrocortisone (61).

IV. SBP IN NONCIRRHOTIC DISEASES

A. SBP in Systemic Lupus Erythematosus (SLE)

SBP has been reported in seven patients with SLE (62–66). SBP in SLE appears to be quite different in its clinical and laboratory characteristics than in the usual cases of SBP. In none of the patients was underlying decompensated cirrhosis present. In three of the seven, pneumococci were cultured from the abdominal fluid; in one β-hemolytic streptococci were responsible, in one both *E. coli* and *Klebsiella* species were recovered, in one *Bacteroides fragilis* was found, and in one no ascitic fluid culture was performed.

Unlike the conventional SBP that occurs in cirrhosis and that is characterized by the preexistence of abundant amounts of ascitic fluid, these patients did not have cirrhosis. SLE had been present from 1 to 8 years, the lupus was active and corticosteroid therapy was being administered. They all had abdominal pain and tenderness. The ascitic fluid was small in amount or absent, even by paracentesis. One had thick yellow pus and one had serosanguinous ascitic fluid. The number of leukocytes did not exceed 300 per cubic millimeter and the number of polymorphonuclear leukocytes was less than 240 per cubic millimeter except for the one patient with purulent ascitic fluid in whom the exact number was not presented.

In SLE bacterial peritonitis appears to reflect the increased susceptibility to infection associated with the underlying collagen vascular diseases and with the administration of adrenocorticosteroid therapy. It appears to differ from conventional SBP in that ascites does not appear to be a prerequisite.

B. SBP in Rheumatoid Arthritis

SBP caused by *Streptococcus pneumoniae* was reported in one noncirrhotic patient with severe rheumatoid arthritis who was being treated with penicillamine (67). This patient has been admitted to the hospital with chills, fever, and leukocytosis without obvious explanation. There was no evidence of cirrhosis and tests of liver function were normal. In the hospital the abdominal pain worsened and laparotomy showed only ''purulent'' peritoneal fluid from which pneumococci were cultured. No perforation was found and the liver appeared normal. No satisfactory explanation of these bizarre events had been discovered. It has been suggested that patients with rheumatoid arthritis are especially susceptible to bacterial infections. This concurrence of SBP and rheumatoid arthritis cannot be considered a valid association, however, until other similar cases are reported.

C. Spontaneous Gonococcal Perihepatitis (Curtis-Fitz-Hugh) Syndrome

Gonococcal peritonitis of the upper abdomen was first described in 1919 (68,69). About 10 years later Curtis associated the presence of "violin-string" adhesions between the anterior surface of the liver and the parietal peritoneum in women with gonococcal pelvic inflammatory disease (PID) (70). A few years later this syndrome, which is known as *gonococcal perihepatitis*, was characterized by right-upper-quadrant pain and, frequently, a perihepatic friction rub. Fitz-Hugh has confirmed the existence and nature of this disorder (71), which has been known as the Curtis-Fitz-Hugh syndrome since that time. This syndrome occurs in 10–15% of patients with PID (72).

As experience with variations of this syndrome increased it was recognized that nongonococcal PID could also give rise to this disorder. Furthermore, the disease is common in patients with intrauterine contraceptive devices (IUCDs) in place, and especially when the PID has developed shortly after insertion of the IUCD (73).

It is postulated that the bacteria pass from the vagina through the Fallopian tubes and then to the subphrenic spaces. Stassen et al. have reported a characteristic example (74). The fact that this disease also occurs in male patients indicates that other routes of transmission, such as hematogenous or lymphatic pathway, may also be possible. The trans-Fallopian route, however, has the tangible ring of truth and of logic. Bacteriologic proof of the trans-Fallopian traverse has been established for gonococci (75). Occasionally, this disorder may be fatal (76). Recently, Chlamydial infections have been thought to give rise to SBP even more commonly than gonococci and often to mimic acute cholecystitis (77).

D. Pregnancy and SBP

Although pregnancy is not a disease, it does represent an altered, nonphysiological state that could conceivably predispose pregnant woman to the development of SBP. Several such cases have been reported (78,79). The first of these occurred in a woman following painless vaginal bleeding, and Group B hemolytic streptococci were cultured from the blood, peritoneum, and vagina (78). Presumably, an ascending infection caused the peritonitis. The second such case is even more complicated (79). In this patient, who had both sickle cell disease and decompensated cirrhosis secondary to non-A, non-B chronic hepatitis, *E. coli* and Klebsiella species were cultured from the blood. It is likely that this case represents true SBP. Nothing in either of these cases suggests that pregnancy per se contributed to the development of the SBP.

E. Iatrogenic SBP and Vasopressin-Induced SBP

We observed two instances of SBP in patients who had been receiving intra-arterial infusions of vasopressin for 12–24 h for management of gastrointestinal bleeding (80). In one, who was bleeding from a peptic ulcer, the infusion was administered into the celiac artery (0.2 units per min); in the other, who was probably bleeding from esophageal varices, it was infused into the superior mesenteric artery (0.4 units per min). These episodes differed from typical SBP in several ways. Both patients developed fever and abdominal pain and tenderness. The diagnosis of SBP was confirmed by peritoneal leukocytosis and by the recovery of bacteria from the ascitic fluid. The cultures, however, were quite atypical for SBP. Instead of the usual isolation of a single aerobic species of organisms, both grew several aerobic bacteria and several anaerobic species. The first case revealed *Escherichia coli, Proteus morgani*, bacteroides, and unidentified gram-positive rods. The second showed *Staphylococcus epidermidis, Bacteroides fragilis*, diphtheroid bacteria, and an alpha-streptococcus.

The syndrome was attributed to the transmural escape from the lumen of the bowel of enteric bacteria induced by vasoconstriction of the arteries to the intestinal tract. Ligation of the superior mesenteric artery results in the escape of intestinal organisms into the blood and lymphatic systems in both clinical and experimental situations (81,82). The local injection of epinephrine also does so (83). Similarly, idiopathic bacterial peritonitis has developed in patients with splanchnic arterial insufficiency. It appears that reducing the arterial blood flow to the intestine may compromise the extremely effective bacterial barrier between the lumen and the lymphatic and blood vessels and may permit the transmural passage of bacteria.

F. Leukopenia-Associated SBP and SBP Triggered by Parvovirus B19

Recently it was observed that a Japanese patient with hepatitis B virus (HBV)–related cirrhosis developed *Klebsiella pneumoniae* SBP one week after an acute infection with parvovirus B19 (84). The viral infection was characterized by chills and high fever (37.2°C) and a sharp drop in the total WBC count to 1,210 per cubic millimeter and in the neutrophil and lymphocyte counts to

544 and 478 per cubic millimeter, respectively. Seven days later the patient complained of severe abdominal pain and tenderness and fever. Paracentesis revealed 12,000 WBC per cubic millimeter in the ascitic fluid. The infection responded promptly to piperacillin. On admission to the hospital 16 days before the viral infection parvovirus B19-genome DNA was absent, but it was detected two days before the fever peak. Anti-B19 IgM became positive on the day of the fever and then increased for several days, after which the anti-B19 IgG titer began to rise. Yamamoto et al. suggested that this classic episode of primary infection with parvovirus B19 triggered the episode of SBP by inducing leukopenia (84). There is no question that an episode of parvovirus B19 occurred, but it is not established that it precipitated the SBP. It will be of great interest to determine what other viral triggers may precipitate SBP. No other triggers have yet been identified although several predisposing factors, such as reduced ascitic fluid protein concentration and perhaps hypothermia, have been identified.

G. Tuberculous Peritonitis (TBP) as a Form of Spontaneous Bacterial Peritonitis

Tuberculosis is an infectious disease that may involve virtually any organ in the body. It frequently involves the organs of the peritoneal cavity (see Chap. 4). Although it is not usually an acute secondary infection, it may act as such. In the most literal sense it satisfies the definition of spontaneous, bacterial peritonitis. First, it develops *spontaneously*. Second, *Mycobacterium tuberculosis* is, indeed, a bacterium. Third, it frequently causes peritonitis, although it may involve many other gastrointestinal tissues as well. Fourth, it is important that SBP be differentiated from TBP in whatever manner possible, because the pathogenesis, prognosis, and therapy of the two infections are completely different from each other. There are many other differences as well. Tuberculous peritonitis has been known for at least several centuries. Over the years tuberculosis has become a widely disseminated infection, no longer being found primarily in the pulmonary tract, but frequently occurring in extrapulmonary locations. At present it is not infrequently localized solely to the abdominal cavity (85), where it may present in a variety of ways. It may mimic any abdominal lesion (86). Because SBP is an acute, highly lethal disease and abdominal tuberculosis is a chronic debilitating and ultimately highly fatal disease, the differentiation is often an important practical matter. Furthermore, TBP is a very different disorder in those patients with chronic liver disease from those without liver disease (87,88) even though it is not a common infection of the peritoneum. The development of multiantibiotic resistant strains of tuberculosis has impeded efforts to control or eradicate this infection.

Shakil and associates studied 64 patients selected on the basis of an increased mononuclear leukocyte cell count in their ascitic fluid (89). They found that 13 had TBP (50%) without cirrhosis (Group 1), 21 had TBP with cirrhosis (Group II), and 26 "control" subjects had cirrhosis and uninfected ascitic fluid (Group III).

In TBP, abdominal distention (94%), abdominal pain (65%), and weight loss (38%) are the predominant presenting symptoms, whereas ascites (100%), fever (74%), and muscle wasting (50%) are the predominant physical signs.

Ascitic fluid cultures for tuberculosis were positive in 45%, peritoneal nodules on laparoscopy were seen in 94%, granulomas were found microscopically in 93%, peritoneal cultures were positive for tuberculosis in 48%, and finally a positive response to therapy was noted in 97%. PPD skin tests are not considered a reliable index of active tuberculosis because many patients with tuberculosis are anergic.

Comparison of Groups I and II (TBP without and with cirrhosis, respectively) showed that those with cirrhosis exhibited higher mean WBC counts (9500 vs. 5400 per cubic millimeter; $p < 0.001$), higher total serum bilirubin concentrations (57 vs. 34 mM per L), lower mean prothrombin times (51 vs. 74%; $p < 0.01$), lower mean ascitic fluid albumin concentrations (1.0 vs. 2.1 g per dl; $p < 0.001$), higher mean serum-ascites to albumin gradients (SAAG) (1.1 vs. 0.6 g per dl; $p < 0.001$) and lower mean lactic dehydrogenase activity levels (208 vs. 344 U per L; $p < 0.05$).

Those observations indicate that about half the patients with tuberculosis have peritoneal involvement and have a high mortality rate if untreated. Further, those who are immigrants and those who develop AIDS are especially susceptible to TBP indicating a high resurgence rate of tuberculosis. Only 15–20% have concomitant pulmonary tuberculosis. Laparoscopy with directed biopsy and histological and bacterial examination are the best ways of establishing the diagnosis of tuberculosis. Blind liver biopsy has a lower success rate and higher morbidity and mortality rates than open or laparoscopy-guided biopsies. The measurement of adenosine deaminase activity in ascitic fluid appears to be a simple and accurate method of making a presumptive diagnosis of TBP when laparoscopy is not available (90). This enzyme, which is involved in the catabolic conversion of adenosine to inosine, is associated with the stimulation of T lymphocytes as part of the response to cell-mediated immunity. Confirmation is achieved by acid-fast stains, the histologic demonstration of granulomas, and, most important, a clinical trial of antituberculous therapy using isoniazid, rifampicin, pyrazinamide, or ethambutol. Tuberculous infections are especially frequent in patients with chronic ambulatory peritoneal dialysis (CAPD).

REFERENCES

1. Conn HO. Spontaneous peritonitis and bacteremia in cirrhotic patients caused by enteric bacteria. Ann Intern Med 60:568–580, 1964.
2. Conn HO, Fessel JM. Spontaneous bacterial peritonitis in cirrhosis. Variations on a theme. Medicine 50:161–197, 1971.
3. Targan SR, Chow AW, Guze LB. Role of anaerobic bacteria in spontaneous peritonitis of cirrhosis. Am J Med 62:387–403, 1977.
4. Bac DJ, De Marie S, Van Blankenstein M. Spontaneous bacteria peritonitis complicating malignancy-related ascites. Dig Dis Sc 41:131–132, 1996.
5. Albillos A, Curvas-Mons V, Millan I. Ascitic fluid polymorphonuclear cell count and serum to ascites albumin gradients in the diagnosis of bacterial peritonitis. Gastroenterology 98:134–140, 1990.
6. Conn HO, Goldfarb J. Spontaneous bacterial peritonitis: an endemic epidemic. In: *Hepatic, Biliary and Pancreatic Surgery*, JS Najarian, JP Delaney, eds., Miami Symposia Specialists, 1980, pp. 441–459.
7. Epstein M, Calia FM, Gabuzda GJ. Pneumococcal peritonitis in patients with postnecrotic cirrhosis. N Engl J Med 278:69–73, 1968.
8. Capron JP, Capron-Chivrac D, Tossou H. Spontaneous *Yersinia enterocolitica* peritonitis in idiopathic hemochromatosis. Gastroenterology 87:1371–1375, 1984.
9. Senejoux A, Cadranel J-F, Benhamou Y. Infection spontanee du liquide d'ascited a *Yersinia pseudotuberculosis* revelatrice d'une probable hemochromatose genetique. Gastroenterol Clin Biol 17:877–885, 1993.
10. Levi Della Vida MV, Campanelli G, Boemi L. *Yersinia enterocolitica* peritonitis in a child with Cooley's disease and splenectomy. Ital J Gastroenterol 14:31–33, 1982.
11. Marx RS, Johnson JE III. *Yersinia enterocolitica* meningitis with septicemia and spontaneous peritonitis. NC Med J 40:691–694, 1979.
12. Melby K, Slordahl S, Gutteberg TJ. Septicemia due to *Yersinia enterocolitica* after oral overdoses of iron Br Med J 285:467–468, 1982.
13. Robins-Browne RM, Rabson AR, Koornhof HJ. Generalized infection with *Yersinia enterocolitica* and the role of iron. Contrib Microbiol Immunol 5:277–282, 1979.
14. Person JL, Anderson DS, Brower RA. Spontaneous bacterial peritonitis in Wilson's disease. Am J Gastroenterol 82:66–68, 1987.
14a. Ariza J, Xiol X, Esteve M, Bañeres FF, Liñares J, Alonso T, Gudiol F. Aztreonam vs. cefotaxime in the treatment of gram-negative spontaneous peritonitis in cirrhotic patients. Hepatology 14:91–98, 1991.
14b. Terg R, Levi D, Lopez P, et al. Analysis of clinical course and prognosis of

culture-positive spontaneous bacterial peritonitis and neutrocytic ascites: evidence of the same disease. Dig Dis Sci 37:1499–1504, 1992.

15. Larcher VF, Manolaki N, Vegente A. Spontaneous bacterial peritonitis in children with chronic liver disease: clinical features and etiologic factors. J Pediatr 106:907–912, 1985.

16. Runyon BA. Spontaneous bacterial peritonitis associated with cardiac ascites. Am J Gastroenterol 79:796–803, 1984.

17. Mal F, Pham Huu T, Benhamou M. Chemoattractant and opsonic activity in ascitic fluid. J Hepatol 12:45–49, 1991.

18. Runyon BA, Morrissey RL, Hoefs HC, Wyle FA. Opsonic activity of human ascitic fluid: a potentially important protective mechanism against spontaneous bacterial peritonitis. Hepatology 5:634–637, 1985.

19. Weinstein MP, Iannini PB, Stratton CW. Spontaneous bacterial peritonitis. Am J Med 64:592–598, 1978.

20. Case Records Mass Gen Hosp: Case 44. NEJM 311:1170–1178, 1984.

21. Pahmer M. Pneumococcal peritonitis in nephrotic and non-nephrotic children. J Pediatr 17:90–106, 1940.

22. Harken AH, Shchat SJ. Gram-positive peritonitis in children. Am J Surg 125: 769–772, 1973.

23. Fowler R. Primary peritonitis. Aust NZ J Surg 26:204–213, 1957.

24. Fowler R. Primary peritonitis: changing aspects 1956–1970. Aust Paediat J 7: 73–83, 1971.

25. Clark JH, Fitzgerald JF, Kleiman MB. Spontaneous bacterial peritonitis. J Pediatr 104:495–499, 1984.

26. Larcher VF, Manolaki N, Vegente A. Spontaneous bacterial peritonitis in children with chronic liver disease: clinical features and etiologic factors. J Pediatr 106:907–912, 1985.

27. Larcher VF, Wyke RJ, Mowat AP, Williams R. Mechanism of yeast opsonisation defect in children with fulminant hepatic failure. Clin Exp Immunol 46:406–411, 1981.

28. Hoefs JC, Runyon RA. Spontaneous bacterial peritonitis. Dis Month 31:1–48, 1985.

29. Runyon BA, Morrissey RL, Hoefs JC, Wyle FA. Opsonic activity of human ascitic fluid: a potentially important protective mechanism against spontaneous bacterial peritonitis. Hepatology 5:634–637, 1985.

30. Such J, Guarner C, Enriquez J. Low C3 in cirrhotic patients predisposes to spontaneous bacterial peritonitis. J Hepatol 6:80–84, 1988.

31. Larcher VF, Wyke RJ, Mowat AP, Williams R. Bacterial and fungal infection in children with fulminant hepatic failure: possible role of opsonisation and complement deficiency. Gut 23:1037–1043, 1982.

32. Kumaravel G, Ramkrishnan MS. Peritonitis in children. J Ind Med Assoc 67: 93–101, 1976.

33. Sen S, Lalitha MK, Fenn AS, Mammen KE. Primary peritonitis in children. Ann Trop Paediat 3:53–56, 1983.

34. Kluger MJ, Kozak W, Conn CA. The adaptive value of fever. Infect Dis Clin North Am 10:1–11, 1996.

35. Dinarello CA. Thermoregulation and the pathogenesis of fever. Infect Dis Clin North Am 10:433–449, 1996.

36. LeCarrer M, Poupon R-Y, Ballet F, Darnis F. Les infections du liquide d'ascite chez le etude clinique et biologique de 36 episodes observes au cours d'une annee. Gastroenterol Clin Biol 4:640–645, 1980.

37. Spivak JL. Disorders caused by heat and cold. In *The Principles and Practice of Medicine*, 21st Ed., A McG Harvey, RJ Johns, VA McKusick, eds., Norwalk, CT: Appleton-Century-Crofts, 1984, pp. 1437–1442.

38. Peduzzi P, Shatney C, Sheagren J. Predictors of bacteremia and gram-negative bacteremia in patients with sepsis. Arch Intern Med 152:529–535, 1992.

39. Chassagne P, Perol M-B, Doucet J. Is presentation of bacteremia in the elderly the same as in younger patients? Am J Med 100:65–70, 1996.

40. Kramer MR, Vandijk J, Rosin AJ. Mortality in elderly patients with thermoregulatory failure. Arch Intern Med 149:1521–1523, 1989.

41. Doherty NH, Fung P, Lefkowitz M, Ellrodt GA. Hypothermia and sepsis. Ann Intern Med 103:308–312, 1985.

42. Bacci L, Schussler GC, Kaplan TB. The relationship between serum triiodothyronine and thyrotropin during systemic illness. J Clin Endocrinol Metab 54:1229–1235, 1982.

43. Tolman KG, Harman CG, Englert E. Jr. Hypothermia in cirrhosis: a cause of renal failure? (Abstr) Gastroenterology 56:1201, 1969.

44. Conn HO. Unpublished observations.

45. Rajan RK. Spontaneous bacterial peritonitis with erythema gangrenosum due to *Escherichia coli*. J Clin Gastroenterol 4:145–148, 1982.

46. Udall DA, Drake DJ Jr, Rosenberg RS. Acute scrotal swelling: A physical sign of primary peritonitis. J Urol 125:750–751, 1981.

47. Conn HO. Sudden scrotal edema. A post-paracentesis syndrome. Ann Intern Med 74:943–945, 1971.

48. Pollack S, Haim S, Enat R. Cutaneous pigmentation: a probable sign of spontaneous bacterial peritonitis. Dermatologica 161:187–190, 1980.

49. Wongpaitoon V, Sathapatayavongs B, Prachaktam R. Spontaneous *Vibrio vulnificus* peritonitis and primary sepsis in two patients with alcoholic cirrhosis. Am J Gastroenterol 80:706–708, 1985.

50. Runyon BA, Hoefs JC. Culture-negative neutrocytic ascites: a variant of spontaneous bacterial peritonitis. Hepatology 4:1209–1211, 1984.

51. Pelletier G, Salmon D, Ink O. Culture-negative neutrocytic ascites: A less severe variant of spontaneous bacterial peritonitis. J Hepatology 10:327–331, 1990.

52. Al Amri SM, Allam AR, Al Mofleh IA. Spontaneous bacterial peritonitis and culture negative neutrocytic ascites in patients with non-alcoholic liver cirrhosis. J Gastroenterol Hepatol 9:433–436, 1994.

53. Tam F, Prindiville T. A comparison of spontaneous bacterial peritonitis and culture negative neutrocytic ascites. Personal communication.

54. Cannady PB, Sanford JP. Negative blood cultures in infective endocarditis: a review. South M J 69:1420–1424, 1976.

55. Runyon BA, Umland ET, Merlin T. Inoculation of blood culture bottles with

ascitic fluid. Improved detection of spontaneous bacterial peritonitis. Arch Int Med 147:71–75, 1987.

56. Conn HO. Unilateral edema and jaundice following portacaval anastomosis. Ann Intern Med 76:459–461, 1972.

57. Sonneck OG. Beethoven: Impressions by His Contemporaries. New York: Dover Publications, 1926.

58. Klein NC, Hargrove KL, Schlesinger MH. Eosinophilic gastroenteritis. Medicine 49:299–319, 1970.

59. Rowland M, Brown RB, Goldman M. Eosinophilic peritonitis: an unusual manifestation of spontaneous bacterial peritonitis. J Clin Gastroenterol 7:369–371, 1985.

60. Noph KD, Sorkin MI, Prowant BF. Symptomatic eosinophilic peritonitis in CAPD. Dialysis and Transplantation 11:309–313, 1982.

61. Leung ACT, Orange G, Henderson IS. Intraperitoneal hydrocortisone in eosinophilic peritonitis associated with continuous ambulatory peritoneal dialysis. Br M J 286:766–769, 1983.

62. Lipsky PE, Hardin JA, Schour L. Spontaneous peritonitis and systemic lupus erythematosus: importance of accurate diagnosis of gram-positive bacterial infections. JAMA 232:929–931, 1975.

63. Case Records Mass Gen: Case 47, NEJM 295:1187–1190, 1976.

64. Shesol F, Rosato EF, Rosato FE. Concomitant acute lupus erythematosus and primary pneumococcal peritonitis. Am J Gastroenterol 63:324–327, 1975.

65. Rozen D, Vanhaeverbeek M, Stenuit R. Polyradiculoneuritis, *Bacteroides fragilis* septicemia and peritonitis in a case of systemic lupus erythematosus. Rev Med Brux 1:395–398, 1980.

66. Rajatanavin R, Pombejara CN, Pekanan P. Spontaneous bacterial peritonitis in systemic lupus erythematosus: a case report. J Med Asso Thailand 64:406–412, 1981.

67. Skau T, Tegner Y. Spontaneous peritonitis and rheumatoid arthritis: a case report. Acta Chir Scand 152:317–318, 1986.

68. Browne MK, Cassie R. Spontaneous bacterial peritonitis during pregnancy. Case report. Br J Obstet Gynecol 88:1158–1160, 1981.

69. Stajano C. La reaccion frenica in ginecologia. Sem Med 27:243–259, 1920.

70. Curtis AH. Cause of adhesions in right upper quadrant. JAMA 99:2010–2021, 1932.

71. FitzHugh T. Acute gonococcic peritonitis of the right upper quadrant in women. JAMA 102:2094–2099, 1934.

72. Onsrud M. Perihepatitis in pelvic inflammatory disease—association with intrauterine contraception. Acta Obstet Gynecol Scand 59:69–71, 1980.

73. Brinson RR, Kolts BE, Monif GRG. Spontaneous bacterial peritonitis associated with an intrauterine device. J Clin Gastroenterol 8:82–84, 1986.

74. Stassen WN, McCullough AJ, Hilton PK. Spontaneous bacterial peritonitis caused by *Neisseria gonorrhoeae*. Gastroenterology 88:804–807, 1985.

75. Kornfeld SJ, Worthington MG. Culture-proved Fitz-Hugh-Curtis syndrome. Am J Obstet Gynecol 139:106–107, 1981.

76. Maloy AL, Meier FA, Karl RC. Fatal peritonitis following IUD-associated salpingitis. Obstet Gynecol 58:397–398, 1981.

77. Shabot JM, Roark GD, Truant AL. *Chlamydia trachomatis* in the ascitic fluid of patients with chronic liver disease. Am J Gastroenterol 78:291–293, 1983.

78. Browne MK, Cassie R. Spontaneous bacterial peritonitis during pregnancy. Case report. Br J Obstet Gynecol 88:1158–1160, 1981.

79. Stauffer RA, Wygal J, Lavery JP. Spontaneous bacterial peritonitis in pregnancy. Am J Obstet Gynecol 144:104–105, 1982.

80. Bar-Meir S, Conn HO. Spontaneous bacterial peritonitis induced by intra-arterial vasopressin therapy. Gastroenterology 70:418–421, 1976.

81. Cirrincione FA, Francona A. Influence of vascular impairment on absorption of bacteria into blood from upper intestinal tract. Proc Soc Exp Biol Med 29:400–401, 1932.

82. Cole WR, Petit R, Brown A. Lymphatic transport of bacteria in surgical infection. Lymphology 1:52–57, 1968.

83. Evans DG, Miles AA, Niven JSF. The enhancement of bacterial infections by adrenaline. Br J Exp Pathol 29:20–39, 1948.

84. Yamamoto T, Ise K, Nunoue T. Parvovirus B19 as a trigger for spontaneous bacterial peritonitis in a patient with cirrhotic ascites. Am J Gastroenterol 91:1857–1859, 1996.

85. Klimach OE, Ormerod LP. Gastrointestinal tuberculosis: A retrospective review of 109 cases in a district general hospital. Quart J Med 221:569–578, 1985.

86. Burack WR, Hollister RM. Tuberculous peritonitis: a study of forty-seven proved cases encountered by a general medical unit in twenty-five years. Am J Med 28:510–523, 1960.

87. Bastani B, Shariatzadeh MR, Dehdashti F. Tuberculous peritonitis—Report of 30 cases and review of the literature. Quart J Med 221:549–557, 1985.

88. Dineen P, Homan WP, Grafe WR. Tuberculous peritonitis: 43 years' experience in diagnosis and treatment. Am Surg 184:717–723, 1976.

89. Shakil AO, Korula J, Kanel GC. Diagnostic features of tuberculous peritonitis in the absence and presence of chronic liver disease: a case control study. Am J Med 100:179–185, 1996.

90. Martinez-Vasquez JM, Ribera E. Adenosine deaminase activity in the diagnosis of tuberculous peritonitis. Gut 27:1049–1053, 1986.

3

Unusual Presentations of Spontaneous Bacterial Peritonitis

Harold O. Conn

Yale University School of Medicine, New Haven, Connecticut, and University of Miami School of Medicine, Miami, Florida

I. INTRODUCTION

Chapter 2 included brief, general descriptions of the clinical variations in which SBP may present. In Chapter 3 we focus on unusual presentations and pathogeneses of SBP. Two variants of SBP, *asymptomatic bacterascites* (ABA) (1) and *culture-negative SBP* (CNSBP), which had briefly been known as culture-negative *neutrocytic ascites* (CNNA) (2), are intriguing, aberrant clinical presentations of SBP.

ABA is defined as the presence of bacteria in the ascitic fluid in the absence of clinical evidence of SBP and in the absence of any intra-abdominal source of infection. ABA was first described, named, and defined by our group at the West Haven Veterans Administration Hospital (WHVAH) in our definitive paper on SBP in 1964 (3). Two other studies of ABA have been reported by Pinzello et al. (4) and by Runyon (5).

Pelletier and his colleagues, however, have written what I consider to be the definitive paper on ABA (1). During the period from 1984 to 1988, 58 ascitic cirrhotic patients were retrospectively identified from the records of Hopital de Bicêtre (Le Kremlin-Bicêtre, France). Thirty-six of them had SBP and 22 had ABA, a ratio of 2.6:1 (Table 3.1). The patients in the ABA group exhibited no clinical features of SBP, i.e., no fever or abdominal signs, but often were malnourished, had bled from the gastrointestinal tract, and had

Table 3.1 Clinical Biological Characteristics in Patients with Asymptomatic BA and SBP

Characteristics	BA (n = 22)	SBP (n = 36)	p Value
Clinical features			
Fever	0	32 (89%)	0.001
Abdominal pain	0	19 (53%)	0.001
Encephalopathy	1 (5%)	18 (50%)	0.01
Gastrointestinal bleeding	3 (14%)	15 (42%)	0.04
Malnutrition	4 (18%)	24 (67%)	0.002
Blood			
WBC (cells/mm^3)	11,713 ± 8,027[a]	10,921 ± 11,313	NS
PMN (cells/mm^3)	9,771 ± 7,656	9,566 ± 6,188	NS
Prothrombin time (% of normal)	53 ± 18	42 ± 16	0.02
Creatinine (mg/dl)	111 ± 61	146 ± 92	NS
Bilirubin (mg/dl)	10.5 ± 11.4	13.8 ± 12.7	0.03
AST (IU/L)[b]	50 ± 33	83 ± 65	NS
Albumin (gm/dl)	2.6 ± 0.5	2.4 ± 0.4	NS
Pugh score	10.9 ± 1.9	12.3 ± 1.4	0.002
Ascitic fluid			
PMNs (cells/mm^3)	30 ± 57	6,660 ± 5,994	0.001
Total protein (gm/dl)	1.1 ± 1.0	1.3 ± 0.7	NS

[a] Values are given as mean ± S.D.
[b] Normal is <30 IU/L.
NS = not significant.
Source: Ref. 1.

encephalopathy, all of which can be attributed to the underlying cirrhosis rather than to SBP. In the SBP group each of these clinical features occurred significantly more frequently than in the ABA group (Table 3.1).

The two groups showed similar concentrations of white blood cells and polymorphonuclear leukocytes (PMN) in the blood, but the mean concentration of PMNs in the ascitic fluid (AF) was 20–25 times greater in the SBP group (p < 0.001). The mean Childs-Pugh score was significantly higher in the SBP group (12.3 vs. 10.9; p < 0.002). The prothrombin time and serum bilirubin and albumin concentrations were significantly more abnormal in the SBP patients. Gram-positive organisms were frequently cultured from the ABA patients and gram-negative bacteria were usually cultured from the SBP patients. The mortality rate was twice as high in the SBP group as in the ABA group (55 vs. 27%; p < 0.05).

It is not clear whether ABA represents (a) an early, preclinical manifestation of SBP, (b) artifactual contamination of the ascitic fluid, or (c) the presence of bacteria in the ascitic fluid without the development of overt infection in the peritoneal cavity. We and several other groups (1,4,5) prefer the transient passage of bacteria as the most logical explanation.

CNSBP is defined as the presence of clinical and/or laboratory evidence of SBP in the absence of any intraabdominal source of infection and of previous antibiotic therapy. Pelletier and coworkers studied a group of patients suspected of having infected ascitic fluid that was similar in size to their group with ABA and that was shown to have CNSBP (2). They compared 38 patients with culture-positive SBP and 15 patients with CNSBP, a ratio of 2.5:1 (Table 3.2). The two groups were similar in clinical and laboratory evidence of SBP

Table 3.2 Clinical and Blood Laboratory Data in Cirrhotic Patients with Culture-Negative Neutrocytic Ascites (CNNA) and Culture-Positive Spontaneous Bacterial Peritonitis (SBP)

	Culture-negative SBP (CNNA)	Culture-positive SBP
Numbers of patients	15	38
Mean (± 1 S.D.) age (yr)	53 ± 9	56 ± 15
Sex ratio (M/F)	10:5	24:14
Previous complications	60%	63%
Fever	67%	82%
Abdominal pain	40%	47%
Digestive hemorrhage	27%	39%
Encephalopathy	33%	50%
Malnutrition	43%	69%
Pugh grading	11.1 ± 2.1	12.4 ± 1.4
White blood cell count (10^9/L)	10 ± 10	9 ± 7
PMN count (10^9/L)	7 ± 7	9 ± 6
Prothrombin time (% of normal)	47 ± 20	42 ± 15
Creatinine (mg %)	1.34 ± 1.10[a]	1.61 ± 1.03[a]
Sodium (mEq/L)	131 ± 5	134 ± 8
Total bilirubin (mg %)	5.1 ± 3.8	8.0 ± 7.3
pH	7.45 ± 0.041	7.43 ± 0.11
Albumin (g %)	2.6 ± 0.4	2.4 ± 0.4
Positive blood culture (%)	13[b]	39[b]

[a] $p < 0.03$.
[b] $p < 0.05$.
Biological data are expressed as mean ± S.D.
Source: Ref. 2.

and of liver disease per se. Each of the clinical signs of SBP occurred slightly more frequently in the SBP group than in the CNSBP group, but these differences were not statistically significant. Both groups were treated with antibiotic agents, i.e., ampicillin plus gentamycin before December 1995 and cefotaxime thereafter. Recovery occurred more frequently in the CNSBP group than in the SBP group (87% vs. 69%) and cumulative survival was higher (p < 0.05).

CNSBP may be the result of the prior administration of antibiotic agents, which in their declining concentrations inhibit the in vitro growth of the bacteria, thus resulting in the clinical findings of SBP, but with sterile cultures. Similarly, the use of too small an aliquot of blood for culture may artifactually prevent the growth of bacteria. Other unknown reasons for the failure to culture the organisms may occur in about 20% of patients with SBP.

The large majority of patients in the CNSBP group showed symptoms and signs suggestive of SBP, but the abnormalities were less severe in the CNSBP group than in the SBP group. Mortality, too, was lower in the CNSBP group. Eighty percent of the CNSBP patients survived the hospitalization compared to 50% in the SBP group (p < 0.05). Runyon and Hoefs (6) and Ink et al. (7) in a similar study made similar observations (7).

Unknown, but probably similar reasons are responsible for the failure to recover bacteria from the blood in subacute bacterial endocarditis in which about 20% of cases are "culture-negative" SBE (8).

A. Clinical Considerations

The spectrum has broadened considerably since its original description. Initially, there was *symptomatic SBP* (9). Soon thereafter asymptomatic or *silent SBP* was recognized (3). At about the same time the syndrome of asymptomatic bacterascites (ABA), which is a positive bacterial culture in the ascitic fluid in the absence of the signs, symptoms, or cultures indicative of SBP, was recognized (3). Finally, *culture-negative SBP* (CNSBP) was described (6). Chu, Chang, and Liaw and their associates in Taiwan have recently analyzed and compared these syndromes with sterile ascites (SA) in a large group of 443 cirrhotic patients with ascites (10).

They classified 8% to 12% of this large group as having each of these variants, i.e., SBP (12%), CNSBP (8%), and BA (11%). Each group was separately analyzed for those patients that were symptomatic and for those that were asymptomatic. About 70% of each of these variants of SBP exhibited signs and/or symptoms compatible with SBP. Furthermore, the hospital mor-

Table 3.3 Results of Ascitic Fluid Examination in Subgroups

Type of ascites	Patients	
	No.	%
Sterile ascites	303	68.4
Spontaneous bacterial peritonitis	55	12.4
Symptomatic	37	8.4
Asymptomatic	18	4.0
Culture-negative SBP (probable SBP)	37	8.4
Symptomatic	26	5.9
Asymptomatic	11	2.5
Bacterascites	48	10.8
Symptomatic	34	7.7
Asymptomatic	14	3.1
Total	443	

tality of these three variations differs. The mortality rate was 20% for the patients with SA and for those with ABA. It ranged, however, from 40% to 55% for patients with SBP, CNSBP, and symptomatic BA. The authors concluded that ABA, when symptomatic, is a *forme fruste* of SBP and, when asymptomatic, represents the clinically insignificant, transient presence of bacteria in the ascitic fluid or, conceivably, a bacterial contaminant. The mortality rate was significantly higher in the symptomatic BA subgroup, i.e., 50% vs. 25% (p < 0.01).

Most of these 443 cirrhotic patients (92%) had nonalcoholic cirrhosis that was probably viral hepatitic in origin, a pattern characteristic of cirrhosis in Taiwan. The results presented in Table 3.3 are valid for nonalcoholic, posthepatitic cirrhosis, but probably differ from those of patients with alcoholic cirrhosis, which is typical of cirrhosis in the West. Conceivably, there may be differences between such complications of the cirrhosis seen in Asian, non-Asian, and other ethnically and geographically defined groups.

Unfortunately, the authors did not separately analyze the symptomatic and asymptomatic subgroups with sterile ascites, who together represent two-thirds of the total group. The absence of these data prevent complete analysis of the value of the symptoms of SBP as a prognostic sign. Furthermore, antibiotic treatment had been given to some of the asymptomatic patients with BA, a fact that makes it difficult to determine the prognostic value of the presence or absence of symptoms.

B. Multiplicity of Infecting Species

More than 70 species of bacteria have been isolated from the AF of patients
with bacteriologically proved SBP (Table 3.4). The infecting bacteria are predominantly species indigent to the human gastrointestinal tract. They are usually aerobic, gram-negative rods, but coccal forms of all types may be present.
They have been arbitrarily divided into (a) aerobic, gram-negative bacilli, (b)
cocci, both gram-negative and gram-positive, (c) anaerobic bacteria, (d) inher-
ently pathogenic bacteria, and (e) miscellaneous species.

Every individual species can be considered as giving rise to an individual
clinical syndrome. These syndromes may be influenced by individual growth
rates of bacteria, by metabolic differences, or by intrinsic aerobic or anaerobic
requirements and by clinical consequences. Some Neisseria such as gonococci
prefer to reside in the genitourinary tract, others such as meningococci favor
infection of the cerebrospinal fluid. Salmonella species tend to reside in the
gastrointestinal or biliary tracts. Pathogens such as *M. tuberculosis* prefer to
hibernate in lymphatic tissues, but have individual preferences in invading
specific tissues. Anaerobic species do not often infect AF, apparently because
of the relatively high oxygen tension there. Chlamydial species are rickettsia-
like organisms that survive a variety of conditions, but the factors that determine their infectivity are unknown.

We have considered some diverse species recovered from patients with
SBP, which are presented below, in roughly the chronological order in which
they were reported. Selected features of these bacteria and characteristics of
their infections will be arbitrarily commented on.

Each previously unreported bacterial species described as the etiological
agent in a patient with SBP can be considered to be a new and unusual presentation of SBP (Table 3.4). Most of them are like peas in a pod and only the
fanciful names of the organisms differ. Most are gram-negative, aerobic organisms and there are few notable clinical or laboratory differences in their clinical syndromes.

Anaerobic bacterial peritonitis is an uncommon syndrome (11), occurring in only about 6% of patients with SBP. *Clostridium perfringens* is
probably the most common of these anaerobic organisms (12), but *Clostridium
tertium* (13), *Fusobacterium necrophorum, Bacteroides fragilis*, and others
have been cultured (14). *Fusobacteria* are remarkable in that they usually, but
not always, produce a foul odor (15). This feature is not very important even
though the ascitic fluid in most instances of SBP is odorless. Indeed, foul
smelling ascitic fluids in SBP are usually attributed to mixed infections, and

Table 3.4 Bacteria Isolated from Patients with SBP

1. Aerobic bacilli
   Acinetobacter calcoaceticus
   Aeromonas hydrophila
   Aeromonas liquifaciens
   Aeromonas sobria
   Arizona hinshawii
   Bacillus providence
   Brucella species
   Campylobacter coli
   Campylobacter difficile
   Campylobacter fetus
   Campylobacter jejuni
   Capnocytophaga ochracea
   Capnocytophaga sanejoux
   Citrobacter species
   Clostridium perfringens
   Enterobacter cloacae
   Escherichia coli
   Haemophilus influenzae
   Klebsiella pneumoniae
   Listeria monocytogenes
   Paracolon species
   Pasteurella multoceda
   Pasteurella ureae
   Plesiomonas shigelloides
   Proteus morgani
   Proteus freundi
   Pseudomonas aeruginosa
   Pseudomonas cepacia
   Pseudomonas paucimobilis
   Pseudomonas stutzeri
   Salmonella species
   Serratia marcesens
   Xanthomatosis maltophilia
   Yersinia enterocolitica
   Yersinia pseudotuberculosis
2. Coccal bacteria
   Enterococcus faecium
   Group B streptococcus
   β-Hemolytic streptococcus

γ-Hemolytic streptococcus
Neisseria perflava
Peptococcus
Peptostreptococcus anaerobius
Propionibacteria species
Staphylococcus aureus
Streptococcus fecalis
Streptococcus milleri
Streptococcus mitis
Streptococcus pneumoniae
Streptococcus pyogenes
Streptococcus sanguis
Streptococcus veridans
3. Anaerobic and micro-aerophilic organisms
   Bacteroides species
   Clostridium faecium
   Clostridium fragilis
   Clostridium tertium
   Clostridium perfringens
   Flavobacterium meningosepticum
4. Pathogenic bacteria
   Mycobacterium avium intracellulare
   Mycobacterium chelonei-like organisms
   Mycobacterium tuberculosis
   Neisseria-gonorrohoe
   Neisseria meningitidis
   Salmonella typhi
   Salmonella typhimurium
5. Miscellaneous organisms
   Candida albicans
   Candida tropicalis
   CDC Group EO-3
   Chlamydia trachomatis
   Monilia sitophilia
   Nocardia asteroides
   Vibrio alginolyticus
   Vibrio cholerae (Non 01)
   Vibrio vulnificus
6. Unspeciated organisms
7. Viral peritonitis

this information may be useful in the differential diagnosis. However, AF is rarely assessed for odor. In the syndrome of vasopressin-induced SBP (16), which is characterized by multiple organisms, both aerobic and anaerobic, it is postulated that the presence of a foul odor may help differentiate "perforated" bacterial peritonitis from the spontaneous type, which is odorless.

The paucity of instances of anaerobic SBP has been attributed to the pO_2 of ascitic fluid in cirrhotic patients, which is approximately that of mixed venous blood (43 Torr) a level that may not be hospitable to strict anaerobic species (17).

Microaerophilic bacteria such as *Campylobacter fetus* "diptheroids," *Peptostreptococcus anaerobus*, and peptococcus have also been cultured in SBP. Other *Campylobacter* species recovered are *C. coli, C. intestinalis,* and *C. jejuni* (18).

Anaerobic and microaerophilic organisms may be associated with pneumocystis intestinalis, i.e., *gas* in the wall of the intestinal tract, which may occasionally be a radiologic sign of diagnostic significance.

Clostridium difficile colitis may closely mimic *Clostridial peritonitis* (19).

C. Unusual Species of Infecting Bacteria

Most of these organisms isolated from the AF of patients with SBP are gram-negative bacteria that are indigenous, enteric bacteria. These include several unusual organisms such as *Campylobacter aeromonas, Capnocytophaga,* and *Acinetobacter* species. Only a few pathogenic species including *Salmonella typhi, Neisseria gonorrhoeae, Neisseria meningitidis, Salmonella typhi,* and *Mycobacterium tuberculosis* have been cultured.

The organisms known to have caused SBP may be grouped into five categories: (1) aerobic gram-negative bacilli, (2) streptococcal organisms, (3) anaerobic bacteria, (4) pathogenic bacteria, and (5) miscellaneous organisms.

However, the appearance of *Yersinia enterocolitica* in a dozen cases of SBP demonstrates that this organism, which was first known for its capacity to induce mucosal colonic ulcerations (20,21), was found to have an even more unusual aspect. It showed great predilection for patients with cirrhosis, especially those with hemochromatosis or other ironic disorders (22,23). This association with the metabolism of iron, on which Yersinial organisms are dependent, renders Yersinial infections a unique species. In addition, this species has a unique aspect, i.e., its capacity to cross react with Brucella organisms to give a positive Widal agglutination test (24). The finding of a positive Widal serologic test has led to the diagnosis of Yersinial infections.

D. Other Uncommon Species Identified

Summarized below are a series of additional bacteria recently recognized as the cause of SBP roughly in the order that they were recovered.

Pasteurella multoceda bacterial peritonitis is a disorder that appears to occur in alcoholic cirrhotic patients who have close contact with animals, particularly cats (25). It may, however, occur in patients who have had no close contact with cats or other domestic animals (25a). Gram-negative bacteria and other species that may cause SBP are usually susceptible to cefotaxime and to other third-generation cephalosporins, which are usually so effective in patients with SBP that they can be given without awaiting cultural confirmation of the infection (25b).

Gonococcal SBP was first reported in 1985 (26), about seven years after the first case of Neisserian SBP had been described, namely meningococcal SBP (27).

SBP caused by *Vibrio vulnificus*, a gram-negative, comma or S-shaped bacterium, was first described in 1985, in two alcoholic cirrhotic patients (28). The disorder, caused by *V. vulnificus*, differed from typical SBP by the appearance of hemorrhagic vesicles and bullae from which *V. vulnificus* was cultured, as well as from the ascitic fluid. At autopsy both patients were found to have hemorrhagic necrosis of the terminal ileum. The mechanism of the ileal necrosis is not understood. The *V. vulnificus* bacteria enjoy growing in seawater and tend to cause infections after the ingestion of fresh shellfish (29,30).

Capnocytophaga ochraceae is an oral, gram-negative, nonflagellated, motile bacterium that grows well in an enhanced CO_2 atmosphere (31,32). It was first reported to be a cause of SBP in 1985.

SBP has been proved to be caused by at least three different species of *Campylobacter*: *C. coli* (33), *C. fetus* (34), and *C. jejuni* (35).

Garcia reported SBP caused by *Salmonella enteritidis* (36) and Pascual described SBP caused by *Enterococcus faecium* (37).

There will be years of investigations required to sort out this diverse bacterial menagerie and to understand the many bizarre clinical relationships and the principles behind them. These calculations, of course, do not include the descriptions of other previously unrecognized causes of SBP.

II. INFECTIONS OF OTHER FLUID COLLECTIONS: SPONTANEOUS BACTERIAL EMPYEMA (SBEmp)

The basic concept of SBP—the spontaneous infection of pre-existing pathophysiologic fluids, such as pleural effusions, presumably by an incidental bacteremia—is a very enticing one.

Pleural effusions, which are as common as ascites, probably become infected in a similar manner. SBEmp was first described by Flaum et al. when Flaum was a house officer at the New Haven Veterans Administration Medical Center (when SBP was originally recognized) and was familiar with the endemic of SBP occurring at that hospital at that time (38). They assumed that SBEmp, like SBP, was pathogenetically a similar disease in an adjacent body cavity, i.e., in pleural fluid (PF).

Xiol and associates prospectively studied the prevalence of SBEmp in the same manner undertaken for SBP as described in Chapter 3 in this book (39). They defined SBEmp as a positive pleural fluid culture or the presence of >500 PMN leukocytes per cubic millimeter PF in the absence of any pneumonic or parapneumonic explanation for such an infection. Thoracenteses were performed at their hospital in all patients with pleural effusions over a four-year period between 1988 and 1992. Bacteriologic, cytologic, hematologic, and biochemical tests were performed on the PF. They included studies of centrifuged PF with direct inoculation of large amounts of PF directly into blood culture media (70 ml "Liquoid" blood culture bottles).

Of the 120 patients who were admitted to the Gastroenterology Service of the Hospital de Bellvitge in Barcelona, Spain, during this period with pleural effusions, 79% also had ascites. Sixteen of the 120 patients (13%) developed SBEmp. These 16 patients had 24 episodes of SBEmp, i.e., 1.5 episodes per patient, a ratio similar to that of SBP. Abdominal pain, which is a common symptom of SBEmp, was associated with SBP in all cases. In 14 of the 24 episodes, SBEmp was associated with SBP, but clearly ascites is not a prerequisite for SBEmp because it was absent in 10 of the episodes (43%). The spectrum of the infecting organisms included *E. coli* in eight episodes, streptococci in four, enterococci in three, *Klebsiella pneumoniae* in two, and *Pseudomonas stutzeri* in one. Six episodes (24%) were culture-negative (CNSBEmp), a percentage similar to that of CNSBP in SBP. Death occurred in 20% of the 24 episodes (83%).

It is probable that the PF was infected by bacteremias rather than by direct contamination of the pleural fluid by ascitic fluid as was suggested in SBEmp in four of 10 patients who did not have SBP. These findings demonstrate the need for thoracentesis in all cirrhotic patients with pleural effusions. Eleven of 16 patients (69%) with SBEmp died during follow-up. Because of the high mortality associated with SBEmp, it should be considered as strong an indication for liver transplantation as SBP even in the absence of SBP (see Chap. 14).

LeVeen and coworkers described serious hydrothorax in 5% of cirrhotic patients with ascites (40). They also described small defects in the diaphragm through which AF entered the pleural cavity. After reduction of portal venous pressure by a peritoneovenous shunt they attempted to obliterate the pleural space by injecting sclerosing agents into it. They obliterated the defects on the upper surface of the diaphragm which tend to rupture into the pleural space, and by doing so eradicated the pleural effusions in about 80% of the patients.

Peritoneovenous shunts are not free of hazard (41), which include disseminated intravascular coagulopathy (DIC), venous thrombosis, and peritoneal fibrosis.

III. UNUSUSAL PRESENTATIONS OF SBP

A. Fibrous Encapsulating Peritonitis (The Cocoon Syndrome)

In their description of a most unusual case of "SBP" in a noncirrhotic patient, Leport et al. described a patient who, in the absence of any history of preceding liver disease, developed pneumococcal bacteremia, but whose ascitic fluid was sterile (42). The patient, a 36-year-old Moroccan woman, who had had no history of alcohol ingestion, abdominal disease, or surgery, developed fever, abdominal pain, and diarrhea. She had given birth to nine children uneventfully. On physical examination she was an obese woman with a temperature of 39°C. Her abdomen was tender, but not otherwise remarkable. There was no pneumoperitoneum. Her laboratory data were normal except for decreased white blood cells of 2300 per cubic millimeter, 63% of which were polymorphonuclear leukocytes. She exhibited elevated serum alkaline phosphatase activity (380 IU) and a decreased serum albumin concentration (2.5 g per dl). Her serum bilirubin and transaminase levels were normal. Serum BUN and electrolyte levels were normal. She had low-grade proteinuria. On admission *Streptococcus pneumoniae* were cultured from her blood, but not from the ascitic fluid. She responded promptly to a 10-day course of penicillin. Thereafter, the fever recurred and was accompanied by rapid distension of the abdomen. Paracentesis yielded turbid ascitic fluid, which was an exudate (5.9 g per dl) that contained innumerable polymorphonuclear WBCs. The ascitic fluid triglyceride level was 450 mg per dl and the plasma level was 165 mg per dl. Chyluria was present. Liver biopsy showed massive steatosis. Ampicillin and clavulanic acid therapy was instituted. Although the fever and hypertriglyceridemia subsided, the ascitic fluid leukocytosis persisted. Laparoscopy showed that thick, dense, nonspecific fibrous deposits covered the small bowel. A liver biopsy revealed massive fatty deposition. The ascites persisted but the patient remained afebrile. Two months later she presented with subacute intestinal obstruction. Laparotomy showed that the abdominal organs were encased in a dense, fibrous capsule that was removed, after which the patient did well. Encapsulating peritonitis has not previously been reported in patients with SBP.

Although the turbidity of the ascitic fluid was presumed to have resulted from a bacterial peritonitis, the presence of hypertriglyceridemia and chyluria suggests that the lipid abnormalities may in some way have been responsible for the encapsulating peritonitis. Chronic encapsulating peritonitis is a rare disorder frequently associated with tuberculosis that is otherwise virtually unknown. Studies for tuberculosis were negative in this patient.

Encapsulating peritonitis had been rarely reported in patients with peritoneovenous shunts (PVS) until Stanley et al. published their systematic autopsy study of 69 patients with PVS (43), 28 of whom (38%) had developed generalized peritoneal fibrosis with cocoon formation. Peritoneal fibrosis was noted at autopsy in only one of their other 485 cirrhotic patients who had not had PVS. Encapsulating peritonitis has also been reported in a patient who had undergone chronic peritoneal dialysis.

Sclerosing peritonitis has been associated with the use of practolol, a first generation adrenergic blocker (44). Recently reports of sclerosing peritonitis after the administration of timolol, a second-generation, nonselective β-blocker (45), have been published. No satisfactory explanation for these bizarre associations has yet been put forth.

It appears that PVS is clearly the most common precipitant of encapsulating peritonitis, and that it is probably *not* related to SBP per se. One may speculate that it is related to disorders that chronically irritate the peritoneal surfaces.

As mentioned above, other nonascitic segregated effusions that may give rise to "spontaneous" bacterial infections include arthritic effusions, which have been associated with *spontaneous bacterial arthritis*, (46,47). Conceivably, meningicoccal meningitis can be considered to be a "spontaneous" variant of the syndrome (48). It, too, has been described, although it would be impossible to differentiate it from the garden variety type of bacterial meningitis if challenged.

By using one's imagination one can create other similar scenarios, such as *spontaneous bacterial cholecystitis* or *empyema* of the gall bladder in a patient with a hydrops of the gall bladder. Similarly, infection of a nonfunctioning urinary bladder could result from the infections of the urinary tract by a random bacteremia (i.e., *spontaneous bacterial cystitis*) in a patient with bladder obstruction.

B. Noncirrhotic SBP

SBP has also occurred in patients with ascites of noncirrhotic origin such as *neoplastic ascites* (49), i.e., the ascites that develops in patients with portal hypertension following metastases to the liver and/or the peritoneum. Actually one can sense that these are pathogenetically two very different phenomena. Metastases to the peritoneum tend to cause a syndrome characterized by blood and neoplastic cells in the ascitic fluid. On the other hand, intrahepatic metastases tend to cause ascites like that of cirrhosis, which is usually free of blood. These two types differ theoretically in their serum-ascites albumin gradients (SAAG) (50). SBP also has been found rarely in patients with cardiac ascites (51) in whom the higher concentrations of protein and complement inhibit the development of the classic type of SBP.

Primary bacterial peritonitis (PBP) is a form of SBP that is almost always seen in infants and children and is usually caused by pneumococci (*Streptococcus pneumoniae*) or group A beta-hemolytic streptococci (GABHS) (54a). PBP is occasionally associated with the streptococcal toxic shock syndrome (STSS), which is defined as signs of shock, the isolation of a GABHS from a normally sterile site (the peritoneal cavity) and abnormalities of at least two organ systems. Watson et al. reported such a patient with hematologic, pulmonary, dermatologic, and coagulation abnormalities. It is postulated that streptococcal exotoxins serve as superantigens that lead to the characteristic greatly enhanced inflammation that occurs in this syndrome.

In 1979 several cases of *primary anaerobic peritonitis* (52,53) were reported, which may have been ascites-free (54).

It has recently been noted that failure to control gastrointestinal hemorrhage (GIH) predisposes patients to bacterial infection (54b). Indeed, the prior occurrence of GIH is not considered a risk factor in the development of SBP (54c).

Bleichner et al. in 1996 (54d) and Soriano et al. in 1992 (54e) pointed out a strong association between GIH and bacterial infection. They recognized that invasive diagnostic and/or therapeutic procedures (54f) that caused transient depression of the reticuloendothelial system (54g) increased bacterial translocation (54h) and were each independent predictors of the failure to control the bleeding, thus providing a rationale for the association. These data also support the concept that infection may be involved in the initiation of

GIH, perhaps via the release of endotoxin into the systemic circulation (54b). Although rational interpretation of these studies supports the prompt use of antibiotics in preventing bacterial infection in general, and SBP in particular, as they are already employed in patients with hypoalbuminemia, with deficient opsonic activity (54h), and with GIH. Clearly GIH and bacterial infection are intimately interrelated by a variety of possible mechanisms that include decreased hepatic arterial blood flow, depletion of complement factors, and/ or saturation of the reticuloendothelial systems.

The explanation for such an association is not known, but certainly these many factors may be involved.

C. Chronic Ambulatory Peritoneal Dialysis (CAPD)

CAPD may be considered either a common variant of SBP or a completely separate syndrome with many features in common (57). Although I consider it to be the latter, it is appropriate to discuss it in detail here. Infection of the peritoneal cavity by bacteria is the major complication of CAPD (55,56).

SBP is a bacterial infection of a pre-existing pathophysiological accumulation of peritoneal fluid, a pathophysiological consequence of portal hypertension that develops almost exclusively in patients with chronic liver disease. On the other hand, CAPD represents infection of an artificial dialysis solution that is repetitively infused into and drained from the peritoneal cavity of patients with chronic renal failure in an attempt to dialyze out abnormally retained metabolic products that are normally excreted in the urine. In both disorders bacteria may infect the peritoneal cavity causing abdominal pain, fever, and other signs of peritoneal inflammation. Although both disorders represent bacterial infections of intraperitoneal fluids and the peritoneum, one occurs "spontaneously" whereas the other usually appears to represent iatrogenic contamination of a synthetic "ascitic" fluid. The "ascitic fluids" in these two syndromes are quite different.

In addition, the nature of the infecting organisms is quite different. In SBP about 70% of episodes are caused by indigenous aerobic gram-negative bacteria and the remainder by gram-positive organisms, usually skin-contaminating bacterial such as coagulase-negative *Staphylococcus aureus*, *Staphylococcus epidermidis*, or *Pseudomonas aeruginosa* (57,58). In SBP the fluids are quite different. The infected dialysate is usually cloudy and shows an increased total protein concentration that reflects to a large degree the complement concentration of the ascitic fluid and tends to be inversely related to the prevalence of bacterial infection. In CAPD there is initially little complement in the dialysis fluid. Furthermore, the numbers of both bacteria and PMNs are much lower in CAPD than in SBP, reducing the random chance of collisions (59). CAPD may occur for the first time after years of dialysis.

Peritoneal macrophages are the predominant phagocytic cells of the peritoneal cavity. This is true in normal subjects and in patients undergoing peritoneal dialysis. Human peritoneal macrophages have been shown to be capable of phagocytizing opsonized *Candida albicans* and *Staphylococcus epidermidis* and of killing opsonized *Salmonella typhimurium* (60). They appear to behave as intact, fully functional phagocytes. However, this capacity does not indicate that the peritoneal cavity of patients on CAPD has adequate phagocytic defenses because the concentration of peritoneal macrophages is insufficient to inactivate all the bacteria that may invade this site. In fact, the concentration of phagocytes in each peritoneal fluid is 10^4 cells per ml (10 cells/cubic millimeter), a concentration which is deemed inadequate for efficient neutralization of the invading organisms (61), although the numbers of cells in peritoneal effluences tend to increase during bacterial peritonitis. The use of commercial dialysis solutions, which have both low pH (5.5) and high osmolality, may interfere with the functions of both macrophages and polymorphonuclear leukocytes. Peritoneal macrophages are fully capable of phagocytizing and killing nonopsonized *Staphylococcus aureus*. Nevertheless the installation of large quantities of dialysis fluids that are devoid of opsonins and that dilute the number of peritoneal macrophages weaken the antibacterial defenses of the peritoneal cavity (62).

A series of previously unreported microbes responsible for SBP have been described in CAPD. These uncommon organisms may reflect the antimicrobial inadequacies of infected intraperitonial-dialysis fluid. These organisms include (a) unspeciated, pleomorphic, nonfermenting, nonmotile, non-spore-forming gram-negative, aerobic, rod-shaped bacilli, which were isolated from the dialysate produced by the dialysis machine and from its tap water supply; (b) *Mycobacterium chelonei*-like organisms; (c) *Pseudomonas cepacia*; (d) *Vibrio alginolyticus*, which is a marine bacterium that can be recovered from fish, crustaceae, and seawater-caused peritonitis in a young man that was probably contracted during a change in peritoneal dialysis fluid after scuba diving; (e) *Nocardia asteroides*, which was found in a patient with disseminated lupus erythematosus and chronic renal failure; (f) *Bacillus providence*, which was recovered from a nephrectomized patient on chronic dialysis; (g) *Candida tropicalis* peritonitis, which was identified in one patient; and (h) *aseptic peritonitis*, which was considered to be endotoxin-induced. Aseptic peritonitis, presumably viral, has also been reported (63).

D. SBP and Prosthetic Devices

A number of prosthetic devices have been associated with the occurrence of SBP and have almost certainly contributed pathogenetically to the development of SBP. These devices include (a) *ventriculoperitoneal shunts* created to decrease the intracranial pressure in patients with hydrocephalus, (b) *indwelling intraperitoneal catheters* used during chronic ambulatory peritoneal dialysis (CAPD), (c) *peritoneovenous shunts* in patients with portal hypertension and ascites, and (d) *intra-uterine contraceptive* devices.

E. SBP in Patients with Ventriculoperitoneal Shunts

Shunts between a brain cavity and the peritoneal space often become infected with gram-positive streptococci—about 25%—and often a bacterial peritonitis ensues. Hubschmann et al. described six patients with SBP characterized by abdominal pain, fever, and leukocytosis (64). Gram-positive organisms were identified in the peritoneal cavity and confirmed bacteriologically by cerebrospinal fluid obtained from the shunts themselves or from the shunt reservoirs. All six were infected by *Staphylococcus epidermidis*. Surprisingly, none had neurologic abnormalities or abnormal findings on lumbar puncture. In a larger, later series Rush et al. found that bacterial infections could ascend from the peritoneal cavity to the brain as well as descend from the cerebrospinal to the peritoneal fluid (65). The ascending infections tended to be caused by gram-negative enteric bacilli whereas the descending infections were usually infected by gram-positive cocci. Septic complications were encountered in 5% to 20% of 300 children with such shunts. Other complications occurred. The shunts sometimes gave rise to CSF ascites, to peritoneal pseudocysts to perforations of the bowel and to bacterial abscesses.

F. SBP in Patients with Intrauterine Contraceptive Devices (IUCD)

SBP may develop in association with IUCDs following salpingitis, endometritis, or even in the absence of overt infection. The use of IUCDs has previously been associated with pneumococcal infections of the genital tract including pneumococcal SBP (66). It is presumed that bacteria from an endometrial nidus of infection can seed the ascitic fluid probably after bacterial migration via the lymph nodes, i.e., bacterial translocation.

G. Other Iatrogenic Types of SBP

"Iatrogenic" is defined as "induced by a physician" or by the physician's actions. "Iatrogenic SBP" can therefore be defined as an episode of SBP induced by a healthcare worker during or as a consequence of a diagnostic or therapeutic procedure. Physicians, surgeons, dentists, nurses, or their colleagues are all capable (and culpable) of inducing SBP in cirrhotic patients. A physician's failure to incise an abscess may induce SBP as an act of omission whereas the bacteremia following such an incision may induce SBP as a complication of commission.

SBP may arise in many ways, but a bacteremia in a cirrhotic patient with portal hypertension, portosystemic collateral vessels and ascites appears to be the most common scenario. Among the procedures cited as possible bacteremogenic procedures are paracenteses, needle sticks, intravenous infusions, surgical procedures, gastrointestinal endoscopic procedures, especially variceal sclerotherapy (67–70), and esophageal dilatation (71). Actually, gastrointestinal hemorrhage, biliary or pancreatic disease, diarrhea, and recent bacterial infections of any organ or system have all occurred significantly more frequently in patients who subsequently developed SBP than in a matched series of cirrhotic patients who did not subsequently develop SBP. Although the rates were higher for patients who had had paracentesis, biliary disease, and pancreatic disease and in patients who developed SBP than in those who did not, these differences were not statistically different. Thus, any procedure in which the skin is broken can be responsible. Some procedures such as endoscopic sclerotherapy (EST) appear to have a special affinity for inducing SBP.

Actually, SBP has been attributed to EST. In 1994 Bac reported no SBP in 172 sessions of prophylactic EST (0%) (before EVH); in four of 720 episodes of elective EST (after HEV) (1%); and in six of 200 emergent episodes of EST (3%) (72). Thus the frequency of SBP is associated both with the urgency of the EST procedure (emergency > elective and elective > prophylactic) and the severity of the cirrhosis. The correlation was so close that they recommended norfloxacin and ofloxacin as prophylactic therapy of cirrhotic patients who had bled from varices. It is still not clear whether the hemorrhage itself or the EST is responsible.

H. TIPS-Associated SBP

TIPS stent-associated SBP has not yet been reported, but it is just a matter of time. The world's literature related to this syndrome consists at the present time of a single article by Sanyal and Reddy (73). Their series of eight patients outlines a precursor syndrome of *spontaneous TIPS peritonitis*, i.e., infectious bacterial TIPSitis. Three of these patients were seen among 215 patients with TIPS at the Medical College of Virginia and at the University of Miami. In addition, the authors mentioned five other cases that had come to their attention.

The syndrome emerging from these eight cases is a relatively simple one. All eight had cirrhosis of various etiologies for which a TIPS had been implanted. Seven of them had Childs-Pugh class B or C cirrhosis. The mean age was 49 years. Three-fourths of them had alcoholic cirrhosis although HCV was involved in some of them. Within a mean period of 9 to 10 months (mean 284 days) of implantation, all had developed fever and often shaking chills with profuse sweating. Most of them complained of aching, right-upper-quadrant abdominal pain and tenderness. None had rebound abdominal tenderness and none had had paracenteses. All had bacteremia, which was monomicrobial in six and polymicrobial in two. *E. coli* was the most common organism isolated (four patients) and *Klebsiella* was the second most common (two patients). A variety of bacteria, including gram-positive streptococci, staphylococci, and *Candida albicans* comprised the others. Seven of the eight were men. CT examination and Gallium scans did not reveal any abnormalities. Doppler ultrasound examinations showed thromboses of the stent or vegetations on the stent, lesions that are difficult to differentiate. The patients responded promptly to appropriate antibiotic therapy and the infections did not recur. This syndrome seems analogous to bacterial endocarditis involving cardiac prostheses. The authors speculate that neointimal hyperplasia may have narrowed the lumen and created turbulence capable of denuding the mucosa and providing a site on which bacteria could be deposited and grow distally toward the stenosis.

Cirrhotic patients with bacteremia are at extremely high risk of developing SBP. It follows, therefore, that patients with TIPS who have a "hole" in the reticuloendothelial filter are at an especially high risk of developing SBP. None of these eight patients actually had SBP.

I. SBP in Acute Liver Disease

SBP has almost always been reported in patients with cirrhosis, i.e., in patients with chronic long-standing liver disease. It was reported in acute liver disease as early as 1982 and occasionally since (74). Recently, Chu and coworkers reported that SBP is very common in "*severe* acute" hepatitis in Taiwan (75). SBP was observed in 26 of 82 consecutive patients with acute, viral hepatitis (32%). Why was SBP so common in this group of patients? Usually SBP occurs in patients with cirrhosis and severe portal hypertension with well-developed portal-systemic shunting. The SBP was monobacterial as in the cirrhotic type, and the infecting bacteria were largely aerobic, gram-negative rods. Were these Taiwanese patients different in some fundamental way? Indeed, they were! The hepatitis in these patients was *very* severe. Prothrombin times were >5 sec prolonged in >90% of them. In fact, they were so prolonged that it was too dangerous to perform liver biopsies in these patients, and so the histological nature of the hepatitis or the possible presence of cirrhosis or some other lesion remains unknown. The patients did not have cirrhosis by ultrasonographic examination, but ultrasonography may miss a multitude of subtle histological signs. Such prolonged prothrombin times are more characteristic of fulminant hepatic failure. Furthermore,the mean serum albumin concentrations were very low, 2.1 g per dl, and the mean protein level in the ascitic fluid was extremely low, <1 g per dl. These concentrations are characteristic of cirrhotic patients in whom SBP is frequently seen. This low protein level is attributed to decreased complement concentrations that reduce the opsonizing capacity of the ascitic fluid. The fact that an additional 17% of the patients had bacteremia suggests that the "hepatitis" may have had extensive adverse effects on the removal of bacteria from both blood and ascites. Actually, the hepatitis itself was quite unusual—the onset of ascites was delayed, appearing one to two months after the onset of illness and the mortality was extremely high (approximately 50%). More than 80% of the patients were HBsAg-positive and were HBsAg carriers with acute exacerbations of the "chronic liver disease." These features are characteristic of the acute viral hepatitis seen in adults in Taiwan (76). Renal failure, gastrointestinal bleeding, and a high fatality rate are characteristic. This type of acute hepatitis appears to be very much like the acute hepatic, "fulminant," late-onset failure described by Gimson et al. (77).

It appears that this report describes a new variant type of viral hepatitis. Whether it is caused by a unique, atypical virus or represents a peculiar genetic predisposition to this disease is not clear. Time may tell.

Wyke and his coworkers reported frequent bacterial and fungal infections, including SBP, in patients with acute fulminant hepatic failure resulting from a variety of causes including viral hepatitis, paracetamol hepatotoxicity, and halothane-induced injury (78,79). They noted that complement concentrations (total C_3, C_4, and C_5) and Factors B & D and complement component and the alternative complement pathways were all reduced, as was the opsonization of heat-killed baker's yeast. Rolando et al. reported a similar series (80).

These findings indicate that the increased incidence of bacterial infection is related to immune-incompetence characterized by impaired phagocytosis of bacteria. A similar pattern has been reported in cirrhotic patients. One may conclude that the lower the complement and protein concentrations of the ascitic fluid, the greater the risk of SBP.

J. Recurrent SBP: The Usual Presentation

The first article that specifically dealt with the high recurrence rate of SBP was published by Tito et al. in 1988 (81). They pointed out that 69% of a group of 75 consecutive patients who recovered from a bout of acute SBP developed recurrent SBP during the first year of follow-up. Moreover, almost one-third of these recurrences were fatal. In a subsequent smaller series Silvain et al. reported a series of 26 survivors of SBP, of whom seven developed recurrences of SBP (27%) (82). The calculated risk of recurrent SBP within one year was 35%. The survival rate in these patients was quite low; it was calculated to be 40% at one year. SBP was responsible for death in 13% of the patients at risk. Although this second report represents a slightly less grim prognosis, the outlook for patients who develop recurrent SBP is extremely poor. Approximately 50% of such patients die of SBP, and 60%, of the survivors of SBP die during the first three years of follow-up. The cumulative survival of the whole series of patients with SBP is about 20% after three years. Furthermore, the overall prevalence of SBP including the initial episode is approximately 80%.

This scenario indicates that the occurrence of SBP is a death knell and suggests that its morbidity and mortality may be reduced by prophylactic antibiotic therapy (83,84), but not eradicated.

The recurrences were largely caused by aerobic enteric bacteria similar to those that caused the original infections. They developed largely in patients with severe Child's class C cirrhosis, especially those with elevated serum bilirubin levels (>4 mg per dl), prolonged prothrombin levels (<45%), and reduced ascitic fluid protein concentrations (<1 g per dl). This depressing prognosis has led to the rational suggestion that all patients who survive an episode of SBP should have liver transplantation as soon as possible since the recurrences appear to occur sooner rather than later. This suggestion is fiscally impractical, of course, but if any other valid indications for liver transplantation exist, patients who survive an episode of SBP will certainly benefit in the long run.

Uncertainty exists about survival rates of SBP survivors after liver transplantation. Survival appears to occur three times as commonly in those patients with orthotopic liver transplants who had had SBP > 30 days prior to orthotopic liver transplants than in those who had not had SBP (85). A recent retrospective analysis suggests that such patients do surprisingly well after liver transplantation (86). Van Thiel and associates retrospectively studied 100 patients who had had orthotopic liver transplantation shortly after SBP. They also studied a matched control group of 20 patients with cirrhosis of similar etiology and severity, but who had not had an episode of SBP. The endpoint of the investigation was the occurrence rate of SBP within 30 days of orthotopic liver transplantation. A diagnosis of post-transplant SBP included all patients who developed a positive, monobacterial ascitic fluid culture or of >50 neutrophils per cubic millimeter in the ascitic fluid in the absence of signs or symptoms of peritoneal infection within 30 days of transplantation.

Of the 100 patients, 32 had been excluded from the analysis because of hepatobiliary problems including primary graft failure. Postoperative sepsis or SBP occurred in six of the 68 patients (8%) studied, and in two of 20 control subjects (10%; p > 0.05). This prevalence is not statistically different from that of the initial prevalence of SBP in ascitic cirrhotic patients.

Although these data appear to indicate that orthotopic liver transplantation does not increase the risk of SBP, it should be kept in mind that this is *not* a randomly selected comparison. The nonrandomized control group had been selected from a much larger group of patients who underwent liver transplantation over a period of seven years. Furthermore, the numbers of patients compared was relatively small. In my opinion the results of this "controlled" trial should not be integrated into our knowledge of SBP until a proper randomized clinical trial with similar results has been reported.

We have included this "usual" presentation of SBP among the unusual ones to emphasize that the recurrence of SBP is a common aspect of the SBP syndrome.

IV. DIAGNOSTIC CONSIDERATIONS

Ideally paracentesis should be performed and cultures and leukocyte counts done in all patients with overt ascites at or shortly after admission to the hospital. This procedure should be repeated whenever the abdominal symptoms appear and/or signs progress.

Properly performed paracentesis (87) is a safe procedure (88). Runyon reported on 229 consecutive paracenteses of large size (60 ml) in 125 patients with overt ascites (88). Two patients with greatly prolonged prothrombin times (6–9 sec) bled into the abdominal wall. Two other patients had persistent peritoneal leaks. There were no other complications except for several small, intra-abdominal wall hematomas. When a vessel in the abdominal wall or a viscus in the intra-abdominal cavity is perforated bleeding may ensue, but such complications are rare. The fear of inducing intraperitoneal infection by diagnostic paracentesis is greatly exaggerated. Cultures of ascitic fluid should be large (10 ml) and inoculated immediately into the culture medium. This procedure more than doubled the yield of positive blood cultures and decreased the time required to make the diagnosis (89).

Although Runyon et al. consider paracentesis to be a safe procedure with a very low complication rate, they found that about 2% of patients bleed after abdominal taps (88). Qureshi et al. reported the aspiration of blood from a large para-umbilical vein in the abdominal wall that measured 5 cm in diameter (89a). Furthermore, they cited several cases of fatal bleeding after paracentesis (89b,c). One additional case of fatal hemorrhage has recently been reported (89d). Certainly, patients should be examined before paracentesis for the presence of Cruveilhier-Baumgartner murmurs, which may warn of such potential dangers.

Hitherto unreported bacteria have been reported as the cause of SBP at the rate of approximately one per year. Six such new organisms have been reported between 1997 and 1999 (90–95).

REFERENCES

1. Pelletier G, Lesur G, Ink O, Hagege H, Attali P, Buffet C, Etienne J-P. Asymptomatic bacterascites: is it spontaneous bacterial peritonitis? Hepatology 14:112–115, 1991.
2. Pelletier G, Salmon D, Ink O, Hannoun S, Attali P, Buffet C, Etienne JP. Culture-negative neutrocytic ascites: a less severe variant of spontaneous bacterial peritonitis. J Hepatol 10:327–331, 1990.
3. Conn HO, Fessel JM. Spontaneous bacterial peritonitis in cirrhosis. Variations on a theme. Medicine 50:161–197, 1971.
4. Pinzello G, Simonetti RG, Craxi A, Di Piazza S, Spano C, Pagliaro L. Spontaneous bacterial peritonitis: a prospective investigation in predominantly nonalcoholic cirrhotic patients. Hepatology 3:545–549, 1983.
5. Runyon BA. Monomicrobial nonneutrocytic bacterascites: a variant of spontaneous bacterial peritonitis. Hepatology 12:710–715, 1990.
6. Runyon BA, Hoefs FC. Culture-negative neutrocytic ascites: a variant of spontaneous bacterial peritonitis. Hepatology 4:1209–1211, 1984.
7. Ink O, Pelletier G, Salmon D. Pronostic de l'infection spontanee d'ascite chez le cirrhotique. Gastroenterol Clin Biol 13:556–561, 1989.
8. Pesanti EL, Smith IM. Infective endocarditis with negative blood cultures: an analysis of 52 cases. Am J Med 66:43–50, 1979.

9. Conn HO. Spontaneous peritonitis and bacteremia in patients caused by enteric bacteria. Ann Intern Med 60:568–580, 1964.

10. Chu CM, Chang KY, Liaw YF. Prevalence and prognostic significance of bacterascites in cirrhosis with ascites. Dig Dis Sci 40:561–565, 1995.

11. Targan SR, Chow AW, Guze LB. Role of anaerobic bacteria in spontaneous peritonitis of cirrhosis. Report of two cases and review of the literature. Am J Med 62:397–403, 1973.

12. Moya Mir, MS, Presa N, Barnadillo R, Martin F, Ciervas-Mons V, Suarez del Villar R. Peritonitis espontánea por *Clostridium perfringens* en tres enfermos cirróticos. Med Clin Barcelona 76:70–72, 1981.

13. Butler T, Pitt S. Spontaneous bacterial peritonitis due to *Clostridium tertium*. Gastroenterology 82:133–134, 1982.

14. Matthews S. Primary anaerobic peritonitis. BMJ 2:90, 903–904, 1979.

15. Willis AT. Aerobic Bacteriology, 3rd Ed., London: Butterworths, 1977, p. 347.

16. Bar-Meir S, Conn HO. Spontaneous bacterial peritonitis induced by intraarterial vasopressin therapy. Gastroenterology 79:418–421, 1976.

17. Sheckman P, Onderdonk AB, Bartlett, RG. Anaerobes in spontaneous peritonitis. Lancet 2:1223–1224, 1977.

18. Ho H, Zuckerman MJ, Polly SM. Spontaneous bacterial peritonitis due to *Campylobacter coli*. Gastroenterology 92:2024–2025, 1987.

19. Drapkin MS, Worthington MG, Chang T-W, Razvi SA. *Clostridium difficile* colitis mimicking acute peritonitis. Arch Surg 120:1321–1322, 1985.

20. Capron JP, Capron-Chivrac D, Tossou H. Spontaneous *Yersinia enterocolitica* peritonitis in idiopathic hemochromatosis. Gastroenterology 87:1373–1375, 1984.

21. Vantrappen GM, Heg HO, Ponette E. Yersinia enteritis and enterocolitis: gastroenterological aspects. Gastroenterology 72:220–227, 1977.

22. Melby K, Slordahl S, Gutteberg TJ. Septicemia due to *Yersinis enterocolitica* after oral overdoses of iron. Br Med J 285:467–468, 1982.

23. Perry RD, Brubaker RR. Accumulation of iron by Yersiniae. J Bacteriol 137: 1290–1298, 1979.

24. Ahvonen P, Jansson E, Aho K. Marked cross-agglutination between Brucellae and a sub-type of *Yersinia enterocolitica*. Acta Pathol Microbiol Scand 75:291–294, 1969.

25. Szpak CA, Woodward BH, White JO. Bacterial peritonitis and bacteremia associated with *Pasteurella multocida*. South Med J 75:801–803, 1980.

25a. Beales ILP. Spontaneous bacterial peritonitis due to *Pasturella multocida* without animal exposure (correspondence). Am J Gastroenterol 94:1110–1111, 1997.

25b. Rimola A, Salmeron JM, Clement G. Two different dosages of cefotaxime in the treatment of spontaneous bacterial peritonitis in cirrhosis: results of a prospective, randomized, multicenter study. Hepatology 21:674–679, 1995.

26. Stassen WN, McCullough AJH, Hilton PK. Spontaneous bacterial peritonitis caused by *Neisseria gonorrhoeae*. Evidence for a transfallopian route of infection. Gastroenterology 88:804–807, 1985.

27. Bar-Meir S, Chojkier M, Groszmann RJ, Atterbury CE, Conn HO. Spontaneous meningococcal peritonitis: a report of two cases. Am J Dig Dis 23:119–122, 1978.
28. Wongpaitoon V, Shapatayavongs B, Prachaktam R. Spontaneous *Vibrio vulnificus* peritonitis and primary sepsis in two patients with alcoholic cirrhosis. Am J Gastroenterol 80:606–708, 1985.
29. Kelly MT, Avery DM. Lactose-positive vibrio in sea water: a cause of pneumonia and septicemia in a drowning victim. J Clin Microbiol 11:278–280, 1980.
30. Johnston JM, Andes WA, Glasser G. *Vibrio vulnificus*. A gastronomic hazard. JAMA 249:1756–1757, 1983.
31. Forlenza SW, Newman MG, Lipsey AI. *Capnocytophaga* sepsis: a newly recognized clinical entity in granulocytopenic patients. Lancet 1:567–568, 1980.
32. Shales DM, Dul MJ, Lerner PI. *Capnocytophaga* bacteremia in the compromised host. Am J Clin Pathol 77:359–361, 1982.
33. Ho H, Zuckerman MJ, Polly SM. Spontaneous bacterial peritonitis due to *Campylobacter coli*. Gastroenterology 92:2024–2025, 1987.
34. Targan SR, Chow AW, Guze LB. Spontaneous peritonitis of cirrhosis due to *Campylobacter fetus*. Gastroenterology 71:311–313, 1976.
35. McNeil NI, Butto S, Ridgway GL. Spontaneous bacterial peritonitis due to *Campylobacter jejuni*. Postgrad Med J 60:487–488, 1984.
36. Garcia V. Spontaneous bacterial peritonitis due to *Salmonella enteritidis* in cirrhotic ascites. J Clin Gastroenterol 12:663–666, 1990.
37. Pascual J. Spontaneous peritonitis caused by *Enterococcus faecium*. J Clin Microbiol 28:1484–1486, 1990.
38. Flaum MA. Spontaneous bacterial empyema in cirrhosis. Gastroenterology 70:416–417, 1976.
39. Xiol X, Castelvi JM, Guardiola J, Sesé E, Castellote J, Perelló A, Cervantes X, Iborra MI. Spontaneous bacterial empyema in cirrhotic patients: a prospective study. Hepatology 23:719–723, 1996.
40. LeVeen HH, Piccone VA, Hutto RB. Management of ascites with hydrothorax. Am J Surg 148:210–213, 1984.
41. Smadja C, Franco D. The LeVeen shunt in the elective treatment of intractable ascites in cirrhosis. A prospective study on 140 patients. Ann Surg 201:488–493, 1985.
42. Leport J, Devars Du Mayne J-F, Hay J-M, Cerf M. Chylous ascites and encapsulating peritonitis: unusual complications of spontaneous bacterial peritonitis. Am J Gastroenterol 82:463–466, 1987.
43. Stanley MM, Reyes CV, Greenlee HB, Nemchausky B, Reinhardt GF. Peritoneal fibrosis in cirrhotics treated with peritoneovenous shunting for ascites. An autopsy study with clinical correlations. Dig Dis Sci 41:571–577, 1996.
44. Cook AIM. Sclerosing peritonitis and practolol therapy. Ann Royal Coll Surg Engl 58:473–475, 1976.
45. Brown P, Baddeley H, Read AE. Sclerosing peritonitis in patients on timolol. Lancet 2:1477–1481, 1974.

46. Pearson RD, Spiva D, Gluckman J. Cirrhosis of liver with septic arthritis due to *Escherichia coli*: unusual locus minoris resistenciae for bacteriemic cirrhosis. NY State J Med 78:1762–1763, 1978.

47. Skau T, Tegner Y. Spontaneous peritonitis and rheumatoid arthritis: a case report. Acta Chir Scand 152:317–318, 1986.

48. Bar-Meir S, Chokier M, Groszmann RJ, Conn HO. Spontaneous meningococcal peritonitis: a report of two cases. Am J Dig Dis 23:119–122, 1978.

49. Isner J, MacDonald JS, Schein PS. Spontaneous *Streptococcus pneumoniae* peritonitis in a patient with metastatic gastric cancer: a case report and etiologic consideration. Cancer 39:2306–2309, 1977.

50. Hoefs JC. Globulin correction of the albumin gradient: correlation with measured serum to ascites colloid osmotic pressure gradients. Hepatology 16:396–406, 1992.

51. Runyon BA. Spontaneous bacterial peritonitis associated with cardiac ascites. Am J Gastroenterol 79:796–797, 1984.

52. Matthews P. Primary anaerobic peritonitis. BMJ 2:903–904, 1979.

53. Scott-McDougal W, Izant RJ, Zollinger RM. Spontaneous anaerobic bacterial peritonitis. Ann Surg 181:310–314, 1975.

54. Harken AH, Shochat SJ. Gram-positive peritonitis in children. Am J Surg 125: 769–772, 1973.

54a. Watson WJ, Powers KS. Primary peritonitis associated with streptococcal toxic shock-like syndrome. Clin Pediatr 38:175–177, 1999.

54b. Goulis J, Armonis A, Patch D, Sabin C, Greensdale L, Burroughs AK. Bacterial infection is independently associated with failure to control bleeding in cirrhotic patients with gastrointestinal hemorrhage. Hepatology 27:1207–1212, 1998.

54c. Pauwels A, Mostefa-Kara N, Debenes B, Degoutte E, Levy VG. Systemic antibiotic prophylaxis after gastrointestinal hemorrhage in cirrhotic patients with a high risk of infection. Hepatology, 24:802–806, 1996.

54d. Bleichner G, Boulanger R, Squara P, Sollet JP, Parent A. Frequency of infections in cirrhotic patients presenting with acute gastrointestinal hemorrhage. Br J Surg 73:724–726, 1986.

54e. Soriano G, Guarner C, Tomas A, Villanueva C, Torras X, Gonzalez D, Sainz S. Norfloxacin prevents bacterial infection in cirrhotics with gastrointestinal bleeding. Gastroenterology 102:1267–1272, 1992.

54f. Blaise M, Pateron D, Trinchet JC, Levacher S, Collignon A, Beaugrand M, Pourriat JL. Systemic antibiotic therapy prevents bacterial infections in cirrhotic patients with gastrointestinal hemorrhage. Hepatology 20:34–38, 1994.

54g. Rimola A, Soto R, Bory F, Arroyo V, Piera C, Rodes J. Reticuloendothelial system phagocytic activity in cirrhosis and its relation to bacterial infections and prognosis. Hepatology 4:53–58, 1984.

54h. Ziegler EJ, McCutchan JA, Fierer J, Glauser MP, Sadoff JD, Douglas H, Braude AL. Treatment of gram-negative bacteremia and shock with human antiserum to a mutant *Escherichia coli*. N Engl J Med 307:1225–1230, 1982.

54i. Runyon BA. Patients with deficient ascitic fluid opsonic activity are predisposed to spontaneous bacterial peritonitis. Hepatology 8:632–635, 1988.

55. Nolph KD, Sorkin M, Rubin J, Argania D, Prowant K, Fruto L, Kennedy D. Continuous ambulatory peritoneal dialysis: three year experience at one center. Ann Intern Med 92:609–613, 1980.

56. Fenton SS, Wu G, Cattran D, Wadgymar A, Allen AF. Clinical aspects of peritonitis in patients on chronic ambulatory peritoneal dialysis. Peritoneal Dialysis Bull 1:S1–S8, 1981.

57. Vas S. Microbiological aspects of peritonitis. Peritoneal Dialysis Bull 1:S11–S14, 1981.

58. Verbrugh HA, Peters R, Peterson PK, Verhoef J. Phagocytosis and killing of staphylococci by human polymorphonuclear and mononuclear leukocytes. J Clin Pathol 31:539–545, 1978.

59. Hammerstrøm J. Human macrophage differentiation in vivo and in vitro: a comparison of human peritoneal macrophages and monocytes. Acta Pathol Microbiol Scand 87:113–120, 1979.

60. Ganguly R, Milutinovich J, Lazzall V, Waldman RH. Studies of human peritoneal cells: a normal saline lavage technique for the isolation and characterization of cells from peritoneal dialysis patients. J Reticuloendothel Soc 27:303–310, 1980.

61. Duwe AK, Vas SI, Weatherhead JW. Effects of composition of peritoneal dialysis fluid on chemiluminescence, phagocytosis, and bactericidal activity in vitro. Infect Immun 33:130–135, 1981.

62. Rubin J, McFarland S, Hellems EW, Bower JD. Peritoneal dialysis during peritonitis. Kidney Int 19:460–464, 1981.

63. Gandhi VC, Kamadana MR, Ing TS, Daugirdas JT, Viol GW, Robinson JA, Geis WP, Hano JE. Aseptic peritonitis in patients on maintenance peritoneal dialysis. Nephron 24:257–259, 1979.

64. Hubschmann OR, Countee RW. Gram-positive peritonitis in patients with infected ventriculoperitoneal shunts. Surg Gyn Obstet 149:69–71, 1979.

65. Rush DS, Walsh JW, Belin R, Pulito AR. Ventricular sepsis and abdominally related complications in children with cerebrospinal fluid shunts. Surg 97:420–427, 1995.

66. Brinson RR, Kolts BE, Monif GRG. Spontaneous bacterial peritonitis associated with an intrauterine device. J Clin Gastroenterol 800:82–84, 1986.

67. Cohen LB, Korsten MA, Scherl EJ. Bacteremia after endoscopic injection sclerotherapy. Arch Intern Med 146:569–571, 1986.

68. Lai K-H, Tsai Y-T, Lee S-D. Spontaneous bacterial peritonitis after endoscopic variceal sclerotherapy. Gastrointest Endosc 32:303–307, 1986.

69. Barnett JL, Elta G. Bacterial peritonitis following endoscopic variceal sclerotherapy. Gastrointest Endoscop 33:316–317, 1987.

70. Schembre D, Bjorkman KJ. Post-sclerotherapy bacterial peritonitis. Am J Gastroenterol 86:481–486, 1991.

71. Botoman VA, Surawicz CM. Bacteremia with gastrointestinal endoscopic procedures. Gastrointest Endoscop 32:342–346, 1986.

72. Bac DJ, deMarie S, Siersema S, Snobl J, van Buren HR. Post-sclerotherapy bacterial peritonitis: a complication of sclerotherapy or of variceal bleeding? Am J Gastroenterol 89:859–865, 1994.

73. Sanyal AJ, Reddy KR. Infective endotipsitis: a newly described complication of transjugular intrahepatic portosystemic shunts. Ann Intern Med, in press, 1998.

74. Meensook C, Rajadanuraks N, Meesangnin C. Spontaneous bacterial peritonitis in acute hepatitis B. J Med Assoc Thailand 73:526–529, 1990.

75. Chu C-M, Chiu K-W, Liaw Y-F. The prevalence and prognostic significance of spontaneous bacterial peritonitis in severe acute hepatitis with ascites. Hepatology 15:799–803, 1992.

76. Chu CM, Sheen IS, Liaw YF. The etiology of acute hepatitis in Taiwan: Acute hepatitis superimposed upon Hb$_s$Ag carrier state as the main etiology in areas with high Hb$_s$Ag carrier rate. Infection 16:233–237, 1988.

77. Gimson AES. Late onset hepatic failure: clinical, serological and histological features. Hepatology 6:288–294, 1986.

78. Wyke RJ, Canalese JC, Gimson AES, Williams R. Bacteraemia in patients with fulminant hepatic failure. Liver 2:45–52, 1982.

79. Larcher VF, Wyke RJ, Mowat AP, Williams R. Bacterial and fungal infection in children with fulminant hepatic failure: possible role of opsonisation and complement deficiency. Gut 23:1037–1043, 1982.

80. Rolando N. Prospective study of bacterial infection in acute liver failure: an analysis of fifty patients. Hepatology 11:49–53, 1990.

81. Tito L, Rimola A, Gines P, Llach J, Arroyo V, Rodes J. Recurrence of spontaneous bacterial peritonitis in cirrhosis: frequency and predictive factors. Hepatology 8:27–31, 1988.

82. Silvain C, Mannant P-R, Ingrand P, Fort E, Besson I, Beauchant M. Récidive de l'infection spontanée du liquide d'ascite au cours de la cirrhose. Gastroenterol Clin Biol 15:106–109, 1991.

83. Gines P, Rimola A, Planas R, Vargas V, Marco F. Norfloxacin prevents spontaneous bacterial peritonitis recurrence in cirrhosis: results of a double-blind, placebo-controlled trial. Hepatology 12:716–724, 1990.

84. Rimola A, Bory F, Terés J, Pérez-Ayuso RM, Arroyo V, Rodés J. Oral nonabsorbable antibiotics prevent infection in cirrhotics with gastrointestinal hemorrhage. Hepatology 5:463–467, 1985.

85. Ukah FO, Harhav H, Kramer D, Eghtesad B, Smimi F, Frezza E, Linden P, Mieles L, Selby R. Early outcome of liver transplantation in patients with a history of spontaneous bacterial peritonitis. Transplant Proc 25:1113–1115, 1993.

86. Van Thiel DH, Hassanein R, Gurakar A, Wright HI, Caraceni P, De Maria N, Nadir A. Liver transplantation after an acute episode of spontaneous bacterial peritonitis. Hepatogastroenterology 43:1584–1588, 1996.

87. Hoefs JC, Runyon BA. Spontaneous bacterial peritonitis. Dis Month 31:1–48, 1985.

88. Runyon BA. Paracentesis of ascitic fluid. A safe procedure. Arch Intern Med 146:2259–2261, 1986.

89. Runyon BA, Umland ET, Merlin T. Inoculation of blood culture bottles with ascitic fluid. Arch Intern Med 147:73–77, 1987.
89a. Qureshi WA, Harshfield D, Shah H, Nechvolodoff C, Banerjee B. An unusual complication of paracentesis. Am J Gastroenterol 87:1209–1211, 1992.
89b. Macdonald GR. Exsanguination, a complication of paracentesis abdominis. Treat Serv Bull 6:383–386, 1951.
89c. Serbin RA: Fatal hemorrhage from paracentesis: a case of Cruveillhier-Baumgarten syndrome. Gastroenterology 30:127–129, 1956.
89d. Minocha A. A fatal case of paracentesis (correspondence). Am J Gastroenterol 94:856, 1999.
90. Yuen K-H, Ng F-H, Mok K-Y, Ng W-F. Monomicrobial nonneutrocytic bacter-ascites due to *Burkholderia pickettii.* Am J Gastroenterol 93:2308–2309, 1999.
91. de Luis DA, Aller R, Boixeda D, Ruiz Del Arbol L, De Argila CM. Spontaneous bacterial peritonitis caused by *Citrobacter diversus*: case report. Clin Infec Dis 24:81–82, 1997.
92. Collazos J, Martinez E, Mayo J. Spontaneous bacterial peritonitis caused by *Streptococcus gordonii.* J Clin Gastroenterol 28:45–46, 1999.
93. Boixeda D, de Luis DA, Mesequer MA, Aller R, Martin de Arguila C, Lopez Santroman A. A case of spontaneous peritonitis caused by *Weeksella virosa.* Eur J Gastroenterol Hepatol 10:897–898, 1998.
94. Vaghjimal A, Sperber K. Spontaneous bacterial peritonitis due to *Corynebacterium* sp. Postgrad Med J 73:319, 1997.
95. Ozakyol AH, Saricam T, Zubaroglu I. Spontaneous bacterial peritonitis due to *Brucella melitensis* in a cirrhotic patient. Am J Gastroenterol 94:2572–2573, 1999.

4

Prevalence of Spontaneous Bacterial Peritonitis

Harold O. Conn
Yale University School of Medicine, New Haven, Connecticut, and University of Miami School of Medicine, Miami, Florida

One of the first questions asked about any newly described disease is, "How common is it?" This is a very logical question, and one that may be difficult to answer early in the history of any syndrome. SBP is no exception, even though it is no longer a new syndrome.

The data collected in an attempt to answer this question are listed in Table 4.1 (1–28). Although only a handful of cases of this discrete, hitherto unrecognized syndrome were described in our initial article on this disease in 1964 (1), the number of patients with SBP that we had seen increased rapidly thereafter (1–4). In retrospect, other individual instances of probable SBP had been described by others as "interesting cases" as early as 1842 (29) and 1893 (30). Until 1964, however, they were not considered to represent a single, full-blown syndrome.

In our definitive article on SBP in 1971 (2), we described 30 episodes of SBP in 26 patients. Later the number increased to about 100 cases based on our series of about 750 cirrhotic patients with ascites over a period of 15 years. In that article (2) we characterized the syndrome and outlined its probable pathogenesis. In addition, we described and defined six patients with *asymptomatic bacterascites* (ABA) and nine patients with typical SBP in which the ascitic fluid cultures were sterile. This latter syndrome is now known as *culture-negative SBP* (CNSBP) or "probable SBP." The term *"culture-negative neutrocytic ascites"* (CNNA), which had been used transiently, has

Table 4.1 Prevalence of SBP, CNSBP, and Bacterascites in Cirrhosis

First author and reference	Year	No. of cirrhosis patients at risk	No. (%) with SBP	No. (%) with CNSBP	No. (%) with BA	Total No. with SBP*
Conn (1)	1964	200	5 (2)	5 (2)	0 (0)	10 (5)
Conn (2)	1971	250	24 (9)	4 (1)	3 (1)	31 (11)
Correia (3)	1975	167	25 (15)	0 (0)	0 (0)	25 (15)
Conn (4)	1980	200	37 (18)	0 (0)	3 (2)	40 (2)
Sanchez-Tapias (5)	1971	120	7 (6)	0 (0)	0 (0)	7 (6)
Le Carrer (6)	1980	242	31 (13)	0 (0)	0 (0)	31 (13)
Kammerer (7)	1982	156	18 (12)	0 (0)	0 (0)	18 (12)
Levy (8)	1982	103	20 (19)	0 (0)	0 (0)	20 (19)
Pinzello (9)	1983	224	27 (21)	6 (3)	1 (1)	34 (15)
Yang (10)	1985	100	10 (10)	0 (0)	0 (0)	10 (10)
Attali (11)	1986	169	18 (11)	14 (8)	8 (5)	40 (24)
Kachintorn (12)	1986	426	30 (7)	4 (1)	0 (0)	34 (8)
Sette (13)	1986	114	11 (10)	4 (4)	0 (0)	15 (13)
Almdal (14)	1987	68	13 (17)	0 (0)	0 (0)	13 (17)
Bercoff (15)	1987	92	10 (11)	0 (0)	0 (0)	10 (11)
Garcia-Tsao (16)	1987	197	35 (18)	0 (0)	0 (0)	35 (18)
Oguto (17)	1988	100	10 (10)	10 (10)	5 (5)	25 (25)
Runyan (18)	1988	119	20 (17)	0 (0)	0 (0)	20 (17)
Abillos (19)	1990	242	41 (17)	0 (0)	0 (0)	41 (17)
Chesta (20)	1991	120	23 (19)	0 (0)	0 (0)	23 (19)
Llach (21)	1992	127	13 (10)	0 (0)	0 (0)	13 (10)
Andreu (22)	1993	110	28 (25)	0 (0)	0 (0)	28 (25)
Conte (23)	1993	265	24 (9)	34 (13)	16 (6)	74 (28)
Fiaccadori (24)	1993	625	34 (5)	10 (4)	0 (0)	44 (7)
Chu (25)	1995	443	55 (12)	37 (8)	48 (11)	140 (32)
Ho (26)	1996	176	68 (39)	9 (5)	0 (0)	77 (44)
Kaymakoglu (27)	1996	80	8 (10)	10 (13)	2 (2)	20 (25)
Puri (28)	1996	70	10 (14)	8 (11)	3 (4)	21 (30)
Total		5225	647 (12)	155 (3)	93 (2)	899 (17)
References 1–14		2539	276 (11)	33 (1)	15 (1)	325 (12)
References 15–28		2686	371 (14)	108 (4)	72 (3)	551 (21)
Total, References 1–28		5225	647 (12)	141 (3)	87 (2)	876 (17)

CNSBP = Culture-negative SBP.
ABA = Asymptomatic bacterascites.
SBP* = SBP plus CNSBP plus ABA.

recently been discarded as being "confusing." For alphabetical symmetry, SBP may be termed *culture-positive neutrocytic ascites* (CPNA).

These three related syndromes are currently considered to represent clinical variants of SBP. In this discussion of the prevalence of SBP we shall consider these variant syndromes both separately and together (Table 4.1). It is appropriate to consider SBP as presenting in several ways: symptomatic or asymptomatic, neutrocytic or nonneutrocytic, and culture-negative or culture-positive. This approach is familiar to physicians who understand the non-A, non-B terminology of viral hepatitis, and who have long been aware that SBP and subacute bacterial endocarditis (SBE), which are parallel syndromes both clinically and pathogenetically, may occur in culture-positive and culture-negative as well as in symptomatic and asymptomatic forms. Both SBP and SBE, which will hereafter be referred to as bacterial endocarditis (BE), may be acute or chronic bacterial infections in which an episode of bacteremia infects a previously abnormal tissue. In the case of SBP, the "tissue" is ascitic fluid, which is abnormal by virtue of its abnormally low concentrations of complement and thereby its deficient opsonizing capacity. In the case of BE the abnormal tissues are deformed or otherwise abnormal cardiac valves or endothelium.

Thus, SBP and BE can be considered "serendipitous" diseases. Serendipity has been defined as "chance and the prepared mind." In this context, *serendipity* is considered to be the summation or potentiation of knowledge induced by a chance observation superimposed on previously acquired information. In such situations a bacteremia, which is a serious infectious episode, gives rise to a much more serious, potentially lethal complication. Another hepatological example of such medical serendipity is the demonstration that the Hepatitis B and C Virions, HBV and HCV, are body tissue–borne viruses. This knowledge has permitted epidemiologists to search for and to find a variety of ways in which these infectious agents can be transmitted, e.g., by blood transfusions by needle sticks, by contamination of abrasions by virus-positive tissue fluids, or in the process of giving birth. Freezers filled with carefully collected and identified specimens of blood, serum, and tissues have provided "libraries" for the retrospective performance and investigations of analyses of such epidemiological features.

I. DEFINITIONS

A number of definitions are needed to simplify the understanding and presentation of these complex relationships.

Prevalence is loosely defined in the *Random House Dictionary of the English Language* as the "extent of occurrence . . . of an event, disease, symptom, sign, cost or other characteristic." It is not limited to a specific unit of time, but it may be restricted to a specific country or type of disease, e.g., alcoholic cirrhosis.

Incidence is more rigorously defined as "the rate of occurrence" of such an event. Incidence, therefore, requires some additional qualifications to permit calculation of the occurrence of the event over a period of time, e.g., per year. Thus, an infection rate, which is an incidence, is expressed as a percentage, such as 6% per year, or as a rate of speed, which involves both distance and time, such as miles per hour, or as an epidemiological rate is expressed as a number per aliquot of patients, e.g., 15 infections per 100,000 population.

It is of interest that the U.S. Food and Drug Administration in its finite wisdom devised the innovative "orphan" drug regulations in which it arbitrarily decided that a disease with a *prevalence* of <200,000 was small enough to justify "orphan" status and thereby to permit more lenient regulations in the requirements for animal investigations and in clinical trials (31). This modification was made presumably to permit small pharmaceutical firms with less capital to compete with large firms in developing new therapeutic agents for relatively small patient populations on more economically level playing fields. The use of "prevalence" rather than the more restrictive "incidence" seems to have been another way in which to level the playing field.

Culture-negative SBP (probable SBP), is the classical syndrome of SBP in which cultures of the ascitic fluid are sterile (32–34). This definition requires the presence of an increased number of polymorphonuclear leukocytes (PMN) (>250 per cubic millimeter) in the ascitic fluid in the absence of bacteria and of "any evidence of an intraabdominal source of infection."

This syndrome may arise from the prior administration of antibiotic agents that remain in the ascitic fluid in a concentration that is sufficient to suppress the in vitro growth of the organisms responsible, but that is insufficient to eradicate the infection completely. It may also represent the failure to detect bacteria because of inadequate aliquots of ascitic fluid being cultured or it may represent the equivalent phenomenon in which 20% false negative blood cultures occur in culture-negative bacterial endocarditis (35). It is intriguing that both of these chronic bacterial infections have culture-negative variants in about the same prevalence, approximately 20%.

Bacterascites (BA) is defined as the presence of culturable bacteria in the ascitic fluid, usually but not necessarily, in asymptomatic cirrhotic patients (36,37). Typically only a single species of bacteria can be cultured in BA, giving rise to the term *monomicrobial, neutrocytic bacterascites. Symptomatic BA*, in which fever, or abdominal symptoms typical of SBP are present, is usually associated with higher levels of total serum bilirubin, lower levels of serum albumin, more prolonged prothrombin times, lower concentrations of ascitic fluid protein and complement, and a lower survival rate than *asymptomatic BA*.

We reviewed all of the published articles in peer-reviewed journals using both a MEDLINE search of the literature on CNSBP, SBP, and BA and their therapy and prognosis and a manual search of the bibliographies of all articles identified as SBP and its variants. All articles that did not present the number of patients at risk, i.e., the number of cirrhotic patients "with ascites," or in whom paracenteses and assessment of the ascites had been performed, were excluded. We accepted the authors' diagnoses of cirrhosis, ascites, SBP, and bacterascites as published because the criteria for these specific diagnoses are not presented in the great majority of articles on SBP. We reviewed all articles in which five or more patients with SBP were reported. Patients with cirrhosis of all etiologies were included. We excluded articles in which recurrent episodes of SBP were included in the calculations presented. We excluded those articles which were qualified as being limited to patients who had developed SBP after a specific procedure such as endoscopic sclerotherapy or who had been part of studies in which prophylactic or therapeutic antibiotic therapy had been administered.

II. RESULTS

We identified 28 articles on SBP in which both the number of cirrhotic patients at risk and the numbers of patients in whom the diagnosis of SBP was established bacteriologically were presented, and from these data we calculated the prevalence of SBP (Table 4.1). When the data about culture-negative SBP were presented by the authors, we calculated the prevalence of this variant of SBP as well. Similarly, if the data about bacterascites were presented, its prevalence was also calculated. Finally, based on all these data the "total" prevalence of SBP was calculated by adding together the numbers of patients with SBP, with CNSBP, and with BA and divided by the total number of patients at risk.

These 28 series, which were usually consecutive series of patients, contained from 68 to 655 patients with a total of 5225 and a mean of 187 patients per series. The percentage of patients in these series with SBP ranged from

2% to 39%, respectively, with a total of 647 patients with bacteriologically proved SBP (12%) (Table 4.1).

These 28 series of patients arranged in chronological order are divided into the first 14 series, which had been published between 1964 and 1987 (1–14), and which included 2539 patients and the second 14 series (15–28), which consisted of 2686 patients that were reported between 1987 and 1996. The prevalence of SBP in the two series were 10.9% and 13.8%, respectively, a statistically significant difference (p < 0.01). This difference demonstrates that the prevalence had increased significantly during these two periods.

We had previously demonstrated that the prevalence of SBP in our personally observed series of cirrhotic patients at the Department of Veterans Affairs Medical Center in West Haven, Connecticut, had progressively increased in the three consecutive seven-year periods which ended in 1964, 1971, and 1978, respectively (4). The prevalence of SBP, which had been based on the number of autopsies performed in cirrhotic patients at our hospital, increased progressively from 3% to 12% to 33% in these three sabbatical periods. This series consisted of a total of 64 patients with SBP.

Culture-negative SBP was reported in a total of 155 patients (3%) and its prevalence increased from 1.2% in the first 14 series (1964–1987) to (4.0%) in the second 14 series (1987–1996) (p < 0.02).

Bacterascites had been reported in 87 patients (2%) and its prevalence increased from 0.6% to 2.6% in the two series, respectively. This difference is probably statistically significant (p < 0.07).

The *total number of patients with "SBP"*, which included SBP plus culture-negative SBP plus bacterascites consisted of 877 patients of whom 17% had SBP, 3% had CNSBP, and 16% had ABA. ABA was reported in 12.8% of the earlier series and 20.5% of the later series (p < 0.01).

Chu and associates in Taiwan, where the Hepatitis B Virus (HBV) is endemic, studied BA in 443 predominantly HBsAg-positive cirrhotic patients with ascites (25). They found that SBP was present in 12.4% of them, CNSBP in 8.4%, and BA in 10.8%. Thus, 32% of these patients showed one or another variant of bacterial peritonitis (BP). Two-thirds of each of these three groups had signs and symptoms that were attributed to SBP. It is not known whether the coexistence of HBV affects the prevalence of SBP or the distribution of the variant syndromes of SBP. The prognosis of the patients with SBP was significantly worse than those with culture-negative SBP as shown by the hospital mortality data (55% vs. 23%; p < 0.01). The patients with asymptomatic BA had similar hospital mortality rates as those with sterile ascites (21% vs. 23%; p > 0.05). Unfortunately, these investigators did not present the prognosis of their patients with *asymptomatic* BA so that the results of a true 2 × 2 table could be assessed.

To determine the prevalence of SBP (i.e., SBP, CNSBP, plus BA) (Table 4.1) we assumed that the presence of SBP, CNSBP, and BA are all indicative of SBP and simply added them together to determine the total numbers of patients with "SBP." We calculated the prevalence of SBP by dividing the total number of patients with SBP by the number of ascitic cirrhotic patients at risk. We did this simple calculation for patients with SBP, with CNSBP, and with BA individually and together to determine the individual prevalences of these three variant syndromes and the overall prevalence of bacterial peritonitis. We excluded patients in whom the bacterial peritonitis was not spontaneous, but which is considered to be the result of a treatable lesion such as a perforation i.e., "secondary" or "perforated" BP.

Clearly, the prevalence of SBP and its variants, culture-negative SBP and BA have all increased significantly in the two series (Table 4.1).

There are many possible reasons for the increasing prevalence. The most important reason is the progressive improvement in bacteriological cultural techniques. Probably the single most important factor is the increasing volume of ascitic fluid implanted into the culture bottles and the freshness of the samples of ascitic fluid, which is assured by adding the blood to be cultured directly to blood culture bottles (38). Initially, the cultures were placed in test tubes, transported to the laboratory and thereafter implanted into the culture media. After it had been shown that fresh samples of ascitic fluid implanted into blood culture bottles yielded a significantly higher percentage of positive cultures, most cultures of ascitic fluid were performed in this manner. In the 1960s and early 1970s the need to perform cultures of the ascitic fluid, even in the absence of overt signs and symptoms of SBP, was not so clearly recognized. The performance of more cultures of ascitic fluid thereafter would have increased the yield of SBP. Other factors have probably contributed as well. Certainly, there have been continual minor technological improvements in the bacterial cultural media and in other aspects of bacteriological cultural techniques, which is an ongoing process. Finally, one must consider the effect of adding several variants of SBP—bacterascites (BA) and culture-negative SBP (CNSBP), which were not always considered to have SBP—to the calculations. At the present time cases of BA and CNSBP are included in studies from which the prevalence of SBP is determined. This calculation makes the prevalence of SBP appear greater than it really is. Perhaps, subtle improvements in cultural techniques for anaerobic and microaerophilic bacteria may also increase the prevalence although no such large increase in the prevalence of bacterial species in SBP has been reported.

Other possible explanations for the apparent increase in prevalence of SBP may reflect the effects of improved therapy of cirrhosis and the increasing use of prophylactic antibiotic therapy which improves survival of cirrhotic patients and increases the number of patients at risk of developing SBP. Improvement in diuretic therapy may permit patients to survive longer, in effect increasing their time at risk of contracting SBP. Similarly, more aggressive therapies of variceal bleeding may increase the risks of developing SBP. The addition of systemic vasopressin to our armamentarium (39), for example, improves the control of variceal hemorrhage and thus increases the number of patients who survive long enough to contract SBP. Similarly, the introduction of endoscopic sclerotherapy has been associated with increased risks of bacteremia and SBP (40). The trend to use large paracenteses as a primary form of therapy of massive ascites results in the loss of enormous amounts of albumin and complement components (41) and may, thereby, increase the risks of SBP (42). No studies have yet proved that large paracenteses increase the prevalence of SBP, but it is a rational consequence of reducing the concentration of complement.

Finally, it is important for physicians to understand that ascites is not a benign, cosmetic disorder, but, rather, that it represents a serious, potentially lethal abnormality, and that a patient with overt ascites should be considered to be a walking culture medium awaiting contamination. Ascites should be evaluated as quickly and as gently as possible. Large paracenteses, which eliminate ascites rapidly, are the most efficient form of treatment, but the large loss of protein and complement may increase the risk of infection (42).

Randomized controlled trials may be required to prove the relative efficacy and the changes induced in the prevalence of SBP by these different forms of therapy.

REFERENCES

1. Conn HO. Spontaneous peritonitis and bacteremia in cirrhotic in Laennec's cirrhosis caused by enteric organisms. Ann Intern Med 60:568–580, 1964.
2. Conn HO, Fessel JM. Spontaneous bacterial peritonitis in cirrhosis: variations on a theme. Medicine 50:161–197, 1971.
3. Correia JP, Conn HO. Spontaneous bacterial peritonitis in cirrhosis: endemic or epidemic? Med Clin No Am 59:963–981, 1975.
4. Conn HO, Goldfarb J. Spontaneous bacterial peritonitis: an endemic epidemic. In: *Hepatic, Biliary and Pancreatic Surgery Symposia Specialists*, HJ Zimmerman, ed., Chicago: Year Book Medical Publishers, pp. 441–452, 1980.
5. Sánchez-Tapias JM, Rodés J, Arroyo V, Bruguera M, Téres J, Bordas JM, Gassull MA, Revert L. Infeccion peritoneal en la cirrhosis hepatica con ascitis. Rev Clin Española 123:375–380, 1971.
6. LeCarrer M, Poupon R-Y, Ballet F, Darnis F. Les infections du liquid d'ascite

chez le cirrhotique: étude clinique et biologique de 36 épisodes observés au cours d'une année. Gastroenterol Clin Biol 4:640–645, 1980.

7. Kammerer J, Dupeyron C, Vuillemin N, Leluan G, Fouet P. Apport des examens cytologiques et bactériologiques du liquide d'ascite cirrhotique au diagnostic de péritonite bactérienne. Med Chir Dig 11:243–251, 1982.

8. Lévy VG, Theis C, Denis C, Denis J. Critères cytologiques de l'infection de l'ascite au cours des cirrhoses. Gastroenterol Clin Biol 6:736–739, 1982.

9. Pinzello G, Simonetti RG, Craxi A, DiPiazza S, Spanò C, Pagliaro L. Spontaneous bacterial peritonitis: a prospective investigation in predominantly nonalcoholic cirrhotic patients. Hepatology 3:545–549, 1983.

10. Yang CY, Liaw YF, Chu CM. White count, pH and lactate in ascites in the diagnosis of spontaneous bacterial peritonitis. Hepatology 5:85–90, 1985.

11. Attali P, Turner K, Pelletier G, Ink O, Etienne JP. pH of ascitic fluid: diagnostic and prognostic value in cirrhotic and noncirrhotic patients. Gastroenterology 90: 1255–1260, 1986.

12. Kachintorn U, Chainuvati T, Chinapak O, Plengvanit U. Spontaneous bacterial peritonitis in cirrhotics: clinical and ascitic fluid findings. Ann Acad Med Singapore 15:222–226, 1986.

13. Sette Jr. H, Mies S, Barros MF, Beltrao L, Raia S. Peritonite bacteriana espontânea. Rev Paul Med 104:292–297, 1986.

14. Almdal TP, Skinhøj P. Spontaneous bacterial peritonitis in cirrhosis. Incidence, diagnosis, and prognosis. Scand J Gastroenterol 22:295–300, 1987.

15. Bercoff E, Durrbach A, Manchon ND, Duranton Y, Senant J, Lecomte N, Bourreille J. La concentration des protides dans l'ascite permet-elle de prévoir la survenue d'une infection du liquide d'ascite? Gastroenterol Clin Biol 11:363–638, 1987.

16. Garcia-Tsao G. Spontaneous bacterial peritonitis. Gastro Clin No Am 21:257–275, 1992.

17. Ogutu EO, Wankya BM, Shah MV, Ndinya-Achola JO. Prevalence of spontaneous bacterial peritonitis at Kenyatta National Hospital. East Afr Med J 68:547–551, 1988.

18. Runyon B. Patients with deficient ascitic fluid opsonic activity are predisposed to spontaneous bacterial peritonitis. Hepatology 8:632–635, 1988.

19. Albillos A, Cuervas-Mons V, Millàn I, Cantón T, Montes J, Barrios C, Garrido A, Escartín P. Ascitic fluid polymorphonuclear cell count and serum to ascites albumin gradient in the diagnosis of bacterial peritonitis. Gastroenterology 98: 134–140, 1990.

20. Chesta J, Brahm J, Poniachik J, Latorre R, Hurtado C, Novoa X, Velasco M. Spontaneous bacterial peritonitis: a frequent and recurrent complication in cirrhotic patients with ascites. Rev Med Chile 119:273–278, 1991.

21. Llach J, Rimola A, Navasa M, Ginès P, Salmerón JM, Ginès A, Arroyo V, Rodés J. Incidence and predictive factors of first episode of spontaneous bacterial peritonitis in cirrhosis with ascites: relevance of ascitic fluid protein concentration. Hepatology 16:724–727, 1992.

22. Andreu M, Sola R, Sitges-Serra A, Alia C, Gallen M, Vila MC, Coll S, Oliver

MI. Risk factors for spontaneous bacterial peritonitis in cirrhotic patients with ascites. Gastroenterology 104:1133–1138, 1993.

23. Conte D, Bolzoni P, Bodini P, Mandelli C, Ranzi ML, Cesarini L, Fraquelli M, Penagini R, Bianchi PA. Frequency of spontaneous bacterial peritonitis in 265 cirrhotics with ascites. Eur J Gastroenterol & Hepatol 5:41–45, 1993.

24. Fiaccadori F, Pedretti G. Peritonite batterica spontanea in corso di cirrosi epatica: Rilievi clinici e considerazioni terapeutiche. Ann Ital Med Int 8:13–17, 1993.

25. Chu C-M, Chang K-Y, Liaw Y-F. Prevalence and prognostic significance of bacterascites in cirrhosis with ascites. Dig Dis Sci 40:561–565, 1995.

26. Ho H, Zuckerman MJ, Ho TK, Guerra LG, Verghese A, Casner PR. Prevalence of associated infections in community-acquired spontaneous bacterial peritonitis. Am J Gastroenterol 91:735–742, 1996.

27. Kaymakoglu S, Eraksoy H, Ökten A, Demir K, Çakaloglu Y, Boztas G, Besisik F. Spontaneous ascitic infection in different cirrhotic groups: prevalence, risk factors and the efficacy of cefotaxime therapy. J Gastroenterol 9:71–76, 1996.

28. Puri AS. Frequency, microbial spectrum and outcome of spontaneous bacterial peritonitis in North India. Indian J Gastroenterol 15:86–89, 1996.

29. Wawruch H. In: Beethoven, Impressions by His Contemporaries, Sonneck OG, ed., New York: Dover Publications, 1967.

30. Charrin V. Peritonite a pneumocoque an moment de la mart. Comptes Rendus Soc Biol 9S:1657–1673, 1983.

31. Federal Register. Such a designation enables small pharmaceutical firms. Vol. 75, Dec. 29, 1992.

32. Runyon BA, Hoefs JC. Culture-negative neutrocytic ascites: a variant of spontaneous bacterial peritonitis. Hepatology 4:1209–1211, 1984.

33. Pelletier G, Salmon D, Ink O, Hannoun S, Attali P, Buffet C, Etienne JP. Culture-negative neutrocytic ascites: a less severe variant of spontaneous bacterial peritonitis. Hepatology 10:327–331, 1990.

34. Al Amri SM, Allam AR, Al Mofleh IA. Spontaneous bacterial peritonitis and culture negative neutrocytic ascites in patients with non-alcoholic liver cirrhosis. J Gastroenterol Hepatol 9:433–436, 1994.

35. Pesanti EL, Smith IM. Infective endocarditis with negative blood cultures: an analysis of 52 cases. Am J Med 66:43–50, 1979.

36. Pelletier G, Lesur G, Ink O, Hagege H, Attali P, Buffet C, Etienne J-P. Asymptomatic bacterascites: is it spontaneous bacterial peritonitis? Hepatology 14:112–115, 1991.

37. Terg R, Levi D, Lopez P, Rafaelli C, Rojter S, Abecasis R, Villamil F, Aziz H, Podesta A. Analysis of clinical course and prognosis of culture-positive spontaneous bacterial peritonitis and neutrocytis ascites. Evidence of the same disease. Dig Dis Sci 37:1499–1504, 1992.

38. Runyon BA, Umland ET, Merlin T. Inoculation of blood culture bottles with ascitic fluid. Arch Intern Med 147:73–75, 1987.

39. Conn HO, Ramsby GR, Storer EH. Selective intra-arterial vasopressin in the treatment of upper gastrointestinal hemorrhage. Gastroenterology 63:634–645, 1972.

40. Cohen LB, Korsten MA, Scherl EJ. Bacteremia after endoscopic injection sclerosis. Gastrointest Endosc 29:198–200, 1983.
41. Quintero E, Gines P, Arroyo V. Paracentesis versus diuretics in the treatment of cirrhotics with tense ascites. Lancet 1:611–612, 1985.
42. Runyon BA, Morrissey RL, Hoefs JC. Opsonic activity of human ascitic fluid: a potentially important protective mechanism against spontaneous bacterial peritonitis. Hepatology 5:634–637, 1985.

5
Tuberculous Peritonitis

Harold O. Conn
Yale University School of Medicine, New Haven, Connecticut, and University of Miami School of Medicine, Miami, Florida

Half of the world's population is infected with *Mycobacterium tuberculosis*, which accounts for 6% of all deaths worldwide. Ten million new cases of tuberculosis are detected annually. In the United States the prevalence of tuberculosis declined steadily by about 5% per year from 1950 to the mid-1980s, after which it dramatically increased by 15–20%. Tuberculous peritonitis (TBP) is an uncommon manifestation of a very common disease. It is currently seen most frequently in developing countries, but therein lies the difficulty. Reliable, clinical observations and sophisticated studies are least likely to be reported from such areas.

I. CLINICAL PRESENTATION

We have synthesized a clinically oriented description of TBP based on a series of 23 articles published in the medical literature between 1960 and 1996 (1–23) (Table 5.1). These articles, which were identified in a MEDLINE search, have been cataloged as tuberculous peritonitis and as abdominal or gastrointestinal tuberculosis. This search was limited to articles published in English and excluded book chapters, articles that appeared in symposia, abstracts, letters to editors, and otherwise non-peer-reviewed articles. We accepted the authors' diagnoses of TBP as correct because few articles presented detailed diagnostic criteria for inclusion in these series. We required that in each of these articles

Table 5.1 Tuberculous Peritonitis: Large Published Series

Ref. No.	Date First	First Author	No. Cases	Country
1	1960	Burack	47	U.S.
2	1962	Hyman	23	U.S.
3	1966	Gonnella	31	U.S.
4	1967	Singh	47	India
5	1967	Sochocky	100	U.S.
6	1968	Levine	30	U.S.
7	1975	Das	68	India
8	1976	Dineen	70	U.S.
9	1977	Karney	30	U.S.
10	1980	Sherman	25	U.S.
11	1981	Geake	74	SA
12	1983	Gilinsky	71	SA
13	1984	Jorge	42	ARG
14	1985	Bastani	30	Iran
15	1985	Klimach	20	ENG
16	1985	Palmer	27	ENG
17	1986	Menzes	43	SA
18	1988	Jakubowski	41	CAN
19	1990	Aguado	37	Spain
20	1992	Bhargava	38	India
21	1992	Manohar	145	SA
22	1996	Lisahora	28	U.S.
23	1996	Shakil	55	U.S.

ARG = Argentina, CAN = Canada, ENG = England, SA = South Africa.

20 or more patients were reported to have TBP. These 23 articles, which included more than 1100 patients, were supplemented by published reviews, case reports, and other peer-reviewed communications on this subject.

Because the articles were written by many authors from many countries for many purposes and from many points of view we have assembled these data into a review of the subject that includes our overall interpretation of the material. We have included data on the clinical presentation of these patients and on criteria for diagnosis, for pathogenesis, for prognosis, and of therapy. These summations approached the subject as an implied comparison of TBP with SBP, the subject matter of this volume, to demonstrate similarities and differences between the two syndromes. The heterogeneity of the clinical material and the large number of unknown details about these data indicate that this summation should be treated as a narrative meta-analysis (24).

It should be pointed out that some of these series of patients were collected over a period of years, as is shown by the subtitle of the first series, "A study of 47 proved cases encountered by a general medical unit in 25 years" (1). However, the prevalence of this disease has varied widely over the past half-century, particularly in the United States, from which about half of the articles and almost half of the patients were derived.

In the United States and Great Britain, TBP is seen most frequently in immigrants from Asia and from developing countries (14,16,23), particularly patients of black and Hispanic origin.

TBP is a disease of paradoxes. It is most likely to occur in indigent, urban patients who live an unrestrained life, but is frequently found in the constrained inhabitants of prisons and reservations (25), who are for practical purposes indigent, but who are healthy and well-nourished and who receive good medical care while they are incarcerated. It occurs usually in patients between the ages of 25 and 45, but is also seen in elderly patients, especially those cared for in nursing homes (17). It is frequently seen in alcoholic patients, especially those with chronic liver disease (23).

It tends to present insidiously (19) as a chronic disease, often with abdominal discomfort and distension. The most common signs and symptoms, i.e., abdominal pain and cramping, diarrhea, fever, anorexia, and weight loss, are nonspecific and resemble those of regional enteritis. The abdominal distention is often caused by overt ascites, which is present in about 85% of patients with TBP (1,23). TBP tends to be more common in women than in men (4,8,14,15,21), but there are many reported exceptions to this generalization.

Abdominal pain is present in more than 90%. Anorexia, weight loss, fever, and gastrointestinal symptoms are each present in about 60% (1). Virtually any other organs may also be involved, although lungs, kidneys, lymph nodes, and the intestinal and genitourinary tracts are involved in descending order of frequency (25).

The recent increase in the prevalence of TBP can be attributed largely to the AIDS epidemic (26), which has changed some of the patterns of tuberculosis, giving rise to many nonpulmonary manifestations and much greater infectivity and virulence, the so-called new tuberculosis (26).

II. AIDS AND TUBERCULOSIS

The concurrence of tuberculosis and AIDS poses particularly difficult diagnostic problems (27). In a series of reports from the United States and Brazil (28,29), more than two-thirds of the patients with AIDS and tuberculosis had extrapulmonary manifestations of tuberculosis. Because tuberculosis in human immunodeficiency virus (HIV)-infected patients causes a progressive deficiency of CD4-T-lymphocytes and poor granuloma formation, frequently reactivation of tuberculosis occurs.

The abdominal manifestations of tuberculosis in patients with AIDS frequently include weight loss, abdominal pain, abdominal masses, disseminated lymphadenopathy, anemia, fever, and diarrhea. Massive gastrointestinal hemorrhage, bowel obstruction, perforation, or abscess formation occur commonly. These complications require differentiation from Crohn's disease, neoplasms, sarcoidosis, blastomycosis, and actinomycosis. Treatment of these combined diseases requires investigation to assess the nature of the tuberculosis and its spread to the gastrointestinal or genitourinary tract or other sites. Sometimes emergency surgical therapy is needed (25). Similarly, the HIV may require systemic therapy because of opportunistic infections of some system or organ in the body. Depending on the site, and types of infections, either medical or surgical therapy or both may be required.

One important aspect of this new type of tuberculosis is the occurrence of multiple drug resistance (30). The occurrence of a miniepidemic of multidrug-resistant tuberculosis by tiny droplet dissemination that developed during a nine-hour airplane flight dramatically demonstrates the infectivity of the new tuberculosis (31,32). It also shows our ability to advance our knowledge about this disorder using up-to-date epidemiological and laboratory methodology.

Although uncommon in the United States and other developed nations, TBP is a frequent cause of ascites in developing countries (1,9,16,22,25), and is a common complication in patients with cirrhosis (1,23,19). It is an especially frequent complication of chronic, ambulatory, peritoneal dialysis (CAPD) (33). This specific syndrome will be discussed in greater detail in this chapter.

TBP may occur at any age but usually does so between the third and fifth decades (25). Although it occurs predominantly in women (5,8), the Fallopian route of infection appears to be uncommon. Abdominal swelling is the most common manifestation (1,16), occurring in more than 80% of patients (1,22). Fever is seen in three-fourths and weight loss and abdominal pain in two-thirds each (23). Chronic diarrhea is reported in only about 15%. Purified protein derivative (PPD) skin tests are usually positive (23) but are frequently negative, especially in patients who are severely ill, often reflecting the paradoxical anergy that occurs in acutely ill patients (34). About half have an abnormal chest X-ray indicative of active tuberculosis (23). Mild anemia is often present (23).

The ascitic fluid is almost always an exudate, i.e., protein concentration of 2.5–3.0 g per dl and the serum-ascites albumin gradient (SAAG) is less

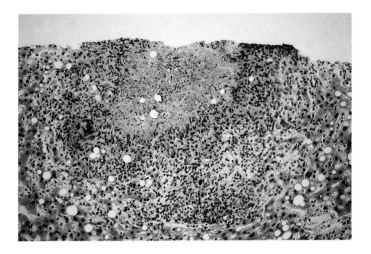

Figure 5.1 Tuberculosis. A large, caseating granuloma with a central zone of caseation necrosis is encircled by scattered epithelioid giant cells and by a dense lymphocytic infiltrate. This lesion was encountered in a young black woman with high fever, a strongly positive tuberculin reaction, and a serosanguinous pleural effusion from which tubercle bacilli were cultured. Acid-fast stain of this section was negative. (From Klatskin G, Conn HO, *Histopathology of the Liver*, New York: Oxford University Press, 1993. Reproduced by permission of the authors and Oxford University Press.)

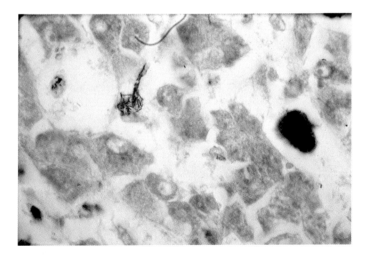

Figure 5.2 *Mycobacterium avian intracellulare* (MAI) infection in AIDS. A clump of acid-fast bacilli is present within a Kupffer cell. (Courtesy of Dr. G. H. Bezahler. From Klatskin G, Conn HO, *Histopathology of the Liver*, New York: Oxford University Press, 1993. Reproduced by permission of the authors and Oxford University Press.)

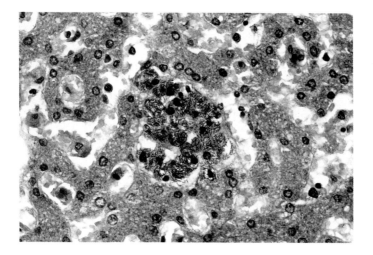

Figure 5.3 Fatal *Mycobacterium avian intracellulare* (MAI) infection in a 29-year-old intravenous drug abuser with AIDS. Multiple hepatic granulomas are composed of foamy, "striated" histiocytes that are filled with MAI bacilli. (Courtesy of Dr. E. C. Klatt. From Klatskin G, Conn HO, *Histopathology of the Liver*, New York: Oxford University Press, 1993. Reproduced by permission of the authors and Oxford University Press.)

than 1.1 g per dl (23,35,36). The leukocyte count ranges from 50 to 4000 per cubic millimeter and consists largely of mononuclear leukocytes (23), unlike SBP, which is characterized by polymorphonuclear leukocytosis (37).

III. DIAGNOSIS

The diagnosis of TBP can be established definitively in one of several ways. First is if the histopathological demonstration of caseating granulomas of the peritoneum with their characteristic epithelioid giant cells and acid-fast bacilli (23) is definitive. Such tissue can be obtained by laparotomy, by laparoscopy with guided-needle biopsy, or by blind-needle biopsy of the peritoneum (38). Samples of liver tissue that contain tuberculous granulomas would seem to be reliable means of making the diagnosis histologically, but the large series reported by Klatskin et al. from the Liver Study Unit at Yale University indicate that it is an unlikely method of making the diagnosis. In 76 consecutive specimens obtained from patients with tuberculosis and hepatic granulomas over a 40-year period, only one showed caseation necrosis (Fig. 5.1; see Color Plate). *M. tuberculosis* was cultured from two others (39) for a total yield of about 3% (39). On the other hand, the organisms responsible for atypical tuberculosis, i.e., *Mycobacterium avium intracellulare* (MAI), in patients with AIDS are widely disseminated in the organs of such patients (Fig. 5.2; see Color Plate), especially in their livers. Indeed, hepatic granulomas from such patients are literally filled with acid-fast positive organisms (Fig. 5.3; see Color Plate).

Second, the bacteriological isolation of *Mycobacterium tuberculosis* from the ascitic fluid is equally diagnostic, although the organisms require five to eight weeks to grow and the false-negative rate is very high. Singh has shown that very large samples, i.e., 1 L of ascitic fluid or more, yield a higher growth of tubercle bacilli than smaller aliquots (40). This phenomenon is similar to the finding that large samples are more efficient than small ones in the diagnosis of SBP (41).

The only other definitive method of documenting the presence of *M. tuberculosis* is the immunological demonstration tuberculous antigen in the ascitic fluid using a specific immunologic technique such as an enzyme-linked immunosorbent assay (ELISA) that is amplified by the polymerase chain reaction (PCR) (42,43). This conceptually simple but technologically sophisticated methodology, which employs an antimycobacterial antibody, has also been used in the diagnosis of pulmonary, pleural, and neurotuberculosis (42–45). This ingenious technique, which can be employed in serum and cerebrospinal fluid, has so far been reported only in the diagnosis of TBP (43). Clearly, it or its descendants will be the methodology of the future for the diagnosis of tuberculosis, especially of TBP.

All other methods employed in the diagnosis of TBP until recently have been nonspecific tests that suggest the diagnosis of TBP, but cannot prove it (Table 5.2). These methods are laboratory tests that in general measure various properties of the ascitic fluid including the specific gravity, the protein, albumin or globulin concentrations, the serum-ascites albumin gradient (SAAG), the number and types of leukocytes, the opsonic index, and the presence and concentration of cholesterol and fibronectin. These studies can differentiate an exudate from a transudate, and can even predict prognosis in the sense that patients with very low serum albumin concentrations (<1.0 g per dl) are

Table 5.2 Laboratory Features of Patients with Tuberculous Peritonitis

	Group I (n = 13)	Group II (n = 21)	P Value
Hematocrit (%)	34 ± 7	31 ± 5	NS
Anemia	10 (77%)	19 (90%)	NS
WBC (10^9/L)	5.4 ± 1.5	9.5 ± 4.7	0.001
Platelets (10^9/L)	313 ± 110	276 ± 146	NS
Serum bilirubin (μmol/L)	7 ± 4	34 ± 36	0.001
Serum ALP (U/L)	211 ± 186	272 ± 191	NS
Serum ALT (U/L)	22 ± 20	27 ± 13	NS
Serum total protein (g/dl)	7.3 ± 14	7.4 ± 12	NS
Serum albumin (g/dl)	2.6 ± 6	2.3 ± 6	NS
Prothrombin time (%)	74 ± 18	51 ± 15	<0.01
As. monocytes	1148 ± 1116	943 ± 676	NS
As. protein (g/dl)	5.3 ± 15	3.0 ± 11	<0.0001
As. albumin (g/dl)	2.1 ± 7	1.0 ± 5	<0.001
SAAG	6 ± 2	11 ± 5	<0.001
As. LDH (U/L)	344 ± 175	208 ± 175	<0.05
As. glucose (mmole/L)	4.9 ± 1.1	5.8 ± 1.9	NS

Values are expressed as arithmetic means ± standard deviation.
Hemoglobin <140 g/L in women.
Serum LDH level (normal range) = 80–250 U/L.
Group I = tuberculous peritonitis without chronic liver disease, Group II = tuberculous peritonitis with chronic liver disease.
WBC = peripheral white cell count, ALP = alkaline phosphatase, ALT = alanine aminotransferase, SAAG = serum-ascites albumin gradient, LDH = lactate dehydrogenase, As. = ascites, NS = no significant difference.
Modified from Ref. 63.

especially susceptible to the development of SBP (46). Obviously they can therefore help differentiate SBP, which is almost always an acute infection with a low albumin concentration, from TBP, which is a chronic disorder with an increased protein concentration (>2.5 g per dl) (9,14,15,23). These measurements may also help identify nephrotic ascites, which characteristically shows hypoalbuminemia and hypogammaglobulinemia (47). Nevertheless, these are secondary or even tertiary methods of diagnosis that do not differentiate TBP from neoplastic ascitic fluid, which is a difficult differential diagnosis.

In this same secondary diagnostic category is the classification of the types of the leukocytes, which are elevated in both SBP and TBP to 250–4000 per cubic millimeter. There is, of course, a clear preponderance of polymorphonuclear leukocytes in SBP (37) compared to TBP, in which mononuclear leukocytes are the predominant cells (9,14,15,23).

Various enzyme levels in ascitic fluid have been proposed as useful measurements in assessing patients for TBP. Among them are lactic dehydrogenase (LDH) and adenosine deaminase activity (ADA) (48). ADA is an enzyme found in leukocytes, erythrocytes, and the cerebral cortex. In body fluids its activity parallels the lymphocyte count in ascitic fluid (49) and is useful in the differential diagnosis of tuberculous pleural effusions and of TBP (50,51). Because reticuloendothelial function is decreased in cirrhosis by virtue of portosystemic shunting, and lymphocyte concentrations may be decreased in patients with AIDS, ADA may show reduced activity in cirrhotic patients and in patients with AIDS. ADA may also be increased in patients with abdominal neoplasms, which renders it less valuable in the differential diagnosis of TBP and peritoneal cancer. Perversely, low ADA activity may thus suggest peritoneal carcinoma. Overall ADA activity is considered to be an insensitive index of TBP (52).

Ascitic fluid cholesterol levels tend to be elevated in patients with malignant disease, and can be used as a reliable differential diagnostic criterion between tuberculous and neoplastic peritoneal involvement (53).

In a recent case report of a clinicopathological conference in the *New England Journal of Medicine* (NEJM) (338:248–254, 1998), the current diagnosis of TBP was reviewed (54). In the patient under discussion the diagnosis was established by the presence of granulomatous inflammation and a positive acid-fast stain of morphologically characteristic bacteria in a Peyer's patch. Although adenosine deaminase in ascitic fluid has been recommended as the method of choice for making this diagnosis, definitive proof of its precision was not presented.

In the case under discussion the diagnosis was made by screening the tissue for fluorescence with auromine O fluorochrome, preferential stained bacteria that were morphologically consistent with *M. tuberculosis*. The bacteria, which had been cultured in selective, liquid isolation media, had the characteristic serpentine beading of *M. tuberculosis* (54). The diagnosis was confirmed by the use of chemiluminescent DNA probes.

IV.   IMAGING IN THE DIAGNOSIS OF TBP

Various imaging procedures have been suggested to be of value in differentiating TBP from other disorders. They include ultrasonography (55), computerized tomography (56–58), and magnetic resonance imaging (59). Unfortunately, although they may be diagnostically valid in groups of patients, they are nonspecific and nondiagnostic in individual patients. They are as useful, however, as real-time ultrasonography, which by its echogenicity is able to differentiate transudates from exudates (60). It may, however, be an overly sophisticated, overly expensive way of doing so.

V.   ASSOCIATION OF TBP WITH OTHER DISEASES

One specific situation in which patients seem to be particularly vulnerable to TBP is the case of patients under therapy with chronic ambulatory peritoneal dialysis for renal disease (61). The reasons for this are not known, but there are many pertinent contributing factors. First, of course, is that patients on dialysis have chronic renal failure, which per se is accompanied by a type of immunoincompetence (62). This abnormality renders the patients susceptible to a variety of infections. Second, the peritoneal fluid of patients with CAPD, which is a diluted, synthetic peritoneal fluid, is a weak imitation of cirrhotic ascitic fluid that is deficient in many of the antibacterial defenses present in "normal" ascitic fluid, including a reduced number of fixed and motile phagocytic leukocytes, and almost certainly a deficiency of both specific and nonspecific oncogenic substances and a decreased protein concentration. These factors are characterized by a relative low concentration of proteins in the ascitic fluid that exhibit decreased opsonization and are associated with high SAAG levels.

In patients undergoing CAPD, chyloperitoneum may suggest lymphatic obstruction and peritoneal fibrosis, which may be a clue to the diagnosis of TBP (7,10).

Shakil et al. have emphasized that patients with TBP and cirrhosis, who usually exhibit a high serum-ascites albumin gradient (SAAG), are especially susceptible to tuberculous peritonitis and other bacterial infections including SBP (63).

VI. TREATMENT OF TUBERCULOUS PERITONITIS

The treatment of TBP can be effectively carried out with the first-line antituberculous drugs: streptomycin, rifampicin, isoniazid, and pyrazinamide. Occasionally, ethambutol, ethionamide, cycloserine, and ciprofloxacin, which are considered second-line antituberculous agents, may sometimes be beneficial in various combinations with first-line agents. When the organisms are resistant to all drugs, desperate therapeutic measures are indicated.

VII. IMMUNOTHERAPY OF TUBERCULOSIS

There have been reports of the addition of *Mycobacterium vaccae* immunotherapy in pulmonary tuberculosis with both drug-sensitive and drug-resistant organisms. Prior et al. administered immunotherapy with *Mycobacterium vaccae* to second-line antituberculous drugs and observed a dramatic cure in a patient with drug-resistant abdominal tuberculosis (64).

At present the treatment of tuberculosis in this new type of tuberculin immunotherapy, particularly of multiple drug-resistant tuberculosis, requires the administration of first- and second-line antituberculous agents or combinations thereof. Because only about one-half of patients with resistance to both rifampicin and isoniazid respond to second-line drugs (65), immunotherapy has been employed. This type of antituberculous immunotherapy differs from the classical immunotherapy of Koch (66), which was designed to promote tissue destruction (67) by the injection of old tuberculin. The new therapy consists of injection of killed *M. vaccae* (68) in association with second-line chemotherapy, which is designed to reinstate antibacterial immunity and to suppress immune mechanisms of tissue destruction (69) and the tuberculosis. This adjunct of chemotherapy, which is not associated with an exacerbation of fever or of prostration, and which appears to be associated with rapid clinical improvement (70), deserves careful controlled evaluation. Clearly, the combination of immunotherapy with drug therapy deserves a trial when other therapies have failed.

VIII. CONCLUSION

Tuberculous peritonitis is a protean disease in terms of its clinical and laboratory manifestations and to some extent in its pathogenesis. The methods of
diagnosis are varied, uncertain, and often slow. Treatment is complex and the
large number of antibiotic agents in use testifies to the lack of an ideal remedy.
The successful management of tuberculous peritonitis requires broad knowledge and the administration of new, imaginative types of treatment.

REFERENCES

1. Burack WR, Hollister RM. Tuberculous peritonitis. A study of forty-seven
    proved cases encountered by a general medical unit in twenty-five years. Am J
    Med 28:510–523, 1960.
2. Hyman S, Villa F, Alvarez S, Steigmann F. The enigma of tuberculous peritoni-
    tis. Gastroenterology 42:1–6, 1962.
3. Gonnella JS, Hudson EK. Clinical patterns of tuberculous peritonitis. Arch Intern
    Med 117:364–366, 1966.
4. Singh MM, Bhargava AN, Jain KP. Tuberculous peritonitis. An evaluation of
    pathogenetic mechanisms, diagnostic procedures and therapeutic measures. N
    Engl J Med 281:1091–1094, 1969.
5. Sochocky S. Tuberculous peritonitis. A review of 100 cases. Am Rev Resp Dis
    95:398–401, 1967.
6. Levine H. Needle biopsy diagnosis of tuberculous peritonitis. Am Rev Resp Dis
    97:889–894, 1968.
7. Das P, Shukla HS. Clinical diagnosis of abdominal tuberculosis. Br J Surg 63:
    941–946, 1976.
8. Dineen P, Homan WP, Grafe WR. Tuberculous peritonitis: 43 years' experience
    in diagnosis and treatment. Ann Surg 184:717–723, 1976.
9. Karney WW, O'Donoghue JM, Ostrow JH, Holmes KK, Beaty HM. The spec-
    trum of tuberculous peritonitis. Chest 72:310–315, 1977.
10. Sherman S, Rohwedder JJ, Ravikrishnan KP. Tuberculous enteritis and peritoni-
    tis: Report of 36 general hospital cases. Arch Intern Med 140:506–508, 1980.
11. Geake TMS, Spitaels JM, Moshal MG, Simjee AE. Peritoneoscopy in the diagno-
    sis of tuberculous peritonitis. Gastrointest Endoscopy 27:66–68, 1981.
12. Gilinsky NH, Marks IN, Kottler RE. Abdominal tuberculosis: A 10-year review.
    S Afr Med J 64:849–857, 1983.
13. Jorge AD. Peritoneal tuberculosis. Endoscopy 16:10–12, 1984.
14. Bastani B, Shariatzadeh R, Dehdashti F. Tuberculous peritonitis—Report of 30
    cases and review of the literature. Quart J Med 56:549–557, 1985.

15. Klimach OE, Ormerod LP. Gastrointestinal tuberculosis: A retrospective review of 109 cases in a district general hospital. Quart J Med 56:569–578, 1985.

16. Palmer KR, Patil DH, Basran GS, Riordan JF, Silk DBA. Abdominal tuberculosis in urban Britain: a common disease. Gut 26:1296–1305, 1985.

17. Menzies RI, Alsen H, Fitzgerald JM, Mohapeloa RG. Tuberculous peritonitis in Lesotho. Tubercle 67:47–54, 1986.

18. Jakubowski A, Elwood RK, Enarson DA. Clinical features of abdominal tuberculosis. J Infect Dis 158:687–692, 1988.

19. Aguado JM, Pons J, Casafont F, Miguel GS, Valle R. Tuberculous peritonitis: a study comparing cirrhotic and noncirrhotic patients. J Clin Gastroenterol 12: 550–554, 1990.

20. Bhargava DK, Shriniwas D, Chopra P, Nijhawan S, Dasarathy S, Kushuwaha AKS. Peritoneal tuberculosis: Laparoscopic patterns and its diagnostic accuracy. Am J Gastroenterol 87:109–112, 1992.

21. Manohar A, Simjee AM, Haffejee AA, Pettengell KE. Symptoms and investigative findings in 145 patients with tuberculous peritonitis diagnosed by peritoneoscopy and biopsy over a five year period. Gut 31:1130–1132, 1990.

22. Lisahora GB, Peters CC, Lee M. Barcia PJ. Tuberculous peritonitis: do not miss it. Dis Colon Rect 39:394–399, 1996.

23. Shakil AO, Korula J, Kanel GC, Murray NGB, Reynolds TB. Diagnostic features of tuberculous peritonitis in the absence and presence of chronic liver disease: a case control study. Am J Med 100:179–185, 1996.

24. Conn HO. Interpretation of data from multiple trials: a critical review. J Intern Med 241:177–183, 1997.

25. Marshall JB. Tuberculosis of the gastrointestinal tract and peritoneum. Clinical reviews. Am J Gastroenterol 88:989–999, 1993.

26. Snider DE Jr, Roper WL. The new tuberculosis. N Engl J Med 326:703–705, 1992.

27. Schamberg A. Intra-abdominal tuberculosis in acquired immunodeficiency syndrome. Diagnosis and management. Int Surg 30:147–151, 1995.

28. Rieder HI, Cauthen GM, Bloch AB. Tuberculosis and acquired immunodeficiency syndrome. Arch Surg 149:1268–1273, 1989.

29. Pitchenik AB, Ertel D. Tuberculosis and nontuberculous mycobacterial disease. Med Clin North Am 76:121–171, 1992.

30. Fischl MA, Daikos GL, Uttamchandani RB, et al. Clinical presentation and outcome of patients with HIV infection and tuberculosis caused by multiple-drug-resistant bacilli. Ann Intern Med 112:184–190, 1992.

31. Kenyon TA, Valway SE, Ihle WW, Onorato IM, Castro KG. Transmission of multidrug-resistant *Mycobacterium tuberculosis* during a long airplane flight. N Engl J Med 334:933–938, 1996.

32. Wedel RP. Airline travel and infection. N Engl J Med 334:981–982, 1996.

33. Cheng IKP, Chan PCK, Chan MK. Tuberculous peritonitis complicating long-term peritoneal dialysis: report of 5 cases and review of the literature. Am J Nephrol 9:155–161, 1989.

34. Snyder N, Bessoff J, Dwyer JM, Conn HO. Depressed delayed cutaneous hypersensitivity in alcoholic hepatitis. Dig Dis 23:353–358, 1978.
35. Hoefs JC. Serum protein concentration and portal pressure determine the ascitic fluid protein concentration in patients with chronic liver disease. J Lab Clin Med 102:260–273, 1983.
36. Runyon BA, Montano AA, Akriviadis EA. The serum ascites albumin gradient is superior to the exudate-transudate concept in the differential diagnosis of ascites. Ann Intern Med 117:215–220, 1992.
37. Conn HO. Spontaneous peritonitis and bacteremia in cirrhotic patients caused by enteric bacteria. Ann Intern Med 60:568–580, 1964.
38. Wolfe JHN, Behn AR, Jackson BT. Tuberculous peritonitis and role of diagnostic laparoscopy. Lancet 1:852–853, 1979.
39. Klatskin G, Conn HO. Histopathology of the Liver. New York: Oxford University Press, 1993 (Vol. I, Text, Vol. II, Photomicrographs).
40. Sing V, Jain AK, Agrawal AD, Gupta S, Khanna S, Khanna AK, Gupta JP. Clinicopathological profile of abdominal tuberculosis. Brit J Clin Pract 49:22–24, 1995.
41. Runyon BA, Umland ET, Mertlin T. Inoculation of blood culture bottles with ascitic fluid: improved detection of spontaneous bacterial peritonitis. Arch Intern Med 147:73–75, 1987.
42. Baig MM, Pettengell KE, Simjee AE, Sathar MA, Vorster BJ. Diagnosis of tuberculosis by detection of mycobacterial antigen in pleural effusions and ascites. S Afr Med J 69:101–102, 1986.
43. Lenoir P, Gilbert L, Vandenplas Y, Alexander M. Tuberculous peritonitis in an adolescent male. Europ J Gastroenterol Hepatol 7:477–480, 1995.
44. Thakur A, Mandal A. Usefulness of ELISA using antigen A60 in serodiagnosis of neurotuberculosis. J Communicable Dis 28:8–14, 1996.
45. Kadival GV, Kameswaran M, Ashtekad MK, Samuel AM. Immunodiagnosis of tuberculosis using polyclonal and monoclonal antibodies. Trop Med Parasitol 41:363–365, 1990.
46. Runyon BA. Low protein concentration of ascitic fluid is predisposed to spontaneous bacterial peritonitis. Gastroenterology 91:1343–1346, 1986.
47. Kark RM, Piarni CL, Pollak VE, Muehrcke RC, Blainey JD. The nephrotic syndrome in adults: a common disorder with many causes. Ann Intern Med 49:751–760, 1958.
48. Segura RM, Pascual C, Oceana I, Martinez-Vazquez JM, Ribera E, Ruiz I, Pelegri MD. Adenosine deaminase in body fluids: a useful diagnostic tool in tuberculosis. Clin Biochem 22:141–148, 1989.
49. Baganha MF, Pego A, Lima MA, Gaspar EV, Pharm B, Cordeiro AR. Serum and pleural adenosine deaminase correlation with lymphocytic populations. Chest 97:605–610, 1990.
50. Voigt MD, Troy C, Lombard C, Kalvaria I, Berman P, Dirsch RE. Diagnostic value of ascites adenosine deaminase in tuberculous peritonitis. Lancet 1:751–754, 1989.

51. Banales JL, Pineda PR, Fitzgerald JM, Rubio H, Selman M, Salazar-Lezama M. Adenosine deaminase in the diagnosis of tuberculous pleural effusions. A report of 218 patients and review of the literature. Chest 99:355–357, 1991.

52. Hillebrand KJ, Runyon BA, Yasmineh WG, Rynders GP. Ascitic fluid adenosine deaminase insensitivity in detecting tuberculous peritonitis in the United States. Hepatology 24:1408–1412, 1996.

53. Sood A, Garg R, Kumar R, Chhina RS, Arora S, Gupta R, Bhatia KL. Ascitic fluid cholesterol in malignant and tubercular ascites. J Assoc Phys India 43:743–747, 1995.

54. Scully RE. Case 3-1998. Case records of the Massachusetts General Hospital. N Engl J Med 338, 248–254, 1998.

55. Kedar RP, Shah PP, Shivde RS, Malde HM. Sonographic findings in gastrointestinal and peritoneal tuberculosis. Clin Radiol 49:24–29, 1994.

56. Ha HK, Jung JI, Lee MS, Choi BG, Lee MG, Kim YH, Kim PN, Auh YH. CT differentiation of tuberculous peritonitis and peritoneal carcinomatosis. AJR 167: 743–748, 1996.

57. Rodriguez E, Pombo F. Peritoneal tuberculosis versus peritoneal carcinomatosis: distinction based on CT findings. Comput Assist Tomography 20:269–272, 1996.

58. Demirkazik FB, Akhan O, Ozmen MN, Akata D. US and CT findings in the diagnosis of tuberculous peritonitis. Acta Radiol 37:517–520, 1996.

59. Murata Y, Yamada I, Sumiya Y, Shichijo Y. Magnetic resonance imaging findings in three patients suffering from abdominal tuberculosis. Rofo 165:192–194, 1996.

60. Malde HM, Gandhi RD. Exudative vs transudative ascites: differentiation based on fluid echogenicity on high resolution sonography. J Postgrad Med 39:132–136, 1993.

61. Huang CH, Chen HS, Chen YM, Tsai TJ. Fibroadhesive form of tuberculous peritonitis: chyloperitoneum in a patient undergoing automated peritoneal dialysis. Nephron 72:708–711, 1996.

62. Golper T, Bennett. W, Jones S. Peritonitis associated with chronic peritoneal dialysis: a diagnostic and therapeutic approach. Dial Transplant 7:1173–1178, 1978.

63. Shakil AO, Korula J, Kanel GC, Murray NGB, Reynolds TB. Diagnostic features of tuberculous peritonitis in the absence and presence of chronic liver disease: a case control study. Am J Med 100:179–185, 1996.

64. Prior JG, Khan AA, Cartwright KA, Jenkins PA, Stanford JL. Immunotherapy with *Mycobacterium vaccae* combined with second line chemotherapy in drug-resistant abdominal tuberculosis. J Infect 31:59–61, 1995.

65. Bogle M, Iseman MD, Madsen LA. Treatment of 191 patients with pulmonary tuberculosis resistant to isoniazid and rifampicin. N Engl J Med 328:527–532, 1993.

66. Koch R. Further communications on a remedy for tuberculosis. Lancet 2:1085–1086, 1890.

67. Eve FS. Impression of the results of Dr. Koch's treatment of tuberculosis. Lancet 2:1149–1151, 1890.
68. Stanford JL, Stanford CA, Rook GAW. Immunotherapy for tuberculosis: investigative and practical aspects. Clin Immunother 1:430–440, 1994.
69. Stanford JL, Rook GAW, Bahr GMP. *Mycobacterium vaccae* in immunoprophylaxis and immunotherapy of leprosy and tuberculosis. Vaccine 8:525–530, 1990.
70. Eternadi A, Parid R, Stanford JL. Immunotherapy for drug resistant tuberculosis. Lancet 340:1360–1361, 1992.

6

Clinical Pathogenesis of Spontaneous Bacterial Peritonitis

Harold O. Conn
Yale University School of Medicine, New Haven, Connecticut, and University of Miami School of Medicine, Miami, Florida

The clinical pathogenesis of SBP was first suggested in two clinical reports about patients with SBP (1,2). The first of these citations is the summary of our first article on SBP written in 1964 (1), when SBP was a rarely recognized clinical entity:

> Patients with decompensated cirrhosis occasionally develop spontaneous peritonitis and bacteremia caused by enteric bacteria. This syndrome is characterized by the abrupt onset of fever, chills, abdominal pain and tenderness, hypoactive bowel sounds, hypotension, and hepatic coma. The diagnosis can be made by the demonstration of turbid ascitic fluid containing increased numbers of polymorphonuclear leukocytes and bacteria and confirmed by the isolation of the enteric organisms from the blood and ascitic fluid.
>
> Five instances of this syndrome are described, and the factors that render cirrhotic patients susceptible to it discussed. This complication, which has rarely been recognized before, is probably not uncommon in decompensated cirrhotics. Since this potentially lethal infection responds rapidly to antibiotic therapy, it is important that it be recognized and treated promptly.

It was apparent at the time this article was written that it was not expected that these few cases would grow so rapidly into the endemic at our hospital and later into the epidemic of SBP that has spread around the world. In this article the salient features of the syndrome were presented and its probable pathogenesis was inferred and implied.

This initial experience was followed by the appearance at our hospital of an additional 25 patients between 1964 and 1971, and which we referred to as "variations on a theme" (2). From this series of patients we were able to flesh out this syndrome and its probable pathogenesis. This was no great feat of clinical wisdom. As each new variation appeared it suggested what form the disorder was taking and what to expect next.

This second article on SBP was based on 32 episodes in 28 patients observed at our hospital and on 46 episodes of what we christened *spontaneous bacterial peritonitis* in 42 additional patients that had appeared in the medical literature between 1893 and 1968 (2). From these 74 patients we synthesized the clinical syndrome, which was unknown prior to publication of our two articles; proposed its widely accepted name (SBP); described its two most common variants, *asymptomatic bacterascites* and *culture-negative SBP*; and proposed its pathogenesis with surprisingly precise insight. The flood of patients with SBP at the West Haven Veterans Administration Medical Center (WHVAMC) continued until we had accumulated a series of 91 bacteriologically proved cases (1–4) plus nine of culture-negative SBP, which we considered to be "probable SBP" (see Table 5.1) and a half-dozen cases of asymptomatic bacterascites (see Table 5.2). We worried that we did not understand precisely how the bacteria passed from the intestinal lumen into the lymphatic and vascular systems, but recognized that *bacterial translocation*, which was first described in 1966 (28), obviously played an important role in its occurrence. We are now very aware that the process of bacterial translocation is a most complex one, and that its many disparate features play the key role in its occurrence and pathogenesis. I predict it will be some years before all of the intricacies of this fascinating phenomenon are understood.

If these articles were to be rewritten today—35 and 40 years later, respectively—they would state that although all of these symptoms and signs are usually seen in SBP, they are not all required to make the diagnosis. Specifically, symptoms such as abdominal pain, chills, and hepatic encephalopathy (HE) and signs such as abdominal tenderness, hypoactive bowel sounds, and hypotension are not all prerequisites for a diagnosis of SBP. In fact, although abdominal pain and fever are present in the large majority (>75%) of such patients, HE may be absent in one-third. Only 10% are free of all signs and only 2% or 3% are truly silent. Similarly, today turbidity of the ascitic fluid is seen in less than half the patients, probably due to a lower threshold of suspicion and to earlier diagnosis. Ascitic leukocytosis, i.e., >250 polymorphonuclear leukocytes per cubic millimeter, and a positive culture remain the primary early and definitive criteria for the diagnosis of SBP.

The second of these articles (2), published in 1971, is based on a series of questions and answers, which we present here verbatim (each followed by comments written in 1999).

I. WHAT ARE THE POSSIBLE ROUTES BY WHICH BACTERIA MAY ENTER THE PERITONEUM?

Organisms can come directly from the *gastrointestinal tract*, from the *blood stream*, from the *lymphatics* or, in females, from the *genital tract*.

The rarest route is through the Fallopian tubes. . . . This route of entry has been implicated by McCartney to explain the predominance of girls with primary peritonitis (5). Obviously, this mechanism played no role in any of our patients, all of whom were male. It is conceivable that this route could have been responsible for some of the women previously reported in the literature.

The most common causes of bacterial peritonitis were perforations of ulcers of the upper gastrointestinal tract or the rupture of abdominal viscera, usually the appendix. Although perforations of the gastrointestinal tract may be silent clinically, they are rarely so, and even when silent they usually exhibit pneumoperitoneum. Despite the greater prevalence of peptic ulcer in cirrhotic patients than in non-cirrhotic patients, in none of the patients reviewed or reported here was there clinical or postmortem evidence of such perforations, and in none of those studied was free air found in the peritoneum radiologically.

Under certain conditions bacteria may enter the peritoneal cavity by traversing the intact intestinal wall. Schweinburg et al demonstrated that in dogs ^{14}C-labeled *E. coli* passed from the bowel into the peritoneal cavity after the introduction of hypertonic solutions into the peritoneum (6). A similar mechanism may explain the enteric bacterial peritonitis which frequently complicates patients undergoing peritoneal dialysis.

In Chapters 7 and 8 of this book, methods by which bacterial translocation (BT) may be induced are discussed. The variety of techniques by which BT can be caused are legion, ranging from the overgrowth of a single species of indigenous bacteria in the intestinal tract, immunosuppression, and thermal injury in which large segments of skin are burned, to hemorrhagic, hypotensive shock, i.e., insufficient blood supply to the gastrointestinal (GI) tract. In addition, specific disorders of the GI tract, such as intestinal or biliary obstruction or portal hypertension, may all give rise to BT. Clearly, bacteria may leave the intestinal lumen by passing between the tight junctions of mucosal cells or via transcellular passage directly *through* intact mucosal cells. BT of different degrees of severity may result in different degrees of bacterial escape to the mesenteric lymph nodes, to portal venous blood, to liver tissue and to the systemic blood. The entry of bacteria, predominantly *Staphylococcus aureus*, *Staphylococcus enteritidis*, and *Pseudomonas aeruginosa*, into the peritoneal cavity during chronic, peritoneal dialysis suggest exogenous contamination rather than transintestinal passage.

> . . . Several abnormalities peculiar to decompensated cirrhosis may decrease local resistance of the intestinal mucosa to bacterial invasion. First, in patients with decompensated portal hypertension, the splanchnic veins and lymphatics are congested. Fluid retention associated with portal hypertension is not limited to the presence of ascites, but may cause edema of all splanchnic tissues, thus affecting adversely the mucosal barrier to bacterial invasion. Consequently, the bowel wall is edematous and often inflamed, and the intestinal mucosa is frequently severely degenerated. Second, diarrhea is frequently present in cirrhosis. Although there is no characteristic intestinal lesion associated with cirrhotic diarrhea, underlying mucosal inflammation or secondary irritation may increase the permeability of the mucosal barrier. Finally, qualitative and quantitative abnormalities in the distribution of intestinal bacteria have been demonstrated in cirrhosis.
>
> The lymphatic system may play an important role in the pathogenesis of spontaneous peritonitis, and several different areas of the lymphatic system may be involved. The engorged intestinal lymphatic system is the prime suspect. . . .
>
> When bacteria penetrate the intestinal mucosa into the submucosal tissues, the intestinal lymphatics carry them to the major lymphatic channels and eventually via the thoracic duct into the systemic circulation. In the ascitic cirrhotic patient both the hepatic and splanchnic lymphatics are distended and hypertrophied and thoracic duct lymph flow, which is derived almost entirely from the hepatic and splanchnic beds, is greatly increased.
>
> It is possible that the hepatic lymphatics themselves may be involved in the pathogenesis of this syndrome. Hepatic lymph is the key to the formation of ascites. In cirrhotic patients with hepatic venous outflow obstruction or in experimental animals with hepatic venous or superior vena caval obstruction, the production of hepatic lymph is increased resulting in the formation of ascites, due largely to the exudation of hepatic lymph directly into the peritoneal cavity. In ascitic patients with bacter-

emia, organisms removed from circulation by the liver may contaminate hepatic lymph and pass through the permeable lymphatic walls into the ascitic fluid. Although there is no experimental evidence to document the passage of bacteria from hepatic blood or reticuloendothelial cells to the lymphatics, the appearance of *E. coli* in the bile of intact guinea pigs and of isolated perfused rat livers after the introduction of *E. coli* into the systemic blood and into the perfusate, suggests that other, even more complex bacterial traverses may take place.

For several reasons the hematogenous route appears to be the most reasonable mechanism to explain the spontaneous bacterial contamination of ascites. First, spontaneous bacteremia is not an uncommon event. Bacteremia occurs after the relatively mild trauma of teeth-brushing or paraffin-chewing in patients with minimal gingival disease or following massage of infected foci such as furuncles, or nonoperative instrumentation of the genitourinary tract. Asymptomatic bacteremias have been found in association with normal menstrual periods and even in apparently healthy subjects (7).

It is possible that portal bacteremias also occur spontaneously, but that the effective hepatic bacterial filter removes the organisms before they reach the systemic circulation. Manipulative examinations of the intestinal tract, either radiologic or endoscopic, or therapeutic enemas in P.S.E. [portosystemic encephalopathy] may precipitate the entry of bacteria into the bloodstream in a manner analogous to teeth brushing. Normally the portal venous blood in man is sterile, but enteric bacteria can often be cultured from the portal blood and liver of dogs. In almost half the patients with ulcerative colitis, however, enteric bacteria can be recovered from the portal venous blood (8). It may be assumed that portal bacteremia also occurs frequently with other disorders in which the intestinal mucosa is eroded. Because of altered bacterial patterns and impaired mucosal barriers, cirrhotic patients may be especially susceptible to spontaneous portal bacteremias.

Second, bacteremia provides a logical common pathway for the great variety of bacteria encountered in patients with spontaneous peritonitis. Other routes of infection, such as unrecognized perforation of the intestinal or biliary tract, direct extension through the diaphragm or passage through the Fallopian tubes, however, must certainly occur. The majority of cases of spontaneous peritonitis can only be explained satisfactorily by the common denominator of a bacteremia. For example, the occurrence of pneumococcal peritonitis in a patient with pneumococcal pneumonia, of streptococcal peritonitis in a patient with erysipelas, or of *E. coli* peritonitis in a patient with a urinary tract infection caused by the same organism all have in common the bacteremia which delivers the organism to the ascitic fluid. One might thus expect to see spontaneous peritonitis caused by any organism which might circulate in the blood of a susceptible patient. In principle this concept is similar to the presumed pathogenesis of subacute bacterial endocarditis except that rheumatic valves are more frequently exposed to streptococci and ascites more commonly to coliform organisms.

II. WHAT ARE THE FACTORS THAT RENDER CIRRHOTIC PATIENTS PARTICULARLY PRONE TO DEVELOP SPONTANEOUS PERITONITIS?

First, is the failure of hepatic removal of bacteria from the blood stream. Many investigators have demonstrated that major vascular abnormalities develop in the hepatic circulation of cirrhotic patients with portal hypertension. McIndoe described the *extrahepatic portal-systemic collateral networks* that shunt portal venous blood around the liver (9). He estimated that more than 80 percent of portal blood may bypass the liver in advanced cirrhosis, and more recent investigations have confirmed this estimate. Other authors have demonstrated that intrahepatic anastomoses between hepatic arteries and portal veins and between portal and hepatic veins exist. Such portal-systemic shunts have been shown to diminish greatly the *hepatic clearance of ammonia* and other substances absorbed from the gastrointestinal tract. In our series of patients the presence of *portal-systemic shunting* was confirmed by abnormal *ammonia tolerance tests*, which closely reflect the degree of portal hypertension, in all patients in whom this test was performed (10). Such shunts are probably also responsible for the decreased extraction of particulate matter by the liver of cirrhotic patients. Presumably, these portal-systemic anastomoses permit circulating bacteria to bypass the hepatic reticuloendothelial filtering system, which has been shown to be the major site of removal of bacteria from the blood. Studies in animals have confirmed the hypothesis that the clearance, of blood-borne bacteria by the hepatic reticuloendothelial system may be diminished in cirrhosis. Decreased hepatic removal of circulating bacteria tends to perpetuate bacteremia and thus afford circulating organisms a greater opportunity to cause metastatic infections at susceptible sites such as ascitic collections. Certainly, primary bacteremia, usually due to coliform organisms, which is a common complication in cirrhosis (11), demonstrates this propensity to bacteremia.

If this concept were correct one would expect that a disease such as subacute bacterial endocarditis (SBE) might be more common in cirrhotic patients than in non-cirrhotic subjects. Indeed, it is our impression that SBE does occur more commonly in cirrhosis, but data to prove this association are probable, but not conclusive (12).

Second, the very abnormalities which cause portal hypertension and induce the development of portal collateral circulation are also responsible for the accumulation of ascites. Although bacterial peritonitis may occur in patients without ascites, it is very rare if it occurs at all.

The relative importance of ascites and of the circumhepatic shunting of blood may be estimated by considering patients with portacaval anastomosis (PCA). One might expect spontaneous peritonitis to be especially common in patients with end-to-side PCA in whom portal-systemic shunting is total. On the other hand, patients with PCA are usually free of ascites because the shunt decreases the portal pressure. Which of these factors prevails? Three of the 28 patients (11%) in our series had end-to-side PCA, a figure slightly but insignificantly smaller than the 16% frequency of PCA in cirrhotic patients at this hospital. All three had massive ascites, itself an uncommon phenomenon in patients with shunts. We have not observed spontaneous peritonitis in any of our patients with PCA in the absence of ascites. Ascites would, therefore, appear to be a more important prerequisite for the development of spontaneous peritonitis than portal-systemic shunting.

HE has been associated with portosystemic shunting of all types—PCA, mesocaval shunts, splenorenal shunts, spontaneous renocaval anastomoses (13), and transjugular intrahepatic portosystemic shunts (TIPS) (14a). The recent report by Rössle et al. (14b) of portosystemic encephalomyelopathy and myelopathy, a syndrome closely related to HE, emphasizes the significance of portosystemic shunting in such disorders.

III. WHAT FACTORS PREDISPOSE TO THE INITIAL BACTEREMIA THAT PRECIPITATES PERITONITIS IN ASCITIC CIRRHOTIC PATIENTS?

There are several factors, which by their great frequency in our series, must be considered to be potential predisposing causes. The role of diarrhea in the production of spontaneous peritonitis, for example, is not clear. Diarrhea, which occurs commonly in cirrhosis (2), may only be coincidentally associated with the peritonitis. It is possible that some of the various causes of diarrhea may be injurious to the mucosa and may permit the escape of intestinal bacteria from the lumen. Diarrhea itself may in some way alter host-bacterial relationships. Diarrhea of diverse etiologies may cause alteration in both the types of bacteria and in the physical distribution of flora in the intestinal tract. Even in acute, experimentally-induced diarrhea in normal subjects coliform organisms may appear as high as the small intestine, where they are not usually present, and may be replaced by enterobacteria as the dominant organisms of the stools (15). Such alterations alone or in combination with the abnormal distribution of intestinal bacteria in cirrhosis could result in the replacement of non-virulent bacteria by invasive organisms.

Neomycin, too, appears guilty by association. Neomycin, by altering the ecologic balance in some undefined way or by injuring the mucosal membrane may change the microbic permeability of the intestinal wall (16). This possibility may be associated with the malabsorptive syndrome and morphologic alterations of the jejunal mucosa induced by neomycin. Other factors such as the almost ubiquitous alkalosis, potassium deficit (17) and the arterial oxygen desaturation of decompensated cirrhosis may subtly alter the delicate balance between the host and its parasites. The installation of alkaline solutions into the duodenum of dogs, for example, may cause the appearance of enteric organisms in the thoracic duct.

Any of these situations may induce BT.

IV. WHAT ARE THE METHODS BY WHICH DEFECTS IN BACTERIAL CLEARANCE CAN BE DETECTED?

The unique occurrence of at least six species of enteric bacteria in the ascites of one of our patients, who was receiving intra-arterial vasopressin therapy for gastrointestinal hemorrhage, suggests the possibility of other pathogenetic features (18). The multiplicity of organisms had immediately suggested gastrointestinal perforation, but exploratory laparotomy and careful postmortem dissection failed to reveal any evidence of such a perforation. This patient, who had received vasopressin directly into the gastroduodenal artery for over 24 hours was shown angiographically to have more than a 50% reduction in the diameter of the artery and, therefore, a disproportionately large decrease in blood flow through that artery. It is tempting to speculate that prolonged arterial constriction or its metabolic consequences, may have permitted the escape of bacteria from the lumen of the intestine. Several investigators in experiments which simulate this situation, have shown that ligation of the superior mesenteric artery results in the escape of bacteria from the upper intestinal tract with the induction of systemic bacteremia. In addition, it has been shown that the local injection of epinephrine, presumably by its vasoconstrictive effect, enhances local bacterial invasion. These authors speculated that local tissue hypoxia, hypercapnia, acidosis or, perhaps, a decrease in exudation of fluids or in diapedesis of leukocytes from the blood were responsible for the increased susceptibility to infection.

The recovery of multiple organisms in this patient is different from the pattern observed in the rest of the patients. Furthermore, this represents the first case of spontaneous peritonitis in which *Bacterioides* and multiple other anaerobic organisms were recovered. The multiplicity of species and their anaerobic nature suggest that transmural migration of bacteria was the probable route of infection of ascitic fluid in this patient, in contrast to the presumed hematogenously-borne peritonitis of the majority of these patients.

This bizarre variation of SBP implies a whole new type of pathogenesis for SBP. Clearly, this multibacterial form of SBP differs completely from the traditional, monomicrobial variety, and opens the way for an alternative pathogenesis of SBP. It also raises questions about why anaerobic bacteria don't cause many more episodes of SBP.

Ulcerative gastrointestinal disorders such as ulcerative colitis and regional ileitis permit the escape of bacteria from the gastrointestinal tract through the ulcerations. Indeed, these diseases are obvious causes of BT and are presumptive causes of SBP (19).

Again, it seems logical that arterial vasoconstriction and mucosal ulceration (19) may give rise to BT and SBP (20) (Chap. 7).

V. IS THERE ANY EXPLANATION FOR THE DISTRIBUTION OF THE SPECIES OF BACTERIA RECOVERED FROM THE PATIENTS WITH SPONTANEOUS PERITONITIS?

Virulence of intestinal bacteria has been defined as the ability to invade the epithelial cell. Whether or not virulence is inherent in the bacteria themselves, or is affected by resistance of the epithelial cells or both is not clear. *E. coli* have been the organisms most commonly responsible. These organisms have exhibited normal cultural characteristics and the expected antibiotic sensitivity spectra. . . .

Certainly some subtypes of *E. coli* and other normal components of the indigent intestinal bacterial flora exhibit a higher order of virulence and are responsible for outbreaks of severe, occasionally lethal food poisoning.

A variety of other aerobic, enteric organisms have been found in other patients. It is remarkable that anaerobic organisms do not play a greater role in spontaneous peritonitis. They are frequently found in secondary peritonitis due, for example, to a ruptured appendix or diverticulum. Obligatory anaerobic bacteria, which make up the large bulk of the intestinal flora, and particularly *Bacteroides*, which is the most common species in the feces of both normal and cirrhotic subjects, have been recovered in only one patient with spontaneous peritonitis, for whom a special pathogenesis has been postulated above. Whether anaerobic organisms do not escape from the intact intestinal lumen, do not survive transit in the bloodstream or do not grow well in large volumes of ascites is not known. These are intriguing problems for investigation.

The second most common organism recovered in SBP is *Streptococcus pneumoniae* (the pneumococcus). The pneumococcus is, of course, a known pathogen, which has, in addition to its pneumoniagenic properties, a special predilection for causing peritonitis in ascitic, nephrotic and cirrhotic patients and also in non-ascitic, non-cirrhotic children (21). The explanation for this propensity is not known.

Furthermore, pneumococcal SBP is not limited to any one type of cirrhosis or to any other specific circumstances.

VI. SUMMARY: CLINICAL PATHOGENESIS OF SBP

1. The sine qua non of SBP is *ascites*, which is derived from the hepatic and splanchnic lymph.
2. The ascitic fluid in patients with advanced cirrhosis is abnormal. It is characterized by *deficient complement* and albumin, which reduce the opsonizing capacity of the ascitic fluid.
3. *Random bacteremias*, which may result from bacterial infections anywhere in the body.
4. *Portosystemic shunting*, both intrahepatic and extrahepatic, decrease the capacity of the *reticuloendothelial system* to remove bacteria from the bloodstream, thus prolonging bacteremia episodes.
5. Enteric bacteria can escape from the intestinal tract by several routes, each of which gives rise to *bacterial translocation*.
   a. *Erosions of the mucosa*, which may be gross in ulcerative diseases such as regional enteritis or ulcerative colitis.
   b. *Transmural passage* of bacteria, which is probably an uncommon phenomenon in intact subjects.
   c. *Vascular or lymphatic* translocation, which may result from bacterial overgrowth, hypotension, endotoxin excess, reduced endotoxin clearance, antibiotic administration, diarrhea, and a variety of immunological dysfunctions such as those induced by hepatic or renal disorders.

     d. *Transfallopian passage* of organisms such as gonococci or Chla-
mydial infestations, which tend to give rise to specific Curtis-
Fitz-Hugh-like syndromes.

6. The *nephrotic syndrome* is associated with an immunodeficiency
state, which tends to give rise to another form of SBP known as
primary peritonitis. Traditionally this disorder was usually a pneumococcal infection, but recently it has become much more like SBP
caused by gram-negative, aerobic enteric organisms.

7. *Chronic ambulatory dialytic peritonitis,* is an SBP-like syndrome,
that is largely caused by skin contaminating bacteria such as *Staphylococcus aureus* and *Staphylococcus enteriditis,* which appears to
be caused by contamination of the synthetic dialysis solutions by
nonenteric bacteria.

Thus many factors, individually and together, may result in SBP, which
for a variety of reasons, including the specific type of infecting bacteria, may
give rise to an almost infinite variety of clinical manifestations.

REFERENCES

1. Conn HO. Spontaneous peritonitis and bacteremia in cirrhotic patients caused
by enteric bacteria. Ann Intern Med 60:568–580, 1964.
2. Conn HO, Fessel JM. Spontaneous bacterial peritonitis in cirrhosis. Variations
on a theme. Medicine 50:161–197, 1971.
3. Correia JP, Conn HO. Spontaneous bacterial peritonitis in cirrhosis: Endemic or
epidemic? Med Clin North Am 59:963–981, 1975.
4. Goldfarb J, Conn HO. Spontaneous bacterial peritonitis: Endemic epidemic. In:
Hepatic Biliary and Pancreatic Surgery, Miami: Symposia Specialists, 1980,
441–450.
5. McCartney JE, Fraser J. Pneumococcal peritonitis. Brit J Surg 36:475–484,
1922.
6. Schweinburg FB, Seligman AM, Fine J. Transmural migration of intestinal bacteria. A study based on the use of radioactive *Escherichia coli.* New Engl J Med
242:747–752, 1950.
7. Reith AF, Squire TL. Blood cultures of apparently healthy persons. J Infect Dis
51:336–342, 1932.
8. Eade MN, Brocke BN. Portal bacteraemia in cases of ulcerative colitis submitted
to colectomy. Lancet 1:1008–1024, 1969.
9. McIndoe AH. Vascular lesions of portal cirrhosis. Arch Path 5:23–43, 1928.
10. Conn HO. Ammonia tolerance in the diagnosis of esophageal varices. Compari-

son of endoscopic, radiologic and biochemical techniques. J Lab Clin Med 70: 442–451, 1967.

11. Tisdale WA. Spontaneous colon bacillus bacteremia in Laennec's cirrhosis. Gastroenterology 40:141–148, 1961.

12. Snyder N, Atterbury CE, Correia JP, Conn HO. Increased concurrence of cirrhosis and bacterial endocarditis. Gastroenterology 73:1107–1113, 1977.

13. Read AE, Sherlock S, Laidlaw J, Walker JG. The neuropsychiatric syndromes and associated with chronic liver disease and an extensive portal-systemic collateral circulation. Q J Med 36:135–150, 1962.

14a. Conn HO, Rössle M. Portosystemic shunts and myelopathy: the first report of spastic paraparesis after TIPS (transjugular intrahepatic portosystemic stent-shunts) and a review of the literature. New Engl J Med, in press, 2000.

14b. Rössle M, Schmidt M, Braune S, Sieger-Stetter V, Ochs A, Langwehrmeier C, Conn HO. Hepatic myelopathy following TIPS implantation: A case report. Eur Ass Study Liver, in press, 1999.

15. Gorbach SL, Neale G, Levitan R, Hepner GW. Alterations in human intestinal microflora during experimental diarrhea. Gut 11:1–4, 1970.

16. Jacobson ED, Chodos RB, Faloon WW. An experimental malabsorption syndrome induced by neomycin. Amer J Med 28:524–530, 1960.

17. Kukral JC, Brandly M, Fritsch BA. Total body composition in cirrhotic patients with metabolic alkalosis, hypokalemia, hyperammonemia and portacaval shunt. Amer J Surg 117:85–94, 1969.

18. Bar-Meir S, Conn HO. Spontaneous bacterial peritonitis induced by intra-arterial vasopressin therapy. Gastroenterology 70:418–421, 1976.

19. Ambrose MS, Johnson M, Burdon DW, Keighley MRB. Incidence of pathogenic bacteria from mesenteric lymph nodes and ileal serosa during Crohn's disease surgery. Br J Surg 71:623–625, 1984.

20. Ferri M, Gabriel S, Gavelli A, Franconeri P, Guguet C. Bacterial translocation during portal clamping for liver resection. A clinical study. Arch Surg 132:162–165, 1997.

21. Fowler R Jr. Primary peritonitis. Aust New Zeal J Surg 26:204–209, 1957.

7

Bacterial Translocation: Studies of Mice and Men

Harold O. Conn
Yale University School of Medicine, New Haven, Connecticut, and University of Miami School of Medicine, Miami, Florida

> *Never been born, never had no father, nor mother, not nothin'.*
> —Topsy in *Uncle Tom's Cabin* by Harriet Beecher Stowe

I. INTRODUCTION

Bacterial translocation (BT)* is defined as the passage of viable bacteria, viruses, or other organisms from the gastrointestinal (GI) lumen to extragastrointestinal sites. The term *translocation* was first employed by Keller and Engley in 1958 to describe the passage of orally administered bacteriophage from the lumen of the intestines of mice to blood or to lymph nodes (1). Wolochow et al. in 1966 were the first to use the term *translocation* to describe the passage of bacteria (*Serratia marcescens*) from the duodena of rats, where they had been inoculated, into the lymph (2). In 1979, Berg and Garlington coined the term *bacterial translocation* to describe the migration of viable, indigenous bacteria from the GI tract to extra-intestinal sites such as the mesenteric lymph nodes (MLN), spleen, liver, kidney, peritoneal cavity, and/or bloodstream (3).

Within the past 25 years, great strides have been made in understanding the mechanisms of translocation. The major mechanisms according to Berg (4) are, "(a) disruption of the ecologic equilibrium that may allow bacterial

---

* A list of the abbreviations used in this chapter is given on p. 143.

overgrowth, (b) deficiencies in host immune defenses and (c) increased permeability of the intestinal mucosal barrier.'' A fourth mechanism of induction is severe trauma that is otherwise unexplained. Everything else known about BT may be considered to be variations on these themes or ''window dressing'' depending on one's point of view.

It is well established that a variety of indigenous bacteria such as *E. coli, Enterococcus faecalis, Klebsiella pneumoniae, Proteus mirabilis,* and *Lactobacillus acidophilus* readily translocate from the GI tract to the MLN of both gnotobiotic and normal animals after the intragastric inoculation of cecal flora (5–8). Obligate anaerobic bacteria such as *Bacteroides* and *Clostridia* effectively compete with and limit the growth of the gram-negative anaerobic bacteria (8). They are also the species least likely to translocate despite their high numbers (10^{10-11} per gram). Aerobic gram-negative bacteria, which tend to translocate more readily, exist in smaller numbers (approximately 10^8 per gram). The mechanisms of this bacterial tolerance and antagonism, respectively, may be related inversely as hypersensitivity to oxygen or lack thereof. Clearly, such findings are compatible with bacterial overgrowth as a major promoting mechanism of BT, although it is not at all clear what is responsible for such overgrowth.

Deficiencies of host immune defenses may permit the escape of bacteria from the bowel lumen by their failure to kill the bacteria before they reach the MLN, which are the first, easily culturable organs in the pathogenetic sequence of BT (9). The MLN have been shown to become contaminated by enteric bacteria before they reach the liver, spleen, blood, or peritoneal cavity (5,6); i.e., the MLN complex is an early stop in the translocation process. Mucosal, cell-mediated, and humoral immunity are probably all involved in preventing this early step in the sequence (10). Secretory IgA, which opsonizes bacteria for clearance by macrophages in the lamina propria and lymph nodes, is probably the first line of defense, followed by the clearance of the opsonized organisms. Immunosuppressive agents such as prednisone and cyclophosphamide are also known to promote BT (11). Other studies support the concept that serum immune factors effectively decrease the passage of bacteria from the MLN to the liver, spleen, and kidney (12). BT was reduced 10-fold from 50% in athymic mice (nu/nu) to 5% (13) in those that have acquired T-cell immunity by thymectomy (14).

Because immunocompromised patients are frequently treated with antibiotic agents, the possibility of synergism between antibiotic and immunosuppressive agents in the translocation process may be important. Owens and Berg and their associates studied the combination of prednisone and/or cyclophosphamide in combination with penicillin and clindamycin (12–14). Penicillin and clindamycin each promoted BT to the MLN, but did not induce spread to other organs. Prednisone and cyclophosphamide each also promoted BT, but to a much lesser degree than the antibiotic agents. The combination of one of these oral antibiotic agents (either) plus one of these immunosuppressive agents (either) promoted the systemic spread of indigenous *Enterobacteriaceae* from the MLN to the peritoneal cavity, thereby inducing spontaneous bacterial peritonitis (SBP). Thus, the combination of agents induced a much more profound escape of organisms from the GI tract to the systemic tissues than either class of drugs alone. Indeed, the combination of agents induced a potentially lethal lesion, which is the equivalent of the rat model of SBP described here.

II. INDUCTION AND ENHANCEMENT OF BACTERIAL TRANSLOCATION IN EXPERIMENTAL ANIMALS

To study the role of the integrity of the intestinal mucosal barrier against the BT of indigenous organisms, Morehouse et al. and others used ricinoleic acid (castor oil), which is known to damage the epithelial cells of the villi when administered directly into the GI canal of experimental animals (15,16) (Table 7.1). A single therapeutic, cathartic dose of ricinoleic acid was given into the stomachs of mice, after which the MLN, spleen, and liver were monitored bacteriologically. The incidence of BT with both facultative and obligate anaerobic bacteria increased with time after the ricinoleic acid, which was also promptly followed by extensive exfoliation of the epithelium of the villi of the proximal small bowel. The BT stopped within seven days after the mucosal epithelium had regenerated.

Hemorrhagic shock, which also produces intestinal mucosal damage and BT in rats (17), was studied in similar fashion. The arterial blood pressure was reduced from 90 to 60 mmHg for 2 h. The rats were sacrificed and their organs cultured after 2 h, by which time BT had already occurred. By light microscopy the intestinal tissues showed ileal and cecal subepithelial edema; by electron microscopy they showed disruption of the tight junctions between epithelial cells. Using a horseradish peroxidase probe, these investigators demonstrated increased intestinal permeability. These studies support the concept that the integrity of the intestinal mucosal barrier is critical to the prevention of BT, which can be induced in a variety of ways. It has been shown that the injury to the mucosa during ischemic shock is mediated by xanthine oxidase-generated superoxide radicals (18). Subsequent studies showed that allopuri-

Table 7.1 Bacterial Translocation in Experimental
Animals

Inducer	Reference
Bacterial overgrowth	12, 56
Biliary obstruction	68–70
Bowel manipulation	79
Burn injury	22, 58
Cold stress	84
Foreign bodies	82
Fulminant hepatic failure (galactosamine)	48, 49
Genetic deficiencies	13, 74
Hemorrhagic shock	17, 19
Hepatic resection (>15%)	33, 45
Immunologic malfunction	64
Immunosuppression	64, 80
Intestinal obstruction	34, 88
Ischemic injury of intestinal tract	18, 36
Malnutrition	43
Multiple "hit" induction	72, 73
Multiple organ failure	29
Pancreatitis	65, 66
Pneumoperitoneum	83
Portal hypertension	50, 51
Senility	84
Total parenteral nutrition	42
Trauma	27, 39

nol, an inhibitor of intestinal xanthine oxidase, reduces the mucosal damage
and BT to the MLN (19) caused by hemorrhagic shock (20).

Thermal injury also promotes intestinal injury and BT of indigenous GI
bacteria in mice and in rats (21). The mucosal damage, like that of ischemic
injury, appears to be mediated by xanthine oxidase (22). The obstructed intestinal tract is associated with many of these same toxicities and mechanisms (23).

Endotoxin-induced shock is also associated with intestinal ischemia and
BT (24) and with multiple organ failure syndrome (MOFS) (24–26). The intravenous or intraperitoneal injection of *E. coli* 026:136 endotoxin promotes the
occurrence of mucosal injury and BT (25), which, like the ischemic shock
syndrome, can be ameliorated by allopurinol. These findings indicate that there
are many ways of inducing BT. Furthermore, many of these diverse mechanisms operate on the same or similar principles.

In investigations of the mechanism of action of endotoxin-induced BT, Deitch et al. studied the structural components of endotoxin, i.e., the core polysaccharide, the polysaccharide side chains, the so-called D-antigens, and lipid A (25). These studies using Salmonella endotoxins showed that BT induction was associated with the terminal-3 sugars of the core polysaccharide or with lipid A. Administration of the active components increased xanthine oxidase activity. The more that is known about the pathogenesis of these interrelated disorders, the more likely it will be to develop BT-suppressing therapies.

The fourth mediator of the pathogenesis of BT is extensive trauma. Trauma and its associated shock are frequently fatal (26). In the United States trauma and shock are the second most common cause of death in patients 21–45 years of age, which is usually mediated by sepsis. Often bacterial contamination of wounds makes this association obvious. However, overwhelming sepsis is often the cause of death in victims of trauma who have not suffered bacterial contamination of their wounds or body cavities and in whom no source of overt infection can be found. This constellation of events is often called the multiple organ failure syndrome (MOFS) and its pathogenesis appears to be directly related to the large amount of dead and injured tissue, which appear to be the equivalent of bacteria as the source of this massive septic response.

In a recent article in *New Horizons* entitled, "Trauma, Shock and Gut Translocation" (27), Deitch and his colleagues introduced some exciting new concepts about BT. They pointed out that sepsis is the most common cause of death among patients who survive serious trauma for more than 48 h, in the absence of overt bacterial contamination of their wounds. Furthermore, in more than half of these fatal cases of sepsis, many of whom die of MOFS, no source of infection was found at autopsy (28). In the absence of overt infection it has been suggested that large amounts of dead or injured tissue may replace bacteria as the stimulus for the septic response. A likely explanation for this paradoxical situation is the failure of gut barrier function, which permits BT after trauma or shock, phenomena well studied in experimental animals (29). Indeed, trauma often induces shock, intestinal ischemia, and endotoxinemia, the key ingredients of all of these syndromes. After thermal injury, decreased blood flow to the GI tract may give rise to gastric ulcerations (Curling's ulcers) and, presumably, to other similar lesions in the lower bowel of both animals (30) and humans (31). It should be kept in mind that every gram of feces contains about 1 mg of endotoxin and 10^8 gram-positive and 10^{10} gram-negative bacteria. Furthermore, translocation of bacteria and endotoxin, both of which are toxic substances, occurs after burns (32), partial hepatectomy (33), intestinal obstruction (34), and many other clinical or experimental disorders. Such lesions appear to show the induction of BT by ischemic perfusion, mediated by xanthine oxidase and prevented by xanthine oxidase inhibition (35). Mucosal injury in these situations appears to be induced by an ischemia-perfusion injury that is also mediated by xanthine-generated oxidants and may be prevented by free-radical scavengers. Conceivably, increased phospholipase A_2 activity and free cellular calcium levels, which are also found in some shock states, may be involved (36). Such lesions can also be induced by the release of cytokines, including tumor necrosis factor (TNF) and interleukin-6 (IL-6) from gut-associated lymphatic tissues (GALT), which comprise more than half of the lymphoid cells in the body (37). There are close relationships between BT and the size of the burn (38), the severity of the shock or trauma (39) and the percentage of the liver excised. Obviously, the mechanisms that may lead to mucosal injury are complex and extensive, but suggest that the therapeutic use of agents that increase gut oxygen levels or that scavenge free radical, intermediate substances may be beneficial (40,41). Similarly, the administration of enteral feeding, which may prevent BT, should be used rather than parenteral feeding, which may induce it (42).

BT has grown like Topsy, rapidly and spontaneously, without precise direction or design. Once the phenomenon of BT had been recognized, it quickly became apparent that it can occur in a broad array of diseases in a wide variety of animal species and can be induced by a whole spectrum of substances and procedures that may appear to have little relationship to each other. This rapidly growing body of medical literature may appear to be an indication that any significant disruption of the normal function of the body, especially of the gastrointestinal track, may induce BT. In an attempt to simplify this ever-growing mass of data, we have separated the data derived from studies in experimental animals (Tables 7.1 and 7.2) from those performed in humans (Table 7.3). Table 7.3 lists specific substances that induce BT. In addition, we have tabulated separately those studies in which attempts to prevent and to diminish BT were performed (see Chap. 8). The more complicated investigations of the prevention or reduction of BT require (a) an experimental model, (b) a substance or procedure that promotes BT, and (c) a substance or procedure that can suppress or prevent BT. Each of these requirements must be controlled. Indeed, each such investigation is like one of a series of controlled studies in which the promoting procedure and its control group are compared with the results of the promoting procedure (or substance) plus the suppressing procedure (or substance) and the results of their controls. Surprisingly, a relatively large number of these promotion–prevention studies in both humans and animals have been performed and published.

Table 7.2 Bacterial Translocation
Associated with Human Disorders

Disease or disorder	Reference
Abdominal trauma	106–109
Acute hepatic resection	95
Bacterial overgrowth	99
Bacterial translocation	104
Colorectal carcinoma	90, 93
Crohn's disease	83
Hematological malignancies	89
Hepatic eschemia	96
Intestinal obstruction	34
Laparotomy	116, 120
Multiple organ failure	124
Nosocomial infection	125
Organ donation	104
Portal vein clamping	96
Thermal injury	121
Total parenteral nutrition	97, 98
Trauma	27, 94
Traumatic shock	94

Table 7.3 Specific Substances That
Induce Bacterial Translocation

Substance	Reference
Antibiotic agents	12
Cyclophosphamide	79, 81
Dexamethasone	57
D-Galactosamine	48, 49
Endotoxin	26, 63
Interleukin-2	61
Octreotid	67
Ricinoleic acid	15, 16
Streptozotocin	56
Zymosan	62

Although BT is quite clear, conceptually, the precise details of its pathogenesis are not nearly so well understood. Do the bacteria pass through the intestinal wall or do they take a more tortuous route, perhaps through the bloodstream? If so, do they traverse the intestinal wall directly? Do they pass between epithelial cells or through them? Studies of specific substances that induce BT are listed in Table 7.3.

In their superb article, J. W. Alexander and colleagues demonstrate that, as Confucius said, a picture is worth a thousand words (43). Their report using electron microscopy (EM) in about 30 photomicrographs, the Confuciun equivalent of 3000 words, solves some of the mysteries of the manner in which BT occurs. Their investigations were performed in Lewis rats and Hartley guinea pigs with Thiry-Vella loops into which ^{14}C-labeled *E. coli*, *Candida albicans*, and Salmonella endotoxin had been introduced after thermal trauma. Thiry-Vella fistulae represent exteriorized, semicircular extensions of the alimentary canal, which are open at both ends, that share the internal milieu of the body but are not in continuity with the lumen of the GI tract. They can be considered to be alimentary anastomoses to nowhere. These studies show clearly that the yeast tend to attach to the mucosal surfaces of epithelial villi (Fig. 7.1) with varying degrees of penetration into the brush order (Fig. 7.2). Microbes can directly penetrate the brush borders of the enterocytes by a unique process, which, by virtue of the absence of surrounding membranous structures, differs from classical phagocytosis (Figs. 7.3 and 7.4). The orga-

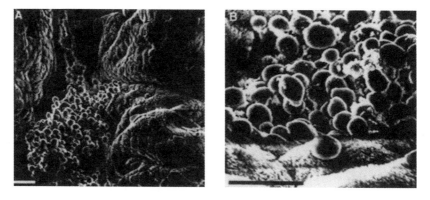

Figure 7.1 A scanning electron micrograph (SEM) of the mucosal surface of Thiry-Villa loops in which *Candida albicans* yeast are attached to some of the epithelial villi 12 hours after 50% surface-area burn injury. The scale bar is 10 μm. (From Ref. 43.)

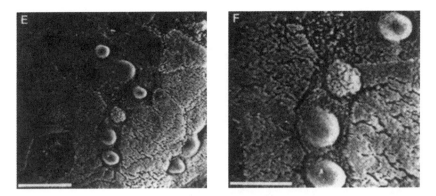

Figure 7.2 Varying degrees of penetration of the candida into the brush border are seen in this scanning electron micrograph (SEM). The scale bar is 5 μm. (From Ref. 43.)

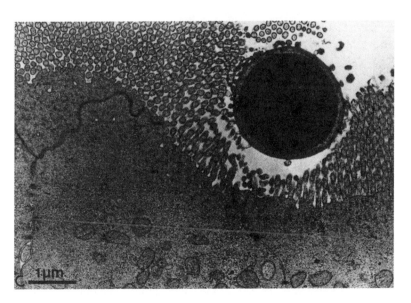

Figure 7.3 In this transmission electron micrograph (TEM), a candida is shown *within* an enterocyte with gross distortion of the plasma membrane and brush border at the presumed site of entry. The scale bar is 1 μm. (From Ref. 43.)

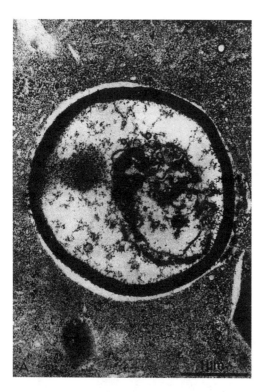

Figure 7.4 An enterocyte, which contains an internalized yeast cell (*Candida albicans*) that is migrating through the mucosa via the intercellular junctions in this transmission electron microscopic photograph. The scale bar is 1 μm. (From Ref. 43.)

nisms can also pass *between* intact enterocytes into the lamina propria. The basal membrane may be disrupted in the process and the cytoplasm of the cell and the yeast extruded. The organisms are usually phagocytosed by macrophages but are also found free in the lymphatic and blood vessels. The yeasts may give rise to daughter cells even after phagocytosis (Fig. 7.5). The *E. coli* translocate directly through the enterocytes rather than between them, whereas endotoxins, which can be identified by monoclonal antibody against the lipopolysaccharides of *E. coli* and *Salmonella minnesota* by fluorescence microscopy, tend to pass between the cells of the lamina propria and of the muscular wall of the bowel by passing *between* the mycocytes. As the authors emphasize, ''These descriptive phenomena provide new insights into the role of the enterocytes and intestinal immune cells in the translocation process.''

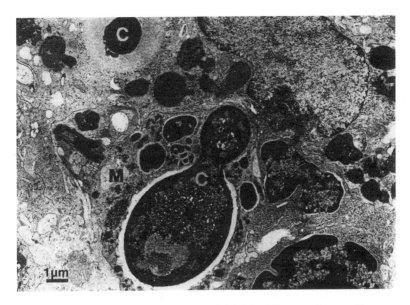

Figure 7.5 Two yeast cells (C), one of which is budding, are shown within a macrophage (M) in a germinal center in a Peyer's patch. The yeast cells appear to translocate frequently through the mucosal epithelium that covers the Peyer's patches. The scale bar is 1 μm. (From Ref. 43.)

With this more graphic picture of BT in mind, let us turn to specific aspects of BT. In 1966, Wolochow et al. had reported for the first time that microorganisms could traverse the intact intestinal wall of normal animals (2). This observation was not completely *de novo*; it was based on their earlier studies in which proteins or small bacteria (*Serratia marcescens* and coliphage II) passed through the normal intestinal wall from the lumen into the extraluminal tissue, a process they termed translocation (44). They found that the frequency of translocation appeared to vary directly with the concentration of bacteria instilled into the duodenum and inversely with the size of the organism. However, size and concentration were not the only variables. For example, Ersoz and associates found greater intestinal permeability in cirrhotic than in noncirrhotic patients using the excretion of 99mTc diethyltriaminepentaacetic acid as a marker, but noted no difference between those with and without SBP (44).

Conceptually, partial hepatectomy induces the classical type of BT. Wang and coworkers reported in 1993 that major hepatectomy, i.e., 70–90%

reproducibly, causes severe BT (45). They attributed the BT to acute liver failure similar in mechanism to the high incidence of bacterial infections that have been observed in humans with acute liver failure (46). Although the serum bilirubin, transaminase, and alkaline phosphatase levels had increased two- to fourfold within 6 h, only a few of the rats were overtly jaundiced, so that the term *liver failure* was being used loosely. *Acute hepatic injury* is a more accurate term. They might just as well have attributed the BT to portal hypertension, which also occurs after major hepatic resections in rats (47), and with other types of acute and chronic portal hypertension. Among the best examples of experimentally induced BT is galactosamine-induced fulminant hepatic injury.

Kasravi and coworkers caused acute hepatic injury by administering *D-galactosamine* (1.1 g per kg body weight intraperitoneally), a well-established hepatotoxin (48,49) in rats. For comparative purpose other groups received either saline as a placebo control or 70% liver resection as a control for hepatic resection-induced BT. At 24 and 28 h, groups of rats had cultures of aortic blood, MLN, liver, spleen, and the small bowel contents, and had histological examinations of the liver performed. The liver injury was characterized by severe, acute confluent hepatic necrosis and three- to fourfold increments in serum bilirubin concentration, alkaline phosphatase, and aminotransferase activity. Similar degrees of hepatic injury were observed in the hepatic resection group but the hepatic injury progressed in the galactosamine group and regressed in the resection group. Portal venous pressure decreased after galactosamine but increased after resection, which indicates that portal hypertension is not the mechanism of BT in both types of injury. BT to MLN, liver, and spleen was noted in all animals with both types of injury at 24 and 48 h. Portal venous pressure and flow were decreased after acute liver injury but were increased after resection findings that suggest that hepatic injury, rather than portal hypertension, was responsible.

To determine whether or not portal hypertension per se is important in BT, Garcia-Tsao et al. studied acute and chronic portal hypertension in the rat model with partial portal vein ligation (50). They assessed the effects of acute portal hypertension two days after ligation when portal-systemic shunting is minimal, and of chronic portal hypertension 15 days after ligation, when extensive portal-systemic shunting simulates cirrhosis. Samples of MLN, blood, liver, and spleen showed that in acute portal hypertension more than 90% had BT to the MLN, compared to about 30% in the control rats. In the chronic portal hypertension model, only one-fourth of the rats had BT to the MLN, and none to the blood, liver, or spleen. The risk of BT seems to have disappeared as the portosystemic shunting increased, presumably due to the disappearance of acute venous congestion, edema, and ischemia. Although portal pressure levels were not measured in these animals, portal hypertension per se does not appear to be the critical factor in the induction of BT. The presence of portosystemic shunting may be a more important factor. Probably, other factors were involved in the BT seen in rats with *E. coli*-C25-mono-associated BT, which is a very different experimental model (51).

Sorell and associates reported BT in Sprague-Dawley rats in which portal hypertension had been induced by calibrated stenosis of the portal vein (52). Fourteen days postoperatively, portal venous pressure levels were measured by cannulation of the ileocolic branch of the superior mesenteric vein. Cultures were taken from the peritoneum, inferior vena cava, MLN, cecum, liver, and spleen. The mean mesenteric vein pressure was 12.7 compared to 7.6 mmHg in the sham-operated control rats. BT of gram-negative bacilli to the MLN and vena caval blood occurred significantly more frequently and with greater numbers of organisms in the portal hypertensive group than in the sham-operated control rats ($p < 0.05$). In addition, hemorrhagic shock, i.e., mean arterial pressure of 40 mmHg or less, was induced in half of the portal hypertensive animals. BT was strikingly increased in the bled animals. They concluded that portal hypertension promotes BT and that hemorrhagic shock enhances these effects.

In 1984, Maejima et al. demonstrated that burn stress promotes BT in mice (53). Pathogen-free mice were subjected to 15% or 30% total body surface burns, which are nonlethal and do not induce BT. After the MLN are colonized with *E. coli* the amount of BT is proportional to the percentage of body surface burned. It has been postulated that indigenous enteric bacteria continually cross the mucosal barrier of the intestine. In normal mice and in those with small burns, those bacteria are eliminated by host immune defense mechanisms. When the surface area burned exceeds 30% BT to MLNs, blood and other organs progressively increases. As burn size increases it is associated with frequent bacteremias, polymicrobial bacteremia, enteric bacteremias, and a much higher mortality rate (54). The occurrence of smoke inhalation injury as well appears to worsen the prognosis.

Ricinoleic acid, the active component of castor oil, is a gastropathic agent that has long been used as a cathartic substance. This substance, which is cytotoxic to gastrointestinal epithelial cells, particularly those of the villus tips, promotes the accumulation of fluid and electrolytes in the intestinal tract. To determine whether such injuries affect BT, Morehouse et al. had administered 50 mg of ricinoleic acid intragastrically to pathogen-free DB-1 mice, a dosage equivalent to that used in humans (15). Within 2 h, the duodenal villi were greatly shortened and showed massive exfoliation of the columnar and goblet cells. Blood and lymphatic vessels in the lumina proper were directly compromised. Within two to four days about 40% of the animals showed translocation of *Proteus mirabilis*, *Lactobacillus acidophilus*, and *Staphylococcus epidermidis* to the MLN, spleen, and liver. These indigenous aerobic organisms were joined in their exodus by endogenous strict anaerobic bacteria. Pathogenic bacteria such as *Salmonella enteritidis* and *Giardia muris* translocate via Peyer's patches (56). This lesion appears to represent overt breaks in the epithelium and may be considered equivalent to the lesions of inflammatory bowel diseases.

Imai and Kurihara reported the results of *streptozotocin (STZ)* in Slc: ddY mice in a single intraperitoneal dose (57). STZ is a diabetogenic agent that suppresses the oral and intestinal flora and results in depressed resistance to bacterial infection. Two weeks after administration BT was noted in MLN, lung, and kidneys from which *E. coli*, *Proteus mirabilis*, and *Staphylococcus epidermidis* were cultured. The diabetes was characterized by hyperglycemia and insulinopenia. The BT induced by STZ is similar to that induced by ricinoleic acid. About 10% of the mice died and the deaths were attributed to aspiration and pneumonia caused by bacterial overgrowth.

Mucosal defense mechanisms include heavy mucus and secretory IgA barriers, which mechanically suppress bacterial adherence to the epithelial cells and diminish BT. Alverdy and Aoys studied the effects of adrenocortioscleroid therapy by administering dexamethasone intraperitoneally 0.8/150 g body weight to Fischer rats for two days and administering saline to a control group (58). They found that the steroid-treated animals exhibited a significant decrease in bile IgA (54 µg per mg protein) compared to 23 µg per mg protein in the saline-treated rats. A similar decrease in the IgA coating of bacteria was observed. In addition, the steroid therapy induced an increase in bacterial adherence (p $<$ 0.01) and of BT to 60%, but not in the saline-treated control group. The accepted hypothesis is that the first step in BT is the adherence of luminal pathogens to the mucosal cell surfaces, and that inhibition of such adherence, which is prevented by secretory IgA and by the mucus barrier, may prevent BT. Thus, dexamethasone permits an increase in the number of bacteria in the cecum and a much higher incidence of BT (60% vs. 0%) than in the control animals. Clearly, steroid therapy decreases resistance to the multiplication of enteric bacteria and their translocation to the MLN.

It is known that oral antibiotic agents such as penicillin, clindamycin, and metranidazol decrease the cecal population of obligate anaerobic bacteria and permit the overgrowth of gram-negative, aerobic bacteria and the development of BT to the MLN (59). It is also known that prednisone administered to mice stimulates the development of BT (60). Berg et al. have shown that use of these three antibiotic agents with corticosteroid administration acts synergistically, stimulating much more BT than either therapy alone, and, in addition, the bacteria translocate to the peritoneum and cause SBP, which was frequently lethal (61). The bacteria responsible in these studies were *Klebsiella pneumoniae*, *Proteus mirabilis*, and *E. coli*, the same organisms that cause the bulk of SBP in humans. Thus, *bacterial overgrowth* plus *immunosuppression* stimulates vigorous bacterial overgrowth and enhances the development of BT. Many other factors are involved in such studies, e.g., interspecies differences between rats and mice. Questions exist about the route bacteria take to translocate from the intestinal lumen and into the lymphatic and vascular systems.

Immunoglobulins, but not *interleukin-2*, significantly reduce the number of bacteria in the plasma of rats treated immediately after intraperitoneal challenge of 2×10^6 microorganisms (*Ps. aeruginosa*, *E. coli*, and *K. pneumoniae*) (62). This effect is associated with an increase in endotoxin. Interleukin did not suppress the bacterial counts, but, instead, enhanced BT (63) and decreased endotoxin levels significantly.

Deitch et al. administered zymosan, which is a component of the cell wall of yeast that activates complement and stimulates neutrophil and macrophage activity intraperitoneally to mice that were normally nourished or malnourished by a low protein diet (0.03% protein) for 21 days (17% protein) (64). Zymosan induced BT to the MLN in the malnourished mice but not in the well-fed animals. The low-protein diet induced mucosal injury, which was more severe the longer the malnutrition existed. Zymosan, which is a nonendotoxin inflammatory agent, causes oxidant-mediated intestinal mucosal injury. The prevention of the zymosan-induced injury, which can be achieved by the inhibition of xanthine oxidase activity by allopurinol, prevents both the mucosal injury and the BT.

Malnutrition thus sets the stage for mucosal intestinal injury, BT, and their consequences. Many other factors are involved; however, this is an example of a ''two-hit'' phenomenon.

Deitch proposed that the ''two-hit'' induction of BT, i.e., after two metabolic insults, such as burn injury and hypotension, together, induces greater deleterious effects than either insult alone and probably plays an important role in the pathogenesis of multiple organ failure (65). Mishima and associates confirmed the synergistic effects of this ''two-hit phenomenon'' in Westar rats with 15% total surface burns and hemorrhagic hypotension, i.e., blood pressure of 30 mmHg (66). These phenomena demonstrate the validity of the ''two-hit'' pathogenesis of BT in which the number of bacteria colony-forming units, i.e., cultured bacteria, cultured from the MLN were significantly greater in rats with burns plus hypotension than with burns or hypotension. This approach makes great sense in interpreting MOFS.

Deitch and Berg and their associates reported experiments in CrL::O [ICR]BR mice in which the effects of *endotoxin* on BT were studied (67). Here, 1- and 2-mg doses of lipopolysaccharide from *E. coli* 026:B6 were injected intraperitoneally, intramuscularly, or subcutaneously. Cultures of blood, MLN, spleen, and liver were obtained aerobically and anaerobically. They found that the incidence of BT to the MLN was directly proportional to the dose of endotoxin. Eighty-eight percent of the mice that received 2 mg by intraperitoneal or intramuscular injection developed BT. Those who did not develop BT received the dose subcutaneously. Both intraperitoneal and intramuscular endotoxin increased transiently the cecal concentrations of enteric bacteria 100-fold after endotoxin. Histological assessment shows that the bowel mucosa appears intact, but that scattered areas of edematous lamina propria and epithelial cell exfoliation can be seen, although no overt breaches in the epithelial barrier were found.

Clearly endotoxin stimulates the occurrence of BT, but the mechanism by which it does so is not clear. Endotoxin has a broad range of biological activities including modulation of the immune system, increasing vascular permeability, impairment of oxygen utilization and cellular metabolism, initiation of disseminated intravascular coagulation, and the production of profound deleterious hemodynamic changes. Whether it stimulates mucosal integrity, increases vascular permeability, or depresses host antibacterial defenses await further investigations. Studies in endotoxin-resistant and endotoxin-sensitive mice did not elucidate the mechanism.

Investigations of host defense mechanisms were performed by Ohsugi et al. (68) in mice, which have impaired T- and B-cell function, and in beige mice, which have impaired NK-cell and polymorphonuclear leukocyte function. After antibiotic decontamination, these mice were inoculated intragastrically with *E. coli*-C25, which causes transient BT for one week, after which the BT disappears. The findings indicate that defense mechanisms other than T and B lymphocytes are important in inhibiting systemic infection from the GI tract.

BT is also a very common manifestation of *acute hemorrhagic pancreatitis*. Tarpila et al. induced acute pancreatitis in Westar rats by the injection of 0.2 ml sterile sodium taurocholate into the pancreatic duct (69). The control group had a sham laparotomy but no intraductal injection. Two days later the laparotomy was repeated and samples were taken for bacterial analysis from the visceral peritoneum, the MLN, macroscopic sites of necrosis in the pancreas, and the contents of the ileum and cecum. Biopsies of the jejunum and ileum were taken for histological examination. All 12 rats in the experimental group developed overt necrotic pancreatitis with fat necrosis and turbid peritoneal fluid. Bacterial overgrowth with both aerobic and anaerobic organisms was present in the ileum and cecum. Histological abnormalities of the endothelium and villous tips were observed. Aerobic cultures from the MLN and pancreas were positive in almost all rats. *E. coli* were the most common organisms recovered. Anaerobic cultures were positive in about half the rats whereas BT was induced in virtually all of the tissues of all the rats.

In a similar experiment, Marotta et al. studied pancreatitis induced by the intrabiliary injection of a trypsin-enterokinase mixture which induced BT in three-fourths of the rats (70). Enemas with rifaxamin (a nonabsorbed, antibiotic agent), enemas with rifaxamin plus lactitol (an intestinal-acidifying, catharsis-inducing nonabsorbed carbohydrate), and control enemas that did not contain any medications were administered. The survival rate was about 50% in the untreated rats, 75% in the rifaxamin group, and 100% in the rifaxamin-lactitol group. The unmedicated enemas had no beneficial effects. This investigation documents the role of colonic bacteria in the mortality of acute pancreatitis, and suggests a therapeutic approach to pancreatitis. Incidentally, the nonabsorbed carbohydrates such as lactulose and lactitol have many beneficial effects other than their antiencephalopathic actions that might be applicable to these experiments (71).

III. OVERVIEW OF THE INDUCTION OF BT IN EXPERIMENTAL ANIMALS

BT has been induced in a variety of ways. To assess them in a rational manner we have classified them according to the major means of induction. These specific substances, injuries, disorders, and procedures are listed in Table 7.1. These methods range from acute injury to the liver caused by D-galactosamine to chronic liver disease induced by carbon tetrachloride or by biliary obstruction, which are attempts to simulate the two most common types of cirrhosis. Closely related are attempts to induce portal hypertension, which is the underlying abnormality of SBP. Some of these techniques are induced by direct interventions such as portal vein clamping or by major hepatic resection, the consequences of which are increments in portal venous pressure and impairment of liver function. Not surprisingly, some of these translocations are mediated by infections such as bacteremia (fungal, lactobacillary), by substances produced during infections (endotoxin, interleukins), or by attempts to impair anti-infectious processes such as the macrophage depletion.

Another direct approach is via the peritoneum. Those reports include the induction of abnormal conditions such as ''irritation'' of the peritoneum by changes in the concentrations of electrolytes of fluids instilled into the peritoneal cavity, which have resulted in transmural migration of bacteria, by manipulation of the intestines, by the introduction of foreign bodies into the peritoneal space, or by the performance of pneumoperitoneum.

Ulcerative gastrointestinal lesions that occur in chronic ulcerative disorders such as ulcerative colitis and Crohn's disease permit the direct entry of enteric bacteria into the lymphatic and vascular systems through holes in intestinal mucosa. It is surprising at first glance that gastrointestinal bleeding is a common method of inducing BT and bacterial infections. Whether this process is related to the decrements in mesenteric arterial blood flow or to breaks in the integrity of the gastrointestinal mucosa or both is not clear. Clearly, the introduction of a variety of bacterial species into the GI tract appear to stimulate bacterial overgrowth in the intestinal tract, which is frequently a prerequisite to BT. A number of other gastrointestinal disorders also predispose to BT. They include intestinal obstruction and biliary obstruction. Intestinal transplantation might be expected to induce BT, and, indeed, it does.

One would anticipate that nutritional disturbances might set the stage for BT, and a number of them have been recognized to do so. Malnutrition is a frequent predecessor of BT. Surprisingly, parenteral nutrition, both total and supplementary, has been identified as such inducers. Some specific diets, including fiber-free diets, have been implicated. Deficiencies of glutamine and of arginine have been identified as specific inducers that can be corrected by supplementary administration of these substances.

A number of medications that act by obvious mechanisms, and others in more subtle, less visible ways have been described (Table 7.2). They include the use of antibiotic agents, which suppress and alter the ecology of enteric bacterial growth and the distribution of organisms in the gut. Adrenocorticosteroids, which affect virtually every physiological mechanism and pathological disorder, have profound effects on BT. Conversely, the administration of antibiotic agents such as the combination of ciprofloxacin and penicillin have been reported to prevent BT.

IV. HUMAN DISORDERS THAT INDUCE BT

Ambrose et al. studied 46 patients with Crohn's disease prior to surgery and compared these results with a control group of 43 patients with a variety of nonulcerative abdominal disorders (72) (see Table 7.2). They were able to culture intestinal bacteria from the mesenteric nodes in 33% of patients with ulcerative lesions compared to only 5% in the control group ($p < 0.01$). Potentially pathogenic bacteria were cultured from the serosa of the Crohn's group twice as frequently as from the control group (p < 0.05). The authors postulated that enteric bacteria escape from the lumen via the ulcerations and account for the frequent mesenteric lymphadenopathy. The common occurrence of BT and the frequent occurrence of fistulae, wound sepsis, and intra-abdominal abscesses in patients with Crohn's disease support this hypothesis.

Deitch reported his results in 42 uninfected patients who underwent laparotomy for a variety of abdominal disorders, 17 of whom had intestinal obstruction and 25 of whom did not (73). Mesenteric lymph nodes were excised for bacteriologic culture at the beginning of surgery in these 42 patients. Ten of the 17 obstructed patients (59%) had positive cultures for enteric bacteria compared to only one of 25 nonobstructed patients (p < 0.01). All of the patients, none of whom had a necrotic bowel, had had perioperative antibiotic agents before surgery. The authors concluded that simple obstruction of the colon or small bowel led to BT by promoting bacterial overgrowth, by increasing intestinal permeability and/or by disrupting the mucosal barrier.

Tancrede and associates studied 55 patients with hematological malignancies and gram-negative bacteremia (74). They found that the organisms isolated were similar to the Enterobacteriaceae and *Pseudomonas* species recovered from the feces of these same patients, and were usually observed in patients with leukopenia. BT had occurred in 45 of the 55 episodes (82%), and may have been associated with immunosuppression or with the treatment of their neoplasms.

Colorectal carcinomas are neoplasms that are associated with BT. This relationship is largely based on a specific association between *Streptococcus bovis* and carcinoma of the colon (75–77). On this basis, Vincent and coworkers undertook a prospective comparison of 20 patients who were to have surgery for colon cancer with 20 control patients with noncolorectal digestive diseases (78). At laparotomy, samples of portal venous blood and samples of pericolonic lymph nodes that were both involved and uninvolved by the neoplasm, portal venous blood, and samples of liver tissue were harvested before antibiotic agents had been administered for bacteriological examination. BT was found in two-thirds of the cancer group and in one-third of the control group (p < 0.05). BT occurred in all involved lymph nodes, but was found uncommonly in the uninvolved nodes (two of 13 samples; 15%) and rarely in the liver (one of 13 samples; 8%). In the control group, bacteria were found frequently in the liver (5 of 6 samples; 83%) and less frequently in the nodes (three of 6 samples; 50%). A much broader spectrum of organisms was found in the cancer group than in the control group (15 species of intestinal organisms compared to two in the control group). These bacteria consisted primarily of Enterobacteriaceae, *Pseudomonas*, *Clostridia*, and streptococci of the same species that had been cultured from a fecal samples taken 24 h before surgery for the same patients. This investigation clearly demonstrates the occurrence of BT and its frequency in this syndrome, and provides some insight into origins of these translocated bacteria and how these abnormalities may develop.

Moore et al. (79) found that acute traumatic shock was associated with bacteremia in 38% (12 of 38) of patients with shock compared with only 11% of the patients without shock (10 of 74). The bacteremias were predominantly caused by gram-negative organisms (79), but only 15% of the mesenteric node cultures were positive. The authors concluded that BT after trauma was infrequent and that enteric BT occurred almost exclusively in terminal patients.

Kanematsu and colleagues noted that there were large increments in portal venous pressure in 65 patients who underwent major hepatic resections (80). In cirrhotic patients the mean pressure rose from 226 to 277 mm saline. Smaller increments were observed in noncirrhotic patients (mean pressure 198 mm saline before resection and 226 mm afterward). The increase in portal venous pressure must almost certainly play a role in the frequent occurrence of BT in patients undergoing large hepatic resections. The critical question is whether is it the loss of hepatic function resulting from the resection per se or from the associated increase in portal venous pressure that is responsible.

In both patients and rats, Wang and coworkers have demonstrated prompt, severe BT after major hepatic resections in which the severity of the BT was related to the amount of liver tissue resected (45,46). However, the largest hepatic resections (approximately 90%) induced liver failure with increased serum bilirubin concentrations and a doubling or tripling of aminotransferase activity, as well as positive cultures of enteric organisms in the blood, MLN, liver, spleen, and kidneys. A severe decrease in arterial blood pressure was also noted. Because shock and acute liver failure are both associated with BT, it is not clear whether the hepatic resections per se or their consequences, e.g., the increase in portal venous pressure, were responsible for the infectious problems.

Hepatic resections also reduce the amount of reticuloendothelial tissue, which, in effect, diminishes the bacteria-clearing capacity of the liver. Since this diminution is roughly proportional to the percentage of the liver substance resected, the effect on BT and on portal pressure increases as the size of the resection increases. Furthermore, large resections also reduce the functional capacities of the liver.

Ferri et al. studied the effects of short-term hepatic ischemia (30 to 60 min) induced by portal triad clamping and vena caval compression above and below the liver during hepatectomy in 15 patients who required hepatic resection of various amounts for a variety of hepatic lesions (81). Bacteriological studies, which consisted of cultures of systemic and portal blood, upper gastrointestinal contents, and MLN, were carried out before and 6 and 24 h after clamping and resection. Preresection cultures were all negative. After the procedure blood cultures were negative, but MLN cultures were positive in almost half the patients. Usually only coagulase-negative staphylococci were cultured. Serious or lethal infections were not seen postoperatively, nor were they related to the BT. Furthermore, the BT could not be related to the resection per se because it is not clear whether the hepatic resections or the clamping procedures per se were responsible for the BT or whether other factors are involved.

Furthermore, total parenteral nutrition (TPN) has been thought to induce BT in animals, and may have induced the BT in some of these patients (82,83). This problem, which had been attributed to bacterial overgrowth in the small bowel in cirrhotic patients (84), was thought to be preventable by enteral feeding, which maintains normal gut flora and immunocompetence and prevents mucosal atrophy (85). Shirabe and associates undertook a controlled investigation of parenteral nutrition in 26 patients who required major hepatic resections for hepatic cancer (86). Although the two groups of 13 patients were similar in underlying disease and the diets they consumed were similar in calories, total amino acids, branched chain amino acids, and carbohydrate, they differed in the amounts of fat consumed. The TPN group had received no fat compared to 4.6 Kcal of fat per Kg body weight per day in the enteral nutrition group. More infections were found in the TPN group (4 vs. 1) than in the enterally fed patients. Although these differences are not statistically significant because of the small numbers of patients studied, they tend to support the studies that found TPN to have adverse effects on BT.

Pierro and coworkers studied the effects of long-term TPN on BT in newborn babies and infants who had undergone surgical procedures and who required parenteral feeding because of gastrointestinal abnormalities (87). After basal cultures of the oropharynx and gut were taken, TPN was begun and blood cultures from both the central and peripheral veins were repeated. The diagnosis of TPN-induced BT was defined as the recovery of the same bacteria from the MLN, blood, or rectum after TPN as had been isolated from the gastrointestinal tract before TPN. Of the 94 infants studied, six of them (6%) developed BT. The BT occurred a median of 58 days after the PN had been begun, and was almost always observed in infants with elevated serum bilirubin levels. The investigators concluded that TPN was associated with enteric BT in a small, but significant percentage of these patients. It is not clear whether hyperbilirubinemia is a prerequisite for BT or was a consequence of the TPN in these patients. Other investigators, however, have not yet been able to confirm that TPN per se does induce BT (88).

Tani and coworkers have described two unusual patients in whom they considered BT of idiopathic origin to have been the cause of septic shock (89). No such case had previously been described in humans. Their first patient, a 67-year-old man with a malignant lymphoma who had previously been treated with radiation therapy, developed septic shock 10 days after a course of chemotherapy that consisted of mitoxantrone, etoposide, prednisone, and carboplatin. He had intense abdominal pain, high fever, severe leukopenia (<300 leukocytes per cubic millimeter), and shock. Exploratory laparotomy showed no intestinal perforation, peritonitis, or any other source of intraabdominal sepsis. *Pseudomonas aeruginosa* were cultured from the blood, MLN, and ascitic fluid. Gram-negative bacilli were seen histologically on the surface of epithelial cells, in the crypts, in the edematous submucosa, and in the villi of the colon. The patient died of sepsis due to a phlegmon of the abdominal wall. These findings represent overt BT with a fatal outcome. The role of the lymphocytic neoplasm in this patient in not known.

The second patient, who was admitted with abdominal pain, developed fever (>40°C) and shock. He was found to have a stenosis of the sigmoid colon that gave rise to severe constipation and a preconstriction megacolon, which was 15 cm in diameter. Laparotomy, performed to relieve a presumed volvulus of sigmoid colon, resulted in a sigmoidectomy, which showed an erosion in the sigmoid colon, and which apparently cured the problem. *Klebsiella pneumoniae* were cultured from the blood and MLN, but no other explanation for the septic shock syndrome was found.

These two cases suggest, but do not prove, that BT itself can give rise to the septic shock syndrome in humans. It remains to be proved unequivocally, however, that BT in the absence of overt, intra-abdominal bacterial infection or bowel perforation can give rise to the septic shock syndrome.

Van Goor found bacterial translocation to be present at the time of transplantation in the tissues of the majority of organ donors who, although not normal, presumably had intact gastrointestinal systems (90). The bacteria isolated in these patients were identical to those cultured from the bowels of the same patients. In addition, endotoxin was detected in more than half of the peritoneal fluids in these patients. Although the precise prevalence of BT in hospitalized patients is difficult to determine, there is considerable evidence that systemic infections frequently originate in the intestinal flora of high-risk patients.

Several other possible instances of BT have been reported in humans.

Reed et al. have reported BT detected at laparotomy in patients after penetrating or blunt abdominal trauma without rupture of the bowel or gross fecal contamination of the abdominal cavity (91). Two MLN were resected from each patient, one of which was used for bacteriologic and one for microscopic examination. These investigators demonstrated that 13 of 15 patients (87%) showed BT of enterobacteria by bacteriologic culture, by electron microscopy, or by both techniques. All four were caused by *Klebsiella* species. The positive bacteriologic isolations were not related to the severity of the trauma, to the accompanying hypotension, or to the outcome. Immunofluorescence, which was positive in 100% in one series, indicated the diagnostic significance of this technique. Of course, many of the patients studied had received antibiotic therapy.

Abdominal trauma was also the focus of prospective investigations by Brathwaite (92) and Peitzman (93) and their associates. Peitzman et al. had studied 25 patients after blunt trauma, none of whom had a primary infection of the peritoneal cavity or a perforation of a hollow viscus. They were relatively young patients (mean age 33) with an average Injury Severity Score (ISS) of 30, and 22 of them had had MLN excised at surgery. All of the nodes were sterile. Almost 40% of the group developed bacterial complications that were not consequences of BT. They also studied four patients with a variety of gastrointestinal diseases, including one each with ulcerative colitis, sigmoid volvulus, small bowel obstruction, and gastrointestinal bleeding, each of which has previously been associated with BT. Three of these four patients, excluding the one with intestinal obstruction, developed BT with enteric bacteria. None of the 25 patients with trauma, which has previously been associated with BT, had developed BT. All 29 patients had received either a first- or second-generation cephalosporin antibiotic agent immediately before surgery. The investigators were surprised by the low yield of BT and assumed that the MLN biopsies had been taken before the organisms had reached the lymph nodes or that the antibiotic therapy had inhibited their growth. Further studies are needed to elucidate this phenomenon.

Several years later Lignau et al. performed a prospective randomized clinical trial (RCT) in noninfected patients who had suffered severe injuries (94). The ISS values (95) ranged from 16 to 74, which includes a broad range of injuries. These patients had not previously received antibiotic therapy, and were expected to require at least 48 h of artificial ventilation and at least three days of care in the surgical intensive care unit (ICU) at the University of Innsbruck. On admission their mean APACHE II score was 15.6, a value that is predictive of a mortality rate of about 20% (96). The treatment group of 80 patients received a solution that contained polymyxin E (100 mg), tobramycin (80 mg), and amphotericin B (500 mg) (PTA) four times a day, whereas the placebo group of 140 patients were given an equal volume of the solvent by nasogastric tube. Another group of 82 patients received polymyxin E, tobramycin, and ciprofloxacin (PTC) (500 mg four times daily). The two treatment groups showed a similar prevalence of pneumonia, of MOFS, of sepsis, and rate of survival, and required a similar number of days of assisted ventilation, but the SID-treated patients showed a reduction in gram-negative aerobic colonization. The investigators concluded that SID indeed reduced bacterial overgrowth in the intestinal tract, but felt that bacterial overgrowth is not the sole link between trauma, sepsis, and organ failure.

Additional recent investigations in critically injured patients, and MOFS were also performed by Tran (97), Moore (98), Stechmiller (99), and their coworkers.

Shannon et al. in a retrospective, controlled clinical trial reported that distal-colon-washout plus ''broad spectrum'' antibiotic agents prevented bacterial sepsis in 27 patients with major trauma such as gunshot, stab wounds, or pelvic fractures (100) and reduced septic infections from 31% to 4% (p < 0.01). The mean ISS was greater in the treatment group than in the control patients. Unfortunately, they never mentioned BT except in the title of the article. Furthermore, they did not indicate whether the control and treatment groups had been selected randomly. Although flawed by the study design and the assumption that BT preceded the infections, this investigation is consistent with the effects of antibiotic therapy and bowel evacuation in the treatment of colonic injury.

In assessing BT in humans one must acknowledge the large, well-designed prospective investigations of MacFie and his associates at the Scarborough Hospital in Yorkshire, England (101). These investigators summarized the results of a number of studies performed at their hospital over a five-year period (102–105). They reported on a total of 449 patients who had undergone laparotomy in whom serosal scrapings from the terminal ileum and a biopsy of ileocecal mesenteric lymph nodes were taken immediately after opening the peritoneum. These specimens were studied by state-of-the-art bacteriologic techniques. These investigators presented their results and proposed six regional avenues of investigation into the pathogenesis of BT: (1) intestinal barrier function, (2) villous morphology, (3) intestinal permeability, (4) microbiology of bacterial translocation, (5) microbiology of the upper gastrointestinal tract, and (6) putative associations between gastric microflora, bacterial translocation, and septic morbidity.

They concluded that BT occurs frequently in surgical patients and is associated with septic morbidity. Furthermore, they showed that three times as many patients with BT developed sepsis as did those who were overtly free of sepsis (41% vs. 14%, p < 0.001). Similarly, patients who were older than 70 years, patients who required emergency surgery, and patients with distal bowel obstruction developed significantly higher rates of BT. Their assessment of villous morphology and dual sugar probes (L-rhamnose and L-lactulose) that were employed as indices of bowel permeability indicates that neither is truly predictive of BT. Indeed, these investigators question whether these probes can even be considered to be reliable indicators of intestinal barrier function. They accept that alterations in the GI microflora may influence BT rates and that the wide variety of organisms that translocate suggests that BT occurs by a nonspecific mechanism that is independent of individual species, and probably reflects the spectrum of the indigenous luminal bacterial flora. Furthermore, they were unable to prove that short periods of TPN had induced the BT, but accept that the incidence of sepsis is greater in patients who require TPN than in those who do not. The presence of obligate anaerobes does not appear to confer protection against BT. Furthermore, *Candida* species are often, but not necessarily, involved in translocation.

They conclude that BT, "probably occurs in healthy individuals but is not clinically significant" in the presence of an intact immune system. In immunocompromised patients and those who are aged or who have distal bowel obstruction, "there is failure to prevent the propagation of viable bacteria from the mesenteric lymph nodes to extraintestinal sites" of sepsis (102). Finally, "BT appears to be an important early step in the promotion of sepsis in debilitated, postoperative patients, rather than the sole initiator." They concluded, therefore, that selective intestinal decontamination is a rational form of therapy.

V.   MISCELLANEOUS BACTERIAL SYNDROMES OF UNCERTAIN PATHOGENESIS IN HUMANS

Several complex, human bacterial syndromes that are clinically quite diverse share important pathogenetic features, namely thermal injury, abdominal trauma, multiple organ failure syndrome, and spontaneous bacterial peritonitis. These topics will be considered together here because they give insights into the interlocking aspects of these otherwise distinct disorders.

A.   Thermal Injury

In an impressive, retrospective investigation, Sittig and Deitch studied the prognostic affects of bacteremia in humans after thermal trauma (106). They reviewed the records of all the patients who had been admitted to the Burn Clinic of the Louisiana State University in Shreveport between 1980 and 1986 with severe burns and who had developed bacteremia. Of the 1108 patients admitted with a mean burn size of at least 22% of the body surface area, 93 (8%) developed bacteremia. The mean size of the burns in the bacteremic patients was 46% of the total body surface area, more than twice the size of the average lesion. Twenty-nine percent of the bacteremic group died compared to only 4% of the nonbacteremic patients ($p < 0.001$). The mean burn size in the patients who died was almost twice as great as in the survivors (71% vs. 39%; $p < 0.002$), and a much higher incidence of inhalation injuries had occurred ($p < 0.002$). Thus, these data do not establish the bacteremogenic effects of burn size per se, although they do suggest that the overall prognosis is inversely associated with burn size. More polymicrobial bacteremias were observed in the fatal cases. The negative risk factors for survival in order of importance were burn size; the presence of gram-negative, enteric bacteremia; the occurrence of polymicrobial bacteremia; and the presence of inhalation injury.

The main cause of death was sepsis in the burn wound itself due to the loss of the skin barrier and the antibacterial and immune defense systems. Clearly, seriously burned patients are immunocompromised as shown by the higher incidence of cross-bacterial contamination in the patients treated on the open wards. BT was not specifically studied in this group of patients.

B. Major Trauma

Although etiologically different from burns, many pathogenetic features of major torso trauma and burns are similar, especially the high incidence of BT. Moore and coworkers at the Denver General Hospital studied 57 patients with emergency trauma; they focused on 20 of them with multiple organ failure who were at greatest risk (79). By definition these were patients who had suffered severe abdominal trauma, who required massive transfusions (>10 units of blood), and/or who had incurred multiple fractures. These 20 patients had portal vein catheters implanted at laparotomy for surveillance of portal and systemic blood cultures and endotoxin assays in the two venous systems. The patients were graded on a 1 to 3 scale for organ failure of the eight component systems: pulmonary, renal, hepatic, cardiac, gastrointestinal, hematologic, central nervous, and metabolic. All the patients had received broad spectrum antibiotic therapy. Twelve of these 20 patients had MLN excised for bacteriologic cultures. Four of the 12 (33%) had BT, two of whom were gram-negative and enteric organisms and two of whom were gram-positive. Because endotoxinemia isn't thought to give rise to numerous inflammatory mediators such as complement fragments, tumor necrosis factor and interleukin-6 were assayed. Complement components and Il-6 were found to be elevated and TNF consistently normal, but none of these assays correlated closely with MOFS. The major infections were intra-abdominal abscesses and pneumonia.

It is generally accepted that gut-derived bacteria or endotoxins are the primary factors in the MOFS, a hyperinflammatory septic state. Although BT is found in only a small fraction of these patients, endotoxinemia appears to be the common bond (107) that recruits active, neutrophilic leukocytes; damages the endothelium; induces the release of cytokines; and triggers the complement and clotting cascades (108). Although the details of these complex disorders are not fully understood, the inflammatory effects of burns and of trauma are much more similar to each other than they are different.

C. Multiple Organ Failure Syndrome

Sepsis induced by the MOFS is one of the major causes of death in critically ill patients (109). MOFS may be the result of massive trauma or inflammation that is caused by bacterial or nonbacterial inflammatory stimulation. It may be associated with respiratory infection, usually by gram-negative aerobic bacteria, but is not necessarily bacterially mediated. It may be prevented by prophylactic antibiotic therapy to suppress bacterial infections and BT.

Goris and associates cited nine investigations of selective intestinal decontamination (SID) in humans in which SID suppressed nosocomial infections (110). Two of these studies were published randomized clinical trials (111,112). Because they did not find a single published report of SID in experimental animals in the literature, they performed a splendid one. In their experimental model, in which zymosan-induced (sterile) peritonitis (ZIP) was used (which has since been validated as a reliable model) they compared the efficacy of trimethoprim (TMP) and streptomycin (SM). The antibiotics were begun five days before the administration of zymosan. TMP was given as 2.5 ml intragastrically (20 mg/L) twice daily for the 12 days of the study. SM was given in equal volumes (25 g/L). The control groups received water instead of the antibiotic solution. The zymosan was administered as a sterile suspension in liquid paraffin (100 mg in 4 ml per 100 g body weight). Daily bacteriologic studies of peritoneal fluid, blood, and stool as well as hematologic and biochemical studies were performed. Specimens of the abdominal organs were taken for histologic examination at death or at the end of the study. TMP eliminated the *Enterobacteriaceae* from the feces throughout the study; SM quickly eliminated the *Enterobacteriaceae*, but these species were quickly replaced by SM-resistant organisms. Surprisingly, survival was better in the SM-treated rats than in those who received TMP. Although the clinical conditions were similar in the TMP and SM-treated rats, more of the TMP rats survived compared to the SM rats (30% vs. 22%; $p > 0.05$).

This study demonstrates that severe local inflammation can induce BT with Enterobacteriaceae and that SID with TMP, and to a lesser extent with SM, effectively prevented the BT. The investigators concluded that the MOFS induced by bacteria, by nonbacterial peritonitis, or by major trauma represent generalized autoinflammatory reactions to massive toxic stimuli. The human and animal investigations complement each other so completely that they permit extrapolation of the experimental, animal data to the human condition.

In a recent article Runyon et al. studied the effect of SID with norfloxacin on BT and SBP in a rat model of cirrhosis, ascites, and SBP (113). Norfloxacin was administered to half the rats in drinking water at night in a dose of 5 mg per kg per day. The appearance of ascites was associated with weight loss, choluria, diarrhea, and lethargy. Death was induced in preterminal rats by methoxyflurane inhalation and ketamine injections. Abdominal paracentesis was performed for ascitic fluid (AF) cell counts and culture of feces and a biopsy of the liver for histologic examination was taken. SBP was defined as a positive AF culture and >250 neutrophilic leukocytes per mm^3, whereas bacterascites (BA) was defined as a positive AF culture and <250 neutrophilic leukocytes per mm^3. Both were considered to represent ''SBP.'' Virtually all 45 rats, 25 of which were receiving norfloxacin and 20 of which were untreated control animals, developed cirrhosis. Ninety-five percent had developed ascites within three to 15 weeks of CCl_4 administration. The norfloxacin greatly decreased the concentration of gram-negative bacteria in the feces ($p < 0.001$) and increased the concentration of enterococci in the stools. One-third of the treated rats grew *Xanthomonas maltophilia* from the stools ($p < 0.01$). Three-fourths of the untreated rats developed SBP compared to one-fourth in the treated group ($p < 0.01$). MLN were positive in 50% of the control and 28% of the norfloxacin-treated rats ($p > 0.05$). The AF of the untreated rats grew *E. coli*, *Pseudomonas aeruginosa*, and *Proteus* organisms; in the treated rats *S. maltophilia*, Enterobacter, and *Acinetobacter* species cultured. Half of the isolated organisms from the norfloxacin-treated rats were resistant to this antibiotic agent. Only 5% of the untreated rats grew resistant organisms. Survival, however, was not increased by norfloxacin, nor was the onset of the SBP delayed. The investigators concluded that BT preceded the development of SBP. If these pathogens are not eradicated by the host defenses, SBP may result. Quinolone resistance, however, may develop rapidly and infections with quinolone-resistant bacteria have been reported (114).

The source of most of the bacteria that induce SBP, like those responsible for the infections in patients after massive trauma and those who are critically ill, appear to be derived from the intestinal tract. The decrease in gram-negative bacteria in rats on SID is associated with an increase in the numbers of gram-positive cocci, usually enterococci. This substitution poses a practical clinical problem because enterococci are usually resistant to the conventional treatment of SBP with third-generation cephalosporin drugs. This resistance raises the specter of having to use aminoglycoside antibiotic agents, which are especially nephrotoxic in cirrhotic patients. Furthermore, the replacement of enterobacteriaceae with *X. maltophilia*, which are also resistant to broad spectrum antibiotic agents, poses a similar dilemma in patients who are receiving norfloxacin for bacterial suppression in patients undergoing bone marrow transplantation (115).

D. SPONTANEOUS BACTERIAL PERITONITIS

Just as ontogeny recapitulates phylogeny, the induction of cirrhosis in rats recapitulates SBP in humans. SBP is a common, lethal bacterial complication of cirrhosis with an incidence of 10–30% and a mortality rate of 15–20% (116). BT has been postulated to be the primary mechanism of passage of the infecting organisms from the gut to the peritoneal cavity, just as it has for gram-negative sepsis in intensive care units, for thermal injury induced sepsis, and for the sepsis associated with chemotherapy. Even though this concept is still not absolutely proven, BT is widely considered to be a paradigm of the pathogenesis of SBP.

BT has been postulated to be the mechanism of passage of the infecting organisms from the gut to the peritoneal cavity, just as it has for gram-negative sepsis in intensive care units, for burn wound sepsis, and for the sepsis associated with chemotherapy.

The rat models of SBP of Runyon and of Llovet and their coworkers, virtually duplicate every detail of SBP in humans (116,117). In both studies Sprague-Dawley rats were rendered cirrhotic by the administration of carbon tetrachloride intragastrically (20 μL per rat). The dose of CCl₄, which was begun at 20 μL per rat, was decreased in rats that were losing weight and increased to 60 μL in those that were not. In this reliable model ascites usually develops within 8 to 12 weeks after CCl₄ has been begun.

Emaciation, lethargy, and choluria developed, and if diarrhea appeared, death usually followed. The rats were sacrificed and ascitic fluid cell count, and cultures of the ascitic fluid, portal venous blood, systemic blood, and mesenteric lymph nodes were examined. More than half the animals that survived the administration of CCl$_4$ developed cirrhosis and ascites (32 of 54; 59%) within two to four months, and 25 of them (78%) developed bacterial translocation. Two-thirds developed SBP, which was defined as a positive bacterial culture from the ascitic fluid and >250 neutrophilic leukocytes per cubic millimeter in the ascitic fluid, or bacterascites, which was defined as a positive culture with the neutrophil count >250 per cubic millimeter in the AF in the absence of any surgically treatable, intra-abdominal infection. Either SBP or BA were considered to represent SBP. The bacteria cultured were usually *E. coli*, *Proteus* species, *Klebsiella oxytocia* occasionally, *Citrobacter freundi*, Group D streptococci, otherwise unidentified gram-negative rods, and rarely enterococci. All the rats with SBP also had positive lymph node cultures, but not all that developed BT exhibited SBP. The lymph nodes in the cirrhotic, translocated animals were significantly larger and darker in color than in those who had not shown BT. Normal control rats or those that had received only one or two doses of CCl$_4$, which had been administered to all animals before the CCl$_4$ was begun, did not develop cirrhosis or translocation. Portal venous blood was positive in one-fourth of the rats with BT, but the systemic blood was always sterile. Thus, BT is not equivalent to and does not guarantee the occurrence of SBP, bacterascites, or bacteremia. Only a single control rat developed BT. These observations suggest that differential bacterial filtration exists along the route from lymph nodes to ascitic fluid to portal venous blood to systemic blood, but there are no clues about where this filtration occurs.

This model, like those induced by extensive burns, severe sepsis, chemotherapy, malnutrition, and hemorrhagic shock, indicates that BT precedes SBP. Furthermore, the bacteriologic species cultured in the rodents are almost identical to those isolated from humans with SBP.

In this model, most of the animals who did not die of acute CCl$_4$ toxicity developed cirrhosis. Of the 32 rats, 31 developed ascites within 8 to 12 weeks (97%) and 25 of them developed BT (78%), almost all with *E. coli* and occasionally with a second organism as well. Sixteen of the 25 (64%) developed SBP or bacterascites. All the rats who developed SBP had positive MLN cultures, but not all rats that exhibited BT developed SBP. Furthermore, portal venous blood was positive in about one-fourth of the animals, but the systemic blood was always sterile. Thus, BT does not necessarily precede the development of SBP or bacteremia. Only a single control rat developed BT.

Many factors may be involved including altered permeability associated with the intestinal edema of portal hypertension and the immune incompetence of cirrhosis.

ACKNOWLEDGMENT

The author acknowledges the generous permission of Dr. J. W. Alexander and his coauthors and editors and the publishers of the *Annals of Surgery* for permission to reproduce Figures 7.1–7.5.

ABBREVIATIONS

AF	Ascitic fluid
APACHE	Acute physiology and chronic health evaluation
BA	Bacterascites
BPIP	Bacteriocidal permeability-increasing protein
BT	Bacterial translocation
CCK	Colecystokinin
DMDP	Dichloromethylene diphosphonate
EIAP	Elevated intraabdominal pressure
GALT	Gut-associated lymphatic tissues
GI	Gastrointestinal
ICU	Intensive care unit
ISS	Injury severity score
IVC	Inferior vena cava
IL 6	Interleukin 6
MLN	Mesenteric lymph nodes
MODS	Multiple organ dysfunction syndrome
MOF	Multiple organ failure
MOFS	Multiple organ failure syndrome
PN	Parenteral nutrition
PTA	Polymyxin E. tobramycin, amphoterin
PTC	Polymixin E. tobramycin, ciprofloxacin
RCT	Randomized clinical trial
SEM	Scanning electron microscope
SID	Selective intestinal decontamination
SBP	Spontaneous bacterial peritonitis
SM	Streptomycin
TEM	Transmission electron microscope
TMP	Trimethoprim
TNF	Tumor necrosis factor
TPN	Total parenteral nutrition
Z	Zymosan
ZIP	Zymosan-induced peritonitis

REFERENCES

1. Keller R, Engley FB Jr. Fate of bacteriophage particles introduced into mice by various routes. Proc Soc Exp Bio Med 109:183–185, 1958.
2. Wolochow H, Hildebrand G, Lamanna C. Translocation of microorganisms across the intestinal wall of the rat: effect of microbial size and concentration. J Infec Dis 116:523–528, 1966.
3. Berg RD, Garlington AW. Translocation of certain indigenous bacteria from the gastrointestinal tract to the mesenteric lymph nodes and other organs in a gnotobiotic mouse model. Infect Immunity 23:403–411, 1979.
4. Berg RD. Bacterial translocation from the gastrointestinal tract. J Med 23:217–244, 1992.
5. Berg RD. Mechanisms confining indigenous bacteria to the gastrointestinal tract. Amer J Clin Nutr 33:2472–2484, 1980.
6. Berg RD. Bacterial translocation from the intestines. Expt Animals 34:1–16, 1985.
7. Berg RD. Bacterial translocation from the gastrointestinal tract. Comp Ther 16:8–15, 1990.
8. Hentges DJ. Role of the intestinal microflora in the defense against infection. In: *Human Intestinal Microflora in Health and Disease*, Hentges DJ, ed., New York: Academic Press, pp. 311–331.
9. Carter PB, Collins FM. The route of enteric infection in normal mice. J Expt Med 139:1189–1203, 1964.
10. Berg RD. Bacterial translocation from the gastrointestinal tracts of mice receiving immunosuppressive chemotherapeutic agents. Curr Microbio 8:285–292, 1983.
11. Gautreaux MD, Deitch EA, Berg RD. Immunological mechanisms preventing bacterial translocation from the gastrointestinal tract. In: *Proceedings of the 10th Int Symp Gnotobiology*, Heidt P, ed., Leiden, The Netherlands, 1990.
12. Berg RD, Wommack E, Deitch EA. Immunosuppression and intestinal bacterial overgrowth synergistically promote bacterial translocation. Arch Surg 123:1359–1364, 1988.
13. Owens WE, Berg RD. Bacterial translocation from the gastrointestinal tract of athymic (nu/nu) mice. Infect Immunity 27:461–465, 1980.
14. Owens WE, Berg RD. Bacterial translocation from the gastrointestinal tracts of thymectomized mice. Curr Microbio 7:169–174, 1982.
15. Morehouse J, Specian R, Stewart J, Berg RD. Promotion of the translocation of indigenous bacteria of mice from the GI tract by oral ricinoleic acid. Gastroenterology 91:673–682, 1986.
16. Gaginella TS, Phillips SF. Ricinoleic acid (castor oil) alters intestinal surface structure. Mayo Clinic Proc 51:6–12, 1976.
17. Baker JW, Deitch EA, Ma I, Berg R. Hemorrhagic shock promotes the systemic translocation of bacteria from the gut. J Trauma 28:896–906, 1988.

18. Parks DA, Bulkley GB, Granger DN, Hamilton SR, McCord JM. Ischemic injury in the cat small intestine: role of superoxide radicals. Gastroenterology 82: 9–15, 1982.

19. Deitch EA, Bridges WR, Baker J, Ma J-W, Ma L, Grisharn M, Granger N, Specian R, Berg R. Hemorrhagic shock-induced bacterial translocation is reduced by xanthine oxidase inhibition or inactivation. Surgery 104:191–198, 1988.

20. Deitch EA, Bridges W, Baker J. Hemorrhagic shock-induced bacterial translocation is reduced by xanthine oxidase inhibition or inactivation. Surgery 104: 191–198, 1988.

21. Deitch E, Maejima K, Berg RD. Effect of oral antibiotics and bacterial overgrowth on the translocation of the GI tract microflora in burned rats. J Trauma 25:385–392, 1985.

22. Maejima K, Deitch EA, Berg RD. Bacterial translocation from the gastrointestinal tract of rats receiving thermal injury. Infect Immun 43:6–10, 1984.

23. Ravin HA, Fine J. Biological implications of intestinal endotoxins. Fed Proc 21:65–68, 1962.

24. Carrico CJ, Meakins JL, Marshall JC, Fry D, Maier RV. Multiple organ failure syndrome. Arch Surg 121:196–208, 1986.

25. Deitch EA, Ma W-J, Ma L, Berg R, Specian R. Endotoxin-induced bacterial translocation: a study of mechanisms. Surgery 106:292–300, 1989.

26. Moore FA, Moore EE, Poggetti R, McAnena OJ, Peterson VM, Abernathy CM, Parsons PE. Gut bacterial translocaton via the portal vein: a clinical perspective with major torso trauma. J Trauma 31: 629–638, 1991.

27. Deitch EA, Rutan FT, Waymack JP. Trauma, shock and gut translocation. New Horiz 4:289–299, 1996.

28. Goris RJ, Beokhorst PA, Nuytinck KS. Multiple organ failure: Generalized autodestructive inflammation. Arch Surg 120:1109–1115, 1985.

29. Deitch EA. Bacterial translocation of gut flora: Proceedings on NIH conference on advances in understanding trauma and burn injury. J Trauma 30 (suppl): S184–S188, 1990.

30. Maejima K, Deitch EA, Berg R. Bacterial translocation from the gastrointestinal tracts of rats receiving thermal injury. Infect Immun 43: 6–10, 1984.

31. Rush BF Jr, Sori AJ, Murphy TF. Endotoxemia and bacteremia during hemorrhagic shock. Ann Surg 207;549–554, 1988.

32. Deitch EA, Macjima K, Berg RD. Effect of oral antibiotics and bacterial overgrowth on the translocation of the GI-tract microflora in burned rats. J Trauma 25:385–392, 1985.

33. Wang X, Andersson R, Soltesz V, Bengmark S. Bacterial translocation after major hepatectomy in patients and rats. Arch Surg 127:1101–1106, 1992.

34. Deitch EA, Bridges WR, Ma JW, Ma L, Berg RD, Specian RD. The obstructed intestine as a reservoir for systemic infection. Amer J Surg 159:394–401, 1990.

35. Deitch EA, Bridges W, Baker J. Hemorrhagic shock-induced bacterial translocation is reduced by xanthine oxidase inhibition or inactivation. Surgery 104: 191–198, 1988.

36. Xu D, Lu Q, Deitch EA. Calcium and phospholipase A appear to be involved in the pathogenesis of hemorrhagic shock-induced mucosal injury and bacterial translocation. Crit Care Med 23:125–131, 1995.

37. Tokay R, Loick HM, Traber DL. Effects of thromboxane synthetase inhibition on postburn mesenteric vascular resistance and the rate of bacterial translocation in a chronic porcine model. Surg Gyn and Obstet 174:125–132, 1992.

38. Ryan CM, Yarmush ML, Burke JF. Increased gut permeability early after burn correlated with the extent of burn injury. Crit Care Med 20:1508–1512, 1991.

39. Brathwaite CEM, Ross SE, Nagele R. Bacterial translocation occurs in humans after traumatic injury: evidence using immunofluorescence. J Trauma 34:586–590, 1993.

40. Zabel DD, Hopf HW, Hunt TK. Transmural gut oxygen gradients in shocked rats resuscitated with heparin. Arch Surg 130:59–63, 1995.

41. Matsuda T, Tamaka H, Reyes RM. Antioxidant therapy using high dose vitamin C: Reduction of postburn resuscitation fluid volume requirements. World J Surg 19:287–291, 1995.

42. Pierro A, van Saene HKF, Donnell SC, Hughes J, Ewan C, Nunn AJ, Lloyd DA. Microbial translocation in neonates and infants receiving long-term parenteral nutrition. Arch Surg 131:176–179, 1996.

43. Alexander JW. The process of microbial translocation. Ann Surg 212:496–512, 1996.

44. Hildebrand GJ, Wolochow H. Translocation of bacteriophage across the intestinal wall of the rat. Proc Soc Exp Biol Med 109:183–185, 1962.

44a. Ersoz G, Aydin A, Erdem S, Yuksel D, Akarca U, Kumanlioglu K. Intestinal permeability in liver cirrhosis. Eur J Gastroenterol Hepatol 11:409–412, 1999.

45. Wang XD, et al. Bacterial translocation in acute liver failure induced by 90 percent hepatectomy in the rat. Br J Surg 80:66–71, 1993.

46. Wang XD, Ar'Rajab A, Andersson R, Soltesz V, Wang M, Svensson M, Bengmark S. The influence of surgically induced acute liver failure on the intestine in the rat. Scand J Gastroenterol 25:31–10, 1993.

47. Rolando N, Harvey F, Brahm J. Prospective study of bacterial infection in acute liver failure: an analysis of fifty patients. Hepatology 11:49–53, 1990.

48. Decker K, Keppler D. Galactosamine hepatitis. Rev Physiol Biochem Pharmacol 71:77–106, 1974.

49. Kasravi FB, Wang L, Wang X-D, Molin G, Bengmark S, Jeppsson B. Bacterial translocation in acute liver injury induced by D-galactosamine. Hepatology 23:97–103, 1996.

50. Garcia-Tsao G, Albillos A, Garden GE, West AB. Bacterial translocation in acute and chronic portal hypertension. Hepatology 17:1081–1085, 1993.

51. Vauthey J-N, Duda P, Wheatley AM, Gertsch P. Portal hypertension promotes

bacterial translocation in rats mono-and non-mono-associated with *Escherichia coli* C25. HPB Surgery 8:95–100, 1994.

52. Sorell WT, Quigley EMM, Jim G, Johnson TJ, Rikkers LF. Bacterial translocation in the portal-hypertensive rat: studies in basal conditions and on exposure to hemorrhagic shock. Gastroenterology 104:1722–1726, 1993.

53. Maejima K, Deitch E, Berg R. Promotion by burn stress of the translocation of bacteria from the gastrointestinal tracts of mice. Arch Surg 119:166–172, 1984.

54. Markley K, Smallman L, Evans C: Mortality of germfree and conventional mice after thermal trauma. Am J Physiol 209:365–370, 1965.

55. Ammon HV, Thomas PJ, Phillips SF. Effects of oleic acid and ricinoleic acids on net jejunal and electrolyte movement. J Clin Invest 53:374–379, 1974.

56. Owens RL, Jones AL. Epithelial cell specialization within human Peyer's patches: An ultrastructural study of intestinal lymphoid follicles. Gastroenterology 66:189–203, 1974.

57. Imai A, Kurihara Y. Endogenous infection in mice with streptozotocin-induced diabetes. A feature of bacterial translocation. Can J Microbiol 30:1344–1348, 1984.

58. Alverdy J, Aoys E. The effect of corticosteroid administration on bacterial translocation. Evidence for an acquired mucosal immunodeficient state. Ann Surg 214:719–723, 1991.

59. Berg RD. Translocation of indigenous bacteria from the gastrointestinal tracts of mice by oral treatment with penicillin, clindamycin or metronidazole. Infect Immun 33:333–352, 1983.

60. Berg RD. Bacterial translocation from the gastrointestinal tracts of mice receiving immunosuppressive chemotherapeutic agents. Curr Micro 8:285–292, 1983.

61. Berg RD. Immunosuppression and intestinal bacterial overgrowth synergistically promote bacterial translocation. Arch Surg 123:1359–1364, 1988.

62. Seifert J, Nitsche D, Gröper H. Influence of immunoglobulin and interleukin 2 on the translocation of microorganisms from gut into blood. J Anat 139:549–552, 1996.

63. Penn RL, Nguyen VQ, Special RD, Steven P, Berg RD. Interleukin-2 enhances the translocation of *Escherichia coli* from the intestines to other organs. J Infec Dis 164:1168–1172, 1991.

64. Deitch EA, Wen-Jing MA, Li Ma, Berg RD, Special RD. Protein malnutrition predisposes to inflammatory-induced gut-origin septic states. Ann Surg 211:560–568, 1990.

65. Deitch EA. Multiple organ failure. Ann Surg 216:117–134, 1992.

66. Mishima S, Yudioda T, Matsuda H, Shimazaki S. Mild hypotension and body burns synergistically increase bacterial translocation in rats consistent with a "two-hit phenomenon." J Burn Care Rehab 18:L22–26, 1997.

67. Deitch EA, Berg R, Special R. Endotoxin promotes the translocation of bacteria from the gut. Arch Surg 122:185–190, 1987.

68. Ohsugi T, Kiuchi Y, Shimoda K, Oguri S, Maejima K. Translocation of bacteria

from the gastrointestinal tract in immunodeficient mice. Lab Animals 30:46–50, 1996.

69. Tarpila E, Nyström P-O, Franzén L, Ihse I. Bacterial translocation during acute pancreatitis in rats. Eur J Surg 159:109–113, 1993.

70. Marotta F, Geng TC, Wu CC, Barbi G. Bacterial translocation in the course of acute pancreatitis: beneficial role of nonabsorbable antibiotic and lactitol enemas. Digestion 57:446–452, 1996.

71. Conn HO. A clinical hepatologist's predictions about non-absorbed carbohydrates for the early twenty-first century. Scand J Gastroenterol 222:88–92, 1997.

72. Ambrose MS, Johnson M, Burdon DW, Keighley MRB. Incidence of pathogenic bacteria from mesenteric lymph nodes and ileal serosa during Crohn's disease surgery. Br J Surg 71:623–625, 1984.

73. Deitch EA. Simple intestinal obstruction causes bacterial translocation in man. Arch Surg 124:699–701, 1989.

74. Tancrede CH, Andremont AO. Bacterial translocation and gram-negative bacteremia in patients with hematological malignancies. J Infect Dis 152:99–104, 1985.

75. Klein RS, Catalano MT, Edberg SC, Casey JI, Steigbigel NH. *Streptococcus bovis* septicemia and carcinoma of the colon. Ann Intern Med 91:560–562, 1979.

76. Klein RS, Recco RA, Catalano MT, Edberg SC, Casey JI, Steigbigel NH. Association of *Streptococcus bovis* with carcinoma of the colon. N Engl J Med 297:800–802, 1977.

77. Roses DF, Richman H, Localio SA. Bacterial endocarditis associated with colorectal carcinoma. Ann Surg 179:190–191, 1974.

78. Vincent P, Colombel JF, Lescut D, Fournier L, Savage C, Cortot A, Quandalle P, Vandemmel M, Leclerc H. Bacterial translocation in patients with colorectal cancer. J Inf Dis 158:1395–1399, 1988.

79. Moore FA, Moore EE, Poggetti RS, Read RA. Postinjury shock and early bacteremia. A lethal combination. Arch Surg 127:893–898, 1992.

80. Kanematsu K, Takenada K, Furuta T, Ezaki O, Sugimachi K, Inokuchi K. Acute portal hypertension associated with liver resection. Arch Surg 120:1303–1305, 1985.

81. Ferri M, Gabriel S, Gavelli A, Franconeri P, Guguet C. Bacterial translocation during portal clamping for liver resection. A clinical study. Arch Surg 132:162–165, 1997.

82. Bower RH, Talamini MA, Sax SC. Postoperative enteral versus parenteral nutrition. Arch Surg 121:1040–1045, 1986.

83. Moore FA, Feliciano DV, Andrassy RJ. Early enteral feeding compared with parenteral, reduces postoperative septic complications. The results of meta-analysis. Ann Surg 216:172–183, 1991.

84. Chesta J, Deflippi C, Deflippi C. Abnormalities in proximal small bowel motility in patients with cirrhosis. Hepatology 17:828–832, 1993.

85. Kudsk DA, Carpenter G, Sheldon GF. Effect of enteral and parenteral feeding of malnourished rats with *E. coli*-hemoglobin adjuvant peritonitis. J Surg Res 31:105–110, 1981.
86. Shirabe K, Matsurnata T, Shimada M, Takenaka K, Kawahara N, Yamamoto K, Nishizaki T, Sugimachi K. A comparison of parenteral hyperalimentation and early enteral feeding regarding systemic immunity after major hepatic resection—the results of a randomized prospective study. Hepatogastroenterology 44:205–209, 1997.
87. Pierro A, van Saene HKF, Donnell SC, Hughes J, Ewan C, Nunn AJ, Lloyed DA. Microbial translocation in neonates and infants receiving long-term parenteral nutrition. Arch Surg 131:176–179, 1996.
88. Sedman PC, MacFie J, Palmer MD, Mitchell CJ, Sagar PM. Preoperative total parenteral nutrition is not associated with mucosal atrophy or bacterial translocation in humans. Br J Surg 82:1163–1167, 1995.
89. Tani T, Hanasawa K, Endo Y, Kurumi Y, Shiomi H, Kidama M, Kushima R, Hattori T. Bacterial translocation as a cause of septic shock in humans: a report of two cases. Jpn J Surg 27:447–449, 1997.
90. van Goor H, Rosman C, Grond J, Kooi K, Wübbels GH, Bleichrodt RP. Translocation of bacteria and endotoxin in organ donors. Arch Surg 129:1066–1067, 1994.
91. Reed LL, Martin M, Manglano R, Newson B, Kocka F, Barrett J. Bacterial translocation following abdominal trauma in humans. Circulatory Shock 42:1–6, 1994.
92. Brathwaite CEM, Ross SE, Nagele R. Bacterial translocation occurs in humans after traumatic injury: incidence using immunofluorescence. J Trauma 34:586–593, 1993.
93. Peitzman AB, Udekwu AO, Ochoa J, Smith S. Bacterial translocation in trauma patients, J Trauma 31:1083–1087, 1991.
94. Lignau W, Berger J, Javorsky F, Lejeune P, Mutz N, Benzer H. Selective intestinal decontamination in multiple trauma patients: prospective, controlled trial. J Trauma Injury and Crit Care 42:687–694, 1997.
95. Baker SP, O'Neill B, Haddon W. The injury severity score: A method for describing patients with multiple injuries and evaluating emergency care. J Trauma 14:187–194, 1974.
96. Knaus WA, Draper EA, Wagner DP. APACHE II: a severity of disease classification system. Crit Care Med 13:818–829, 1985.
97. Tran DD, Cuesta MA, Van Leeuwen PA, Nauta JJ, Wesdorp RL. Risk factors for multiple organ system failure and death in critically injured patients. Surgery 114:21–30, 1993.
98. Moore FA, Moore EE, Poggetti R, McAnena OJ, Peterson VM, Abernathy CM, Parsons PE. Gut bacterial translocation via the portal vein: a clinical perspective with major torso trauma. J Trauma 31:629–638, 1991.
99. Stechmiller JK, Treloar D, Allen N. Gut dysfunction in critically ill patients: a review of the literature. Am J Crit Care 6:204–209, 1997.

100. Shannon FL, Moore EE, Moore FA, McCroskey BL. Value of distal colon washout in civilian rectal trauma—reducing gut bacterial translocation. J Trauma 28:989–994, 1988.
101. MacFie J. Bacterial translocation in surgical patients. Ann Royal Coll Surg Eng 79:183–189, 1997.
102. Sedman PC, MacFie J, Sagar P, Mitchell CJ, May J, Mancey-Jones B, Johnstone D. The prevalence of gut translocation in humans. Gastroenterology 107:643–649, 1994.
103. Sedman PC, MacFie J, Palmer MD. Preoperative total parenteral nutrition is not associated with mucosal atrophy or bacterial translocation in humans. Br J Surg 82:1663–1667, 1995.
104. O'Boyle C, MacFie J, Mitchell CJ. The microbiology of bacterial translocation in humans. Gut, in press.
105. O'Boyle C, Macfie J, Dave K. Alterations in intestinal barrier function do not predispose to translocation of enteric bacteria in gastroenterological patients. Br J Surg, in press.
106. Sittig K, Deitch EA. Effect of bacteremia on mortality after thermal injury. Arch Surg 123:1367–1370, 1988.
107. Rush BF, Sori AJ, Murphy TF. Endotoxemia and bacteremia during hemorrhagic shock. Ann Surg 207:549–554, 1988.
108. Wilmore EW, Smith RJ, O'Dwyer ST. The gut: a central organ after surgical stress. Surgery 104:917–923, 1988.
109. Goris RJA, Boekholtz WKF, van Bebber IPT, Nuytinck JKS, Schillings PHM. Multiple-organ failure and sepsis without bacteria. Arch Surg 121:897–901, 1986.
110. Goris RJA, van Bebber IPT, Mollen RME, Koopman JP. Does selective decontamination of the gastrointestinal tract prevent multiple organ failure? An experimental study. Arch Surg 126:561–565, 1991.
111. Kerver AJH, Rommes JH, Mevissen-Verhage EAE. Previous colonization and infection in critically ill patients: a prospective randomized study. Crit Care Med 16:1087–1093, 1988.
112. Ulrich C, Harinck-de Weerd JE, Bakker NC, Jak ZK, Doorn Ridder VA. Selective decontamination of the digestive tract with norfloxacin the prevention of ICU-acquired infections: a prospective randomized trial. Intensive Care Med 15:424–431, 1989.
113. Runyon BA, Borzio M, Young SU, Squier S, Guarner C, Runyon MA. Effect of selective bowel decontamination with norfloxacin on spontaneous bacterial peritonitis, translocation, and survival in an animal model of cirrhosis. Hepatology 21:1719–1724, 1995.
114. Novella NK Soriano G, Gana J, Andreu M, Ortiz J, Coll S, Sabat M. Prophylaxis of the first spontaneous bacterial peritonitis in cirrhotic patients. (Abstract). Hepatology 20:115A, 1994.
115. Khardori N, Reuben A, Rosenbaum B, Rolston K, Body GP. *In vitro* suscepti-

bility of *Xanthomonas (Pseudomonas) maltophilia* to newer antimicrobial agents. Antimicrob Agents Chermother 34:1609–1610, 1990.

116. Kaymakoglu S, Eraksoy H, Ökten A, Demir K, Çalangu S, Çakaloglu Y, Boztas G, Besisik F. Spontaneous ascitic infection in different cirrhotic groups: prevalence, risk factors and the efficacy of cefotaxime therapy. Eur J Gastrol & Hepatol 9:71–76, 1996.

117. Runyon B, Squier S, Borzio M. Translocation of gut bacteria in rats with cirrhosis to mesenteric lymph nodes partially explains the pathogenesis of spontaneous bacterial peritonitis. J Hepatol 21:792–796, 1994.

118. Llovet JM, Rodriguez-Iglesias P, Moltinho E, Planas R, Bataller R, Navasa M, Menacho M, Pardo A, Castells A, Cabre E, Arroyo V, Gassull M, Rodes J. Spontaneous bacterial peritonitis in patients with cirrhosis undergoing selective intestinal decontamination. J Hepatol 26:88–95, 1997.

8

Prevention of Bacterial Translocation

Harold O. Conn
*Yale University School of Medicine, New Haven, Connecticut, and
University of Miami School of Medicine, Miami, Florida*

I. INTRODUCTION

A large number of reports of investigations that deal with the induction of
BT* have been published. It appears, however, that BT can be prevented in
at least as many ways as it can be induced (see Chap. 7). The great variety
of agents, substances, and procedures employed to induce BT in these experiments and the many hypotheses, therapies, and preventive measures utilized
render simple, rational classification extremely difficult. We have therefore
arbitrarily arranged them in a functional order based primarily on the primary
preventive mechanisms used. Some of these investigations present both multiple promoters and "preventers" rather than a single promoter and a single
preventive principle for each experiment.

Studies of the prevention of BT are more complicated investigations
than those that study the induction of BT. An induction study simply requires
a susceptible animal and an inducing agent or procedure. Each prevention
study requires an experimental model in which the agent, substance, or procedure that promotes BT be compared with the promoting agent *plus* a suppressing agent or procedure that suppresses or prevents BT. Both of these
requirements must be controlled. Indeed, each such "prevention" study is like

---

* A list of the abbreviations used in this chapter is given on p. 143.

one of a series of controlled investigations in which the promoting procedure and its control group are compared with the results of the promoting procedure *plus* the suppressing procedure. Surprisingly, a large number of these promotion–prevention studies have already been performed and published.

It is reasonable to assume that substances and/or procedures with actions opposite to those identified as promoters of BT may be tried as inhibitors of BT. If, for example, BT were caused by the overgrowth of bacteria in the intestinal tract, it is reasonable to assume that antibiotic agents that suppress bacterial overgrowth may be able to inhibit BT. Indeed, such studies have been published.

II. SUPPRESSION OF INTESTINAL FLORA ANTIBIOTIC AGENTS IN PREVENTION OF BT

Brook and Ledney studied the effects of irradiation-induced BT and their prevention by antibiotic agents by using groups of 60 mice (C$_3$H/HeN) that were given 8.2 Gy of ^{60}Co radiation (1) (see also Table 8.1). They observed an 85% mortality rate in the control group, a 77% mortality rate in those treated with ofloxacin (p < 0.05), and only an 8% rate in those who received both ofloxacin and penicillin (p < 0.001). Enterobacteriaceae and streptococci were recovered from the livers of the control mice. A decrease in the number of Enterobacteriaceae was noted in the ofloxacillin-treated group, and a reduction in the number of streptococci were noted in the penicillin-treated patients. The numbers of both types of bacteria were reduced in the mice that received both antibiotic agents. These observations demonstrate that this type of BT can be prevented by antibiotic therapy, and provide much food for thought.

Goris et al. studied the preventive effect of selective intestinal decontamination (SID) on zymosan-induced BT and on the multiple organ failure syndrome (MOFS) in rats that had received zymosan (2), which causes intense peritoneal inflammation and simulates BT. Zymosan was administered intraperitoneally in a dose of 4 mg suspended in liquid paraffin to 250–300 g Wistar rats. SID was instituted using trimethoprim (TMP) (2.5 ml of a 20 g/L solution) intragastrically twice daily for five days preceding the administration of zymosan and once daily for the next 12 days. This antibiotic agent suppressed Enterobacteriaceae but had little effect on other bacteria. The control rats received sterile water instead of the TMP solution. In a second study the rats were given streptomycin (SM) (2.5 ml of a 25 g/L solution) on the same schedule as the TMP solution. Fecal cultures demonstrated that both

Table 8.1 Prevention of Bacterial Translocation I: Administration of Antibiotic Agents

First author	Ref. No.	Animal species	Induction of BT	Prevention of BT	Results of therapy
Brook	1	Mice	Irradiation	Ofloxacin (Of) Penicillin (Pen) Of plus Pen	Reduces mortality Decreases enterobacteria Decreases streptococci Decreases enterobacteria and strepto-cocci
Goris	2	Rats	Zymosan	Trimethoprim Streptomycin	Suppresses bacteria growth Increases motility
Yao	3	Rats	Burn (70%)	SID: Polymyxin, Tobramycin, 5-Flucytosine	Attenuates cell-mediated immune dysfunction Suppresses intestinal bacteria
Marotta	4	Rats	Pancreatitis (intrabiliary trypsin/enterokinase)	Rifaximin (Enema) Rifaximin plus lactitol	Decreases blood endotoxin levels Decreases infection of MLN, AF Decreases histologic injury
Privitera	5	Pigs	Small bowel/liver trans-plantation	Pefloxacin	Reduces enterobacteria Reduces streptococci
Runyon	6	Rats	Cirrhosis	Norfloxacin	Reduces SBP Decreases gram-negative bacteria Survival unchanged
Shannon	9	Humans	Rectal trauma, extra-peritoneal	Proximal colostomy Distal colon washout Broad spectrum antibiotic	Decreases septic mortality Decreases bacterial sepsis Suppresses cecal bacteria

antibiotic programs were effective, but that TMP was more so because of recolonization with SM-resistant bacteria in the SM-treated group. On the other hand, the survival rate was higher in the SM-treated animals. The emergence of SM-resistant species so rapidly is, of course, an undesirable consequence of such therapy.

Yao et al. reported that selective intestinal decontamination with polymixin E, tobramycin, and 5-flucytosine administered together ameliorated burn injury and BT in Sprague-Dawley rats (3). These findings suggest that BT may be a manifestation of cell-mediated immune dysfunction, which can be attenuated by SID, presumably by virtue of its antibiotic activities.

Marotta et al. studied the effects of the suppression of enteric bacteria in four groups of Wistar rats in which acute necrotizing pancreatitis was induced by the intrabiliary injection of a trypsin-enterokinase mixture (4). Group I (control) received no treatment. Group II rats received daily enemas (30 ml) containing 20 mg/kg rifaximin. Group III received the rifaximin enema plus lactitol (0.5 g/kg). Group IV (control) was given daily saline enemas. Animals were sacrificed after 6, 12, 24, and 72 h. Ascitic fluid (AF), mesenteric lymph nodes (MLN), pancreas, spleen, arterial and portal venous blood, and bile were cultured. Both enema-treated groups showed a significant increase in survival. Blood endotoxin levels progressively increased in the untreated rats (Groups I and IV) but were suppressed in the treated groups (II and III). The AF was frequently infected with enteric organisms. BT was present in nodes close to the pancreas. Histologic evidence of damage to the pancreas was less severe in the rifaximin-treated groups. Rifaximin enemas were effective in minimizing the increase in endotoxin concentrations, in suppressing the infections of AF and MLN, and in preventing histologic injury. Lactitol, which also alters the intestinal bacterial population, may also have anti-BT activity.

Privitera and colleagues found that parenteral fluoroquinolones, such as pefloxacin, administered postoperatively, prevented BT in Landrace pigs after small bowel transplantation or liver-small bowel transplantation (5). Pefloxacin, a systemic fluoroquinolone antibiotic agent, reduced the endoluminal bacterial counts of enterobacteria and enterococci. The number of animals studied reported is small and the duration of follow-up is short. Further studies of this complex model are needed.

Runyon and his coworkers studied the effects of selective bowel decontamination (SID) with norfloxicin in Sprague-Dawley rats with carbon tetrachloride-induced cirrhosis (6). All rats had ascites and were prone to develop BT and/or SBP and to die. The rats were given either norfloxacin in drinking water or plain water. Seventy percent of the untreated rats developed bacterial peritonitis compared to 28% of the antibiotic-treated animals (p < 0.02). Although BT was reduced from 50% in the untreated group to 28% of the treated animals, this difference was not statistically significant. Gram-positive organisms were isolated from the MLN in 100% of the episodes of SBP, and in 71% of the MLN in the untreated animals compared to only 10% of the MLN in the treated group. Survival was similar in the two groups. Although norfloxacin greatly reduced the numbers of gram-negative bacteria in the stools and the rate of developing SBP, it *increased* the risk of developing gram-positive BT and peritonitis. It did not improve survival, however. The investigators expressed concern about the isolation of *Xanthomonas maltophilia* from the stool and ascitic fluid of the treated rats and of *Enterobacter* and *Acinetobacter* from their lymph nodes (7). These organisms, which are often found in immunosupressed individuals, are extremely antibiotic-resistant. In a related investigation by Lignau et al. in humans with severe trauma, SID with multiple broad-spectrum antibiotic agents was shown to reduce intestinal bacterial colonization but did not reduce the rates of MOFS (8). It appears that SID may not be the whole answer to the SBP and postsurgical sepsis problems.

Shannon et al., in a retrospective study of the value of washout of the human distal colon after extraperitoneal rectal trauma plus antibiotic therapy, reported that BT was reduced by proximal colostomy and intraoperative washout of the distal, rectosigmoid colon plus broad spectrum antibiotic therapy (9). They concluded that this procedure reduced septic morbidity. Unfortunately, they never mentioned in the article how many patients in the treatment and control groups had actually developed BT, or how the diagnosis of BT was established. Furthermore, they never indicated whether the control and treatment groups were selected randomly. From the wording in the article, I suspect not. Consequently, the reader should keep these caviats in mind.

Clearly, antibiotic agents can suppress BT induced in a variety of ways in a variety of animal species. Numerous antibiotic substances are effective. Prophylactic SID is effective especially in preventing BT and SBP. In situations in which antibiotic agents have been used in combination with other antibacterial approaches, such as the mechanical removal of the bacteria, the antibiotic treatment appears to be the predominant factor in the prevention of BT.

III. ARGININE AND RELATED DIETARY ADDITIVES WITH ANTIENDOTOXIN PROPERTIES IN THE PREVENTION OF BT

Endotoxin has been shown to induce BT in Sprague-Dawley rats (10) (see Table 8.2). However, there is an antidote for endotoxin-induced BT. Adjei

Table 8.2 Prevention of Bacterial Translocation II: Administration of Antiendotoxin-Suppressing Substances

First author	Ref. No.	Animal species	Induction of BT	Prevention of BT	Results of therapy
Adjei	11	Mice	Endotoxin	Arginine (2%, 4%)	Reduces rate of BT Reduces mortality Reduces colony count
Gennari	13	Mice	Bacterial overgrowth (E. coli) Burn (30%)	Arginine Glutamine and/or fish oil	Enhances bacterial killing Improves mucosal barrier function
Gianotti	14	Mice	Cecal ligation Cecal puncture Bacterial overgrowth Burn (70%) Blood transfusion	Nα NL-Arg	Improves survival Increases bacterial killing
Gonce	17	Guinea pigs	Endotoxin	Arginine	Enhances bacterial killing
Sorrels	18	Rats	Endotoxin	Aminoguanidine	Decreases BT
Rannekampff	19	Mice	Burn	BPIP	Decreases BT Inhibits endotoxin

and his associates studied the effects of an arginine-supplemented diet (11) because arginine has been shown to have beneficial immunomodulating activity in infected animals (12). In their endotoxin-induced BT model in mice, they demonstrated that arginine (2% and 4%) reduced the percentage of BT induced by *E. coli*-derived lipopolysaccharide (endotoxin) from 100% in the untreated control group to about 60% in the 2% arginine group and to about 40% in the 4% arginine group. Furthermore, mortality rates and colony counts in the MLN, spleen, and cecum were all significantly decreased by arginine supplementation (p < 0.05). They speculated that arginine enhances the clearance of translocated microorganisms and results in improved survival.

Gennari et al. induced BT in BALB/c mice that had been maintained on the AIN-76A semipurified diet, after which they were challenged by gavage with 10^{10} *E. coli*, by homologous blood transfusions, which leads to immunosuppression and increased susceptibility to infection, and by a burn injury of 30% of the body surface (13). The mice were maintained on the basal diet supplemented by either (a) fish oil (FO) plus glutamine, (b) arginine plus glutamine, or (c) FO plus arginine. Four hours after burn injury the animals were sacrificed and assessed for BT in MLN, spleen, and liver. Quantitative colony counts were performed to assess the number of the gavaged bacteria recovered.

Although all of the dietary-supplemented animals showed improved outcomes in this gut-derived sepsis model, the mechanisms of improvement differed. Mice supplemented with FO plus glutamine exhibited decreased BT to the liver and spleen. Mice supplemented with arginine plus glutamine had an increased capacity to kill translocated bacteria in the liver. Mice supplemented with FO plus arginine had improved mucosal barrier function and decreased BT as well as enhanced microbial killing. The beneficial effects of arginine supplementation appear to be clear. However, the model used by Gianotti et al. (14) is very complex. BT and gut-derived sepsis were induced by cecal ligation and puncture of the cecum, plus gavage with 10^{11} *E. coli* plus a 20% burn injury. It is not clear how much of the BT is related to the bowel ligation alone, how much to the bowel puncture, how much to the transfusions, how much to the instillation of *E. coli*, and how much to the burn injury. Admittedly these six injuries together are collectively a very potent stimulus to BT. This is "six-hit BT" (15,16). I don't know how such complex injuries can be reliably reproduced by other investigators. Furthermore, I'm not sure how the results of these multiple injuries can be interpreted.

Gianotti and coworkers found that the BT-induced by cecal ligation and puncture plus *E. coli* gavage plus burn injury plus allogeneic, homologous blood transfusion in BALB/c mice was reduced and survival enhanced (20% to 56%) by arginine supplementation (14). The use of an arginine inhibitor of nitric oxide synthesis (Nω-nitro-L-arginine) (NNA) diminishes the beneficial effects of arginine especially in the killing of the translocated organisms measured by ^{14}C tagging of *E. coli*.

Unfortunately, these studies do not indicate the significance of these improvements in terms of mouse mortality and/or morbidity. Furthermore, as a clinician I have no way of knowing how these results can be applied to the human condition. I assume that it is better to have never translocated bacteria than to have translocated them and then killed them promptly. As I assess this problem, it seems to me to be an equivalent response to the question, "Is it better to have loved and lost than never to have loved at all?" Sophisticated, well-organized investigations such as this seem to me to be impractical exercises. I'm not sure how to apply these beautiful data other than to design follow-up studies to try to answer the clinical questions definitively.

Endotoxin is, however, a double-edged sword since it increases BT and upregulates nitric oxide synthase (NOS), which may promote BT or enhance microbial killing (17). To determine the effect of inhibiting NOS activity by administering aminoguanidine, Sorrells et al. (18) gave rats endotoxin alone and noted BT in 100%. Rats that received aminoguanidine with the endotoxin showed inhibition of NO production and a 50% decrease in BT (18). NO administered for prolonged periods, however, promotes BT by inducing cellular injury and gut barrier failure. Theses paradoxical results, which are confirmed by bacteriologic and histologic studies, seem to be the result of using different NOS inhibitors. This type of research can become very complicated.

Bactericidal permeability-increasing protein (BPIP) is a potent bactericidal, permeability-inhibiting, and lipopolysaccharide (endotoxin)-neutralizing protein that was found by Rannekampff in the granules of neutrophilic leukocytes (19). A recombinant protein that corresponds to the amino terminal 23 kD fragment of this protein ($rBPI_{23}$) has been shown to neutralize plasma endotoxin levels, to decrease BT, and to increase survival of mice after one-third body surface burn injuries (20). Rannekampff and coworkers demonstrated that $rBPI_{23}$ (10 mg/kg body weight) administered intraperitoneally to CF-1 mice before and for several hours after the burn prevented BT ($p < 0.005$), which had been assayed by culturing the MLN, in the majority of the burned mice. The mechanism of BPIP, a potent bacteriocidal substance that reduces but does not abolish BT, is not known, but it appears to reduce intestinal injury by inhibiting the effects of endotoxin. It is believed that endotoxin's most lethal BT-inducing effects are mediated by its disruption of the intercellular tight junctions between intestinal cells (21). Whether the anti-BT effects of BPIP are due to its bactericidal action, its antiendotoxinic activity, or both is not clear.

Gennari and Alexander reported that hyperoxia improved gut barrier function and preserved gut morphology in BALB/c mice that were gavaged with *E. coli* (10^9 organisms) and subjected to a 20% skin burn (22). Short-term hyperoxia (4 or 8 h of 100% oxygen) induced slight improvement in survival on the first day. Long-term hyperoxia (8 h of 100% oxygen plus five days of 40% oxygen) significantly improved survival (30% to 70%; $p < 0.05$) (Fig. 8.1) presumably by improving gut barrier function. In addition, BT was reduced and the clearance of bacteria from lymph nodes and liver was increased by hyperoxia. Ulceration of the villous tips, shortening of the villi, and loss of mucosal mass were all prevented or reduced by short-term hyperoxia.

Lactulose is a nonabsorbed disaccharide (galactosidofructose) that is metabolized in the intestinal tract by enteric bacteria, creating an acidified intestinal lumen and its contents. The acidification has bacteria-suppressing properties. In addition, lactulose has anti-endotoxin effects that may prevent or ameliorate BT (23).

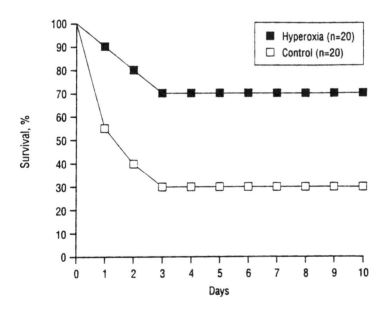

Fig. 8.1 Survival in mice after skin burn (20%) and enteral challenges with *E. coli* by gavage after long-term oxygen administration (8 h 100% oxygen plus 40% oxygen for 5 days). Survival was significantly greater from the third day onward. (From Ref. 22.)

Lactulose has also been used effectively to suppress BT induced by surgical trauma. In this study it decreased the numbers of gram-negative aerobes and facultative anaerobes and increased the number of lactobacilli ($p < 0.001$). These changes were accompanied by an increase in the mucosal height of the terminal ileum and cecum, which is compatible with proliferation of the ileal mucosa, one of the many metabolic effects of lactulose (23,24). It is associated with the metabolism of its component monosaccharides to short-chain fatty acids (SCFA), which stimulate the proliferation of the mucosal epithelium (25). The intestinal luminal acidification is soothing to the postoperative intestinal mucosa (26). In addition, it eradicates chronic *Salmonella* and *Shigella* carrier states (27), it prevents diverse infections in hospitalized patients (28), it decreases the amount of deoxycholate in bile (29), it reduces the recurrence rate of adenomatous colonic polyps (30), it antagonizes endotoxins after ischemic hepatic necrosis (23,31), and it prevents renal dysfunction after obstructive jaundice, which is one of the disorders that stimulates BT (32). In my opinion these antiendotoxinic effects of lactulose are the most likely explanation for these beneficial effects of lactulose on BT and its various consequences, but its antibacterial effects may provide supplementary benefits.

Lactulose has also been used effectively to treat the BT that results from surgical trauma, which ranges in severity from gentle manipulation of the intestinal tract (33) to blunt trauma (34) or intestinal ligation (35). Lactulose, which is effective in the treatment of hepatic encephalopathy and other intestinal disorders, has cathartic, antibacterial, and endotoxin-inhibiting properties, all of which may be beneficial in preventing BT.

IV. SUPPRESSION OF INTESTINAL BACTERIAL FLORA

Özçelik and associates in Istanbul compared the effects in Sprague-Dawley rats with surgical manipulation (or sham surgery) which received either lactulose (2 ml of a 33% solution) or saline intragastrically starting three days before surgery (36) (see Table 8.3). The surgical trauma consisted of laparotomy followed by palpation and compression of the gastrointestinal tract from duodenum to rectum for several minutes. (I predict that it will be difficult to standardize and calibrate manual ''compression'' of the intestinal tract.) Forty-eight hours later portal venous blood, MLN, liver, and spleen were removed and cultured. Cecal pH was reduced from 7.8 to 6.9 in the control and lactulose groups, respectively. BT was significantly increased in the MLN and portal

Table 8.3 Prevention of Bacterial Translocation III: Reduction in Intestinal Bacterial Overgrowth

First author	Ref. No.	Animal species	Induction of BT	Prevention of BT	Results of therapy
Özçelik	36	Rats	Surgical trauma	Lactulose	Decreases cecal pH Reduces BT in MLN, PB Decreases cecal enterobacteria Increases cecal lactobacilli
Mao	42	Rats	Methotrexate Elemental diet	Lactobacilli Fermented oat base	Reduces BT Restores normal microecology Decreases mucosal weight
Wang	44	Rats	Hepatectomy (90%)	Cholecystokinin	Accelerates transit time Suppresses bacterial overgrowth Prevents BT
Wang	45	Rats	Hepatectomy (90%)	Cisapride	Restores normal intestinal motility Enhances acetylcholine activity Prevents BT
Fuller	60	Mice	Bacterial overgrowth E. coli C25	Immunostimulation	Reduces BT Causes splenomegaly
Wang	62	Rats	Hepatectomy (90%)	Dextran 70	Reduces BT Suppresses E. coli overgrowth Decreases endothelial permeability

blood in the surgical trauma group ($p < 0.01$), but was greatly reduced by lactulose in the MLN and portal blood. The bacteria involved were largely gram-negative, aerobic bacteria. In the lactulose-treated rats there was a significant decrease in cecal gram-negative aerobes and anaerobes ($p < 0.01$) and a significant increase in lactobacilli ($p < 0.01$). Fermentation of lactulose by enteric bacteria stimulates the growth of SCFA that induces proliferation of the intestinal mucosa (37). Lactulose is a simple, effective method of suppressing this type BT. It is not clear how it affects BT induced in ways other than alterations in the intestinal bacterial ecology, but it deserves clinical investigation.

Methotrexate (MTX), a chemotherapeutic agent that promotes BT and endotoxemia, increases the number of *Enterobacteriaceae*, a potentially pathogenic species of bacteria. MTX, which also decreases the ratio of *Lactobacilli* to *Enterobacteriaceae* in the bowel, is a potentially pathogenic alteration (38). The administration of *Lactobacilli* appears to offer nutritional and therapeutic benefits (39) in chemotherapy-induced enterocolitis and in ulcerative and pseudomembranous colitis (40). In previous studies *Lactobacillus plantarium* was shown to stimulate colonization of human intestinal mucosa (41) and *Lactobacillus reuteri* R2LC to be antagonistic to intestinal inflammatory diseases. Furthermore, oats, which are high in fiber content, have beneficial effects in patients with inflammatory bowel disease, especially after fermentation by these two lactobacillary strains, which gives rise to a product called "oat base." This liquid substance, which is acidic ($pH < 4$), contains 4.2% β-glycans and 2.8% proteins.

Mao and associates studied the effects of oat base in rats given a continuous infusion of an elemental diet plus *L. plantarium* and *L. reuteri*, with and without fermentation and the intraperitoneal injection of MTX (20 mg per kg) (42). The lactobacilli plus oat-base combination diminished weight loss and intestinal permeability and increased the epithelial mucosal mass in enterocolitic rats. The lactobacilli alone reduced BT and restored the intestinal microecology to normal. Both substances decrease endotoxin levels. Clearly, *Lactobacilli* and fermented oat-base, alone or together, have potent anti-BT and restorative properties for the diseased bowel. Once again, however, too many therapies with too many methods of action, like too many cooks, may spoil the culture broth.

A. Cholecystokinin in Reduction of BT

It is well known that subtotal hepatectomy (90%) precipitates BT, slows intestinal transit time, and permits the overgrowth of enteric bacteria (43). Wang and his coworkers gave cholecystokinin (CCK) intravenously to rats after hepatectomy and showed that it accelerated intestinal transit time, *decreased* bacterial overgrowth in the intestines, and reduced BT (44).

B. Prevention of BT by Cisapride

Bacterial overgrowth with an increase in pathogenic aerobic bacteria and a decrease in anaerobic bacteria and lactobacilli is thought to give rise to gut barrier failure, which is characterized by BT. Impaired intestinal motility follows major hepatic resections, and bacterial overgrowth and, ultimately, leads to BT. Wang et al. studied Sprague-Dawley rats after 90% hepatectomy, which induces hypomotility and stimulates BT (45). They administered cisapride, a 5-hydroxytryptamine agonist that in dose of 6 mg/kg intravenously stimulates intestinal motility. Sham-operated rats served as controls, all of which developed BT to the MLN and two-thirds of which developed BT to the systemic circulation. None of the cisapride-treated animals, which have enhanced acetylcholine activity and normal intestinal motility, developed BT. It was concluded that cisapride maintains the integrity of the intestinal barrier. Clearly, cisapride can prevent the BT associated with major hepatic resection.

V. REDUCTION OF MACROPHAGE VOLUME IN PREVENTION OF BT

Tokyay et al. challenged BT head on (46): ''What would happen to BT if the MLNs were excised?'' they asked. They compared minipigs after mesenteric lymphadenectomy with sham-operated animals after 40% third-degree burns (see Table 8.4). The adenectomy prevented BT, although some bacteria were recovered from the AF. These studies suggest that BT occurs at least in part via mesenteric lymphatic channels.

How is the process of BT affected by the excision of the mesenteric lymph nodes prior to thermal injury? This question is, to my mind, overly simplistic because it is probable that not all of the mesenteric nodes can be excised. Perhaps, removal of most of the nodes is sufficient. Nevertheless, such studies have been performed only in minipigs (46). The design was complex. The burned animals (Group I) had a 40% third-degree burns with the MLN intact. In Group II, the MLN were excised surgically immediately after the burn. Sham burns were inflicted on a third group (Group III) and a fourth group had had the MLN excision without the burn injury (Group IV). In Group I bacteria were cultured from several organs: from 62% of the MLN and lungs,

Table 8.4 Prevention of Bacterial Translocation IV: Reduction of Macrophage Activity

First author	Ref. No.	Animal species	Induction of BT	Prevention of BT	Results of therapy
Tokyay	46	Minipigs	Burn (40%)	Mesenteric lymphadenectomy	Prevents BT Decreases infected ascitic fluid
Spaeth	47	Rats	Endotoxin	Splenectomy	Decreases BT
Silva	48	Rats	Bacterial overgrowth	Peyer's patch ligation	Increases BT in portal vein Decreases BT in MLN

50% of the spleens, 38% of the liver and kidneys, 25% of the peritoneal fluid specimens, and 12% of the portal blood samples. No such spread was seen in either group without MLN excision (Groups II and IV), although these groups had a high rate of BT to AF (approximately 85%). Peritoneal translocation was significantly less frequent when the MLN had been excised. These observations suggest that SBP is not primarily a lymph-transmitted infection, although it is one route of infection and that can be partially prevented by removal of MLN. The immunocompetence of the host is probably a more important factor, however. It should be kept in mind that indigenous flora from the bowel can frequently be cultured from the MLN of patients with Crohn's disease.

Splenectomy is known not to stimulate BT in mice (47). On the other hand, splenectomy appears to enhance resistance to BT in Harlan mice that is induced by *E. coli* 0111:Bd endotoxin (48). BT was increased from 23% in the splenectomized mice to 59% in the sham-splenectomized mice and to 73% in the in operated control group. Why should splenectomy diminish BT? Perhaps it is related to the suppression of endotoxin.

The spleen plays an important role in the defense mechanisms against infection. Asplenic patients have long been known to be susceptible to encapsulated organisms, and it is thought that this effect enhances the clearance of circulating bacteria. More recently, it has been recognized that the spleen plays a modulatory role in the antibacterial defenses of the gut. Splenectomy itself causes a very small induction of BT to MLN (5–10%). Moreover, the administration of endotoxin induces BT to MLN in about 60% of the patients. However, endotoxin plus splenectomy causes BT in 23% (p < 0.01) and a 2 to 4 log increase in cecal gram-negative bacilli. Thus, the mechanism is not clear. The spleen is the site of antibody and complement production, and is the source of mediators that regulate cell populations and phagocytosis by macrophages. It also inhibits xanthine oxidase, which may give rise to an ischemia-induced injury and BT, both of which are mediated by xanthine oxidase-generated oxygen free radicals. Splenectomy may also limit endotoxin-induced intestinal mucosal injury. Endotoxin may augment or suppress xanthine oxidase under specific conditions. After splenectomy it may stimulate host bacterial immune responses. Whatever the mechanism(s), splenectomy does inhibit BT.

Silva et al. studied the role of the surgical ligation of Peyer's patches on BT (48). After ligation of Peyer's patches and the instillation of *E. coli* R6 (2×10^8 per ml) into the intestinal lumen to stimulate bacterial overgrowth, BT increased to the portal vein and decreased to the MLN. However, the authors state that none of the differences was statistically significant. In "Statistics According to Conn,'' nonsignificant differences are not true differences, and such ''differences'' should be ignored until sufficient numbers of studies are performed to achieve statistical significance. Therefore, it remains unclear whether or how Peyer's patches are involved in BT. Furthermore it is not clear to me how effective ''ligation'' of Peyer's patches is. Are 90% of the patches ligated, or 10%? What percentage of Peyer's lymphocytes and macrophages are removed by Peyer's patchectomy?

VI. PREVENTION OF BT BY MISCELLANEOUS SUBSTANCES OR PROCEDURES

A variety of substances, such as dehydroepiandrosterone, allopurinol, and phosphotidylcholine; diets, such as low-protein, high-cellulose diets; and metabolic states, such as hyperoxia, have all been shown to prevent BT. Because the substances vary greatly in type and the diets vary in content and no single explanation or exact mechanism of action is known, they are grouped under the rubric ''miscellaneous,'' and are presented in arbitrary order in Table 8.5. A short discussion of the investigations in which these modalities have been shown to prevent BT are presented for each.

Because adrenocorticoids enhance BT it is logical to consider antisteroidal approaches to the prevention of BT. Gennari and Alexander demonstrated in mice that dietary supplementation with dehydroepiandrosterone (DHEA) (25 mg/kg/d) reversed the immunosuppression induced by prednisone (10 mg/kg/d) in BALB/c mice following *E. coli* gavage plus 20% total body surface burns (49). Both arginine and glutamine as well as DHEA were capable of enhancing the killing of translocated bacteria. Such studies have important applications in the prevention of infections in steroid-treated patients. Survival rates were increased from about 35% to 70–80%.

Schimpl and associates studied the effects of allopurinol on BT in Sprague-Dawley rats with portal hypertension induced by calibrated portal vein constriction or by common bile duct ligation (50). They compared the effects of allopurinol, a competitive xanthine oxidase inhibitor (50 mg/kg intraperitoneally 24 and 2 h before examination) in operated animals and in sham-operated control animals that were studied with and without allopurinol. In the sham- and nonoperated groups, BT to the spleen and MLN occurred. Allopurinol decreased BT in the portal hypertensive and bile duct-ligated groups ($p < 0.05$). In addition, they studied intestinal mucosal malondialdehyde levels as indices of lipid peroxidation and PMN-derived myeloperoxi-

Table 8.5 Prevention of Bacterial Translocation V: Miscellaneous Antibacterial Translocation Procedures

First author	Ref. No.	Animal species	Induction of BT	Prevention of BT	Results of therapy
Gennari	22	Mice	Bacterial overgrowth E. coli gavage	Hyperoxia	Reduces mortality Enhances bacterial clearance from MLN Decreases loss of mucosal mass
Gennari	49	Mice	Prednisone, burn (20%) E. coli gavage	Dehydroepiandrosterone Arginine, glutamine	Reverses susceptibility to infection Restores normal microecology Improves survival
Schimpl	50	Rats	Portal hypertension Common bile duct constriction	Allopurinol	Decreases BT Decreases BT Reduces malondialdehyde Reduces myeloperoxidase
Schimpl	51	Rats	Portal hypertension Common bile duct constriction	Antioxidant vitamins (vitamin C, vitamin E)	Reduces oxidative metabolism Decreases BT Preserves endotoxin absorption
Wang	52	Rats	Liver resection (90%)	Phosphotidylcholine Phosphotidylinositol	Maintains intestinal barrier
Wang	53	Rats	Liver resection (90%)	Ethylhydroxyethylcellulose	Prevents BT
Bovee-Oudenhoven	55	Rats	Salmonella	Calcium supplements	Decreases BT Reduces urinary NO Precipitates iron
Fuller	60	Mice	E. coli C25	Immunostimulation (Propionibacterium acnes)	Reduces BT Induces splenomegaly
Wang	62	Rats	Liver resection (90%)	Dextran	Decreases BT Minimizes endothelial permeability
Okuyama	88	Rabbits (neonatal)	Absence of breast milk	Epidermal growth factor	Decreases BT Increases goblet cells in intestine

dase as evidence of activation of bacterial inflammation, both of which were reduced by allopurinol. The investigators urged caution in interpretation because rats and humans are so different. The difference is probably not so great as it appears.

Schimpl et al. compared the effects of antioxidant vitamins on the presence of BT in Sprague-Dawley rats with (a) portal hypertension induced by calibrated partial portal vein ligation, (b) complete portal vein ligation, and (c) sham-operated rats. Peritoneal visceral fluid, portal venous blood, vena caval blood, MLN, spleen, liver, and ileal contents were individually cultured 28 days after laparotomy (51). The portal hypertensive rats developed significantly greater numbers of gram-positive organisms, and the bile duct-ligated rats exhibited much greater numbers of both gram-positive and gram-negative bacteria in the ileal cultures induced by the overgrowth of *E. coli*, *Proteus* species, lactobacilli, *Pasturella*, and enterococci. BT was found in the portal hypertensive rats in the MLN and spleen and in the bile of bile duct-ligated animals. Portal pressure levels were elevated to a similar degree in the portal hypertensive and bile duct-ligated rats, i.e., 19 mmHg compared to 7 mmHg in the sham-operated control rats. Liver enzyme levels were increased after bile duct ligation in both the vitamin-treated and vitamin-free groups.

Vitamin C (10 mg/kg) and vitamin E (10 mg/kg) were administered subcutaneously to half the animals in each subgroup; the other half received saline. Vitamins C and E are antioxidant substances that appear to prevent lipid peroxidation. The authors concluded that BT is caused by bacterial overgrowth *plus* increased oxidative metabolism. The oxidative metabolism can be prevented by the antioxidant substances.

As indicated in Table 8.5, Schimpl et al. demonstrated in portal hypertension that vitamin E and vitamin C, oxidant substances, suppress BT in Sprague-Dawley rats (51) and believe that these substances protect against free-radical-mediated damage by decreasing glutathione (GSH) in the liver and by decreasing hepatic arterial perfusion. The treated animals showed reduction in intestinal lipid peroxidation, which the investigators considered to be a measure of oxidative cell injury. In addition, these studies suggest possible roles of lipid peroxidation or of glutathione synthesis and of both in the pathogenesis of BT and its inhibition.

A.   Phospholipids in Prevention of BT

Wang and associates have shown that BT after hepatectomy in Sprague-Dawley rats can be decreased by the administration of phospholipids (phosphotidylcholine and phosphotidylinositol) (52). Presumably, these effects are mediated by maintaining the integrity of the intestinal barrier.

Wang et al. have also shown that ethylhydroxyethyl cellulose prevents the BT induced by large hepatic resections (90%) in rats (53). Although the mechanism of this effect is not known, it might be caused by the bacterial degradation in the intestinal tract of the cellulose moiety of this substance.

Why does water-soluble ethylhydroxyethyl cellulose (EHEC) prevent BT following major hepatic resection? The studies of Wang et al. show that EHEC, which is a nonionic surfactant, inhibits the adherence of bacteria on the surfaces of the distal small intestinal and colonic enterocytes. Oral administration of EHEC is more effective than intravenous. EHEC coats the surfaces of enterocytes and bacteria and alters their characteristics so that they are more hydrophilic and mutually rejective, and also diminishes the phagocytic capacities of intestine macrophages. EHEC also stimulates peristalsis, which diminishes the time available to induce BT. Furthermore, the cellulose moiety of the molecule is apparently metabolized by enteric organisms and thus decreases intestinal pH, and, like lactulose, shortens the intestinal transit time and reduces bacterial overgrowth, thus decreasing endotoxin production, each of which may contribute to the prevention of BT.

B. Calcium in Prevention of BT

Bovee-Oudenhoven et al. studied the effects of dietary calcium supplementation in rats on low (20 mmol/kg), medium (60 mmol/kg), and high (180 mmol/kg) $CaHPO_4$ diets because dietary calcium is thought to decrease the cytotoxicity of intestinal contents by the precipitation of cytotoxic surfactants (54). In this way they attempted to determine the effect on the infectivity of the oral administration of 5×10^8 *Salmonella enteritidis* BT, which was measured by *Salmonella* counts in MNN, Peyer's patches, and spleen (55). They found that high calcium diets improved resistance to colonization. BT measured by bacterial counts reduced the severity of gut-derived systemic infections. BT was measured by bacterial counts in the MLN and by the excretion of urinary nitric oxide, which is an oxidation product of bacteria in intestinal tissue. The mechanism of this effect is uncertain although the precipitation of iron by the calcium is a reasonable explanation.

Other dietary supplements may have similar or even opposite effects on BT and bacterial colonization. In fact, even the absence of the specific components of diet may affect these phenomena. Both individual components or their absence, as well as the routes by which they are administered, may affect these phenomena. The effect of the parenteral administration of foodstuffs is an especially good example. Total parenteral nutrition is fraught with hepatic hazards including cholestasis, cholelethiasis, hepatic fibrosis, biliary cirrhosis and, ultimately, hepatic failure. It is surprising that TPN solutions when administered both enterally and parenterally may promote BT (56,57), and sometimes these effects may be related both directly or inversely to the duration of administration of the diet.

C. Prevention of BT by Nonspecific Immunostimulation

BT develops in immunosuppressed mice in genetically athymic mice and in neonatally thymectomized mice (58). Because the grafting of thymus tissue into genetically athymic mice (nu/nu), which are deficient in T-cell-mediated immunity, inhibits the BT in immunosuppressed animals, Fuller and Berg investigated the effects of nonspecific immunostimulation in specific pathogen-free (SPF) mice that had been decontaminated with streptomycin and penicillin. These mice were inoculated with *E. coli* C25 in their food and water, which induced BT of the MLN, from which *E. coli* C25 were cultured (59).

These mice were "monoassociated" with *E. coli* C25 exclusively, i.e., *E. coli* C25 inhabited their intestinal tracts. Such monoassociation itself can lead to BT with the monoassociated organism.

Immunostimulation, which was induced by the administration/orally of parenterally killed *Propionibacterium acnes*, is a potent immunomodulator (59), causes marked splenomegaly, and reduced the incidence of BT from 75% to 41% of the mice inoculated (p < 0.01) (60). Immunostimulation with formalin-killed *P. acnes* may "immunize" such animals against other bacterial species as well (61).

D. Dextran in Prevention of BT

Wang and coworkers reported that subtotal hepatectomy (90%) in rats induced a decrease in mean arterial pressure, and increase in the number of *E. coli* in the distal small intestine and BT. Dextran 70 decreased the percentage of animals with BT. These abnormalities were associated with increased endothelial permeability and could be prevented by the administration of intravenous dextran 70. Therefore BT was prevented by intravenous dextran, which maintained the integrity of the gut vascular endothelial barrier (62).

VII. EFFECT OF OBSTRUCTIVE JAUNDICE ON BT

It is well known that obstructive jaundice increases susceptibility to BT (63,64) and to infection (65,66) (Table 8.6). The susceptibility to infection is

Table 8.6 Prevention of Bacterial Translocation VI: Various Methods of Suppressing Obstructive Jaundice-Induced BT

First author	Ref. No.	Animal species	Induction of BT	Prevention of BT	Results of therapy
Schimpl	50	Rats	CBDL	Allopurinol	Reduces BT Reduces inflammation
Schimpl	51	Rats	CBDL	Vitamin C Vitamin E	Reduces BT Decreases GSH Decreases hepatic perfusion
Cakmakci	67	Rats	CBDL	External bile duct drainage	Reduces serum bilirubin Reduces BT Reduced endotoxin absorption
Slocum	71	Rats	CBDL	Presence of bile in intestinal tract	Prevents BT
Ding	73	Rats	CBDL	Cholic acid, Deoxycholic acid, or Whole bile	Prevents BT
Ding	74	Rats	CBDL	MTPEA[a]	Reduced BT
Ding	75	Rats	CBDL	Portal decompression	Reduces BT
Karsten	77	Rats	CBDL	Biliary decompression	Reduces BT
			E. coli inoculation into CBD		

[a]MTPEA, muramyltripeptidephosphatidylethanolamine; CBD, common bile duct; CBDL, common bile duct ligation; GSH, glutathione.

thought to reflect impaired reticuloendothelial (RE) function. To determine the mechanism of action, Cakmakci et al. studied common bile duct ligation (CBDL) in albino rats with and without bile diversion, i.e., venting of the obstructed bile (67). When internal biliary drainage was used, BT occurred much more commonly than in the undrained animals. Thus, they demonstrated that the absence of bile in the intestinal tract appreciably enhances BT to the abdominal organs, but not to the lungs or blood. Three-fourths of the bacteria responsible are indigenous, aerobic, gram-negative bacteria. Quantitative cultures showed that the distribution of the normal cecal bacterial flora are not appreciably altered by the CBDL. Serum bilirubin levels are increased after CBDL, but not in bile-diverted animals. Furthermore, endotoxins are bound by bile salts in the intestinal tract (68) and endotoxinemia is common in obstructive jaundice. Internal drainage of the bile decreased the absorption of endotoxin and serum endotoxin levels (69) whereas external drainage did not (70). Slocum et al. demonstrated that the absence of intestinal bile promotes BT (71). Whatever the precise mechanism, it seems clear that the absence of bile from the intestinal tract plays a major role in the increased BT and sepsis of obstructive jaundice (72) and, probably, in intestinal obstruction as well. Stated conversely, the presence of bile in the intestinal tract prevents BT.

Ding and associates studied various inhibitors of BT in obstructive jaundice. They reported that the oral administration of cholic and deoxycholic acid and whole bile inhibited both BT and endotoxin absorption in rats with CBDL (72,73). In related studies in a CBDL rat model of obstructive jaundice, Ding et al. reported that muramyl tripeptide phosphatidylethanolamine (MTPEA), a macrophage immunostimulant inhibits BT (74).

Ding and associates demonstrated increased BT in Sprague-Dawley rats after CBDL (75). Two weeks after CBDL, the rate of BT was higher than in the unobstructed controls. At that time choledochoduodenostomy was performed, and promptly after biliary decompression the incidence of BT progressively decreased, so that three weeks after decompression the BT was no longer evident. The incidence of BT showed a highly significant correlation of serum alkaline phosphase activity and the rate of BT. Clearly, obstructive jaundice induces BT and the relief of the obstruction corrects it.

Obstructive jaundice may cause disruption of tight junctions of epithelial cells in the biliary tract and may diminish the secretion of IgA into the bile (76). Such changes are characteristic of what occurs in BT, and may help explain the frequency of bacterial cholangitis in biliary obstruction. Karsten et al. (77) performed CBDL in Wistar rats, half of which were then decompressed by choledechojejunostomy. Then 10^8 E. coli were inoculated in retrograde fashion with the CBD at 5- and 20-cm water pressures, well within the levels observed in obstructive jaundice, and two weeks later the bile, lymph, and blood were cultured (77). They found that BT from the biliary tree to the bloodstream had occurred. BT to the lymphatic system was observed much more frequently to the lymph than to the blood. Presumably, the lymph, which originates in the spaces of Disse, passes into the lymphatics through the thoracic duct and into the systemic circulation. All preinoculation cultures were sterile; all postinoculation cultures were positive for *E. coli*. The number of colony-forming units were significantly higher in the animals inoculated at the higher pressure level. This finding indicates that the reflux of bacteria into the lymphatic system occurs before and at lower pressure levels than reflux into the bloodstream.

The studies summarized in Tables 8.5 and 8.6 indicate that the BT induced by CBDL can be prevented in a variety of ways: by decompressing the biliary system; by administering antioxidant vitamins or allopurinol, a xanthine oxidase inhibitor; by replacing whole bile or primary bile acids in the intestinal tract; or by administering MTPEA, a macrophage immunostimulant. There are many ways to skin this particular cat.

VIII. DIETARY PROTEIN IN THE INDUCTION AND PREVENTION OF BT

A. Introduction

The relationship of dietary protein intake and BT is one of the most complex and controversial aspects of medicine (Table 8.7). Both too little and too much protein have been shown to induce BT. Casafont and colleagues have shown that protein malnutrition gives rise to BT and SBP whereas a normal diet prevents both BT and SBP (78) (Fig. 8.2). Casafont and colleagues (78) and Nettelbladt et al. (78a) have shown that protein malnutrition and brief fasting, respectively, may give rise to BT and/or SBP, whereas a normal diet of cellulose, also known as bulking fiber, prevents these phenomena (Table 8.7). Nelson and coworkers have demonstrated that high-protein diets are associated with BT (79). Casafont had studied Sprague-Dawley rats with CCl_4-induced cirrhosis that were given 0.7 g protein per day of a standard rat chow diet and compared them with rats fed ad lib diets (78). BT occurred in 95% of the malnourished and in 29% of the well-fed animals ($p < 0.01$) (SBP occurred in similar percentages in both groups). These findings parallel long-held observations that malnutrition is one of the causes of cirrhosis, and that high-protein diets are a common cause of hepatic encephalopathy.

Table 8.7 Prevention of Bacterial Translocation VIII: Diet Therapy

First author	Ref. No.	Animal species	Induction of BT	Prevention of BT	Results of therapy
Casafont	78	Rats	Malnutrition	Normal diet	Reduces BT
			Cirrhosis		Reduces SBP
Nelson	79	Guinea pigs	High protein (20%)	Low protein diet (5%)	Reduces BT
			Sepsis		
Barber	80	Rats	Endotoxin	Normal diet	Reduces BT
Sedman	84	Humans	TPN (prelaparotomy)	Normal diet	Reduces BT
Spaeth	85	Mice	TPN (IV)	Cellulose	Reduces BT
			TPN (oral)	Cellulose	Reduces BT
Spaeth	86	Mice	TPN (oral)	Bulk forming agents	Reduces BT
				(Cellulose)	Increases stool volume
				(Kaolin)	Increases cecal levels of E. coli
Go	87	Rabbits	Formula-fed	Breast milk	Prevents BT
Okuyama	88	Rabbits (newborn)	Formula-fed	Epidermal growth factor	Prevents BT
					Increases goblet cells
Nakasaki	89	Rats	TPN	Proteoglycan	Reduces BT
Nettelbladt	78a	Rats	TPN	Cellulose	Reduces BT

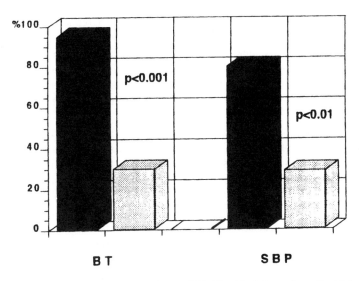

Fig. 8.2 Dietary protein intake vs. BT. The black bars show the high percentages of BT and SBP noted in malnourished rats compared to the much lower percentage in normally fed animals (stippled bars). Thus, normal nutrition greatly decreases both BT and SBP. (From Ref. 78.)

Nelson had compared low (5%) and high (20%) protein diets in septic guinea pigs that were being inoculated with *E. coli* and *Staphylococcus aureus* intraperitoneally (79). The low-protein diets resulted in less BT, fewer translocated bacteria, and greater survival than the high-protein diets.

Using a defined formula diet that was free of both fiber and glutamine in Wistar rats, Barber et al. induced BT and increased susceptibility to endotoxin associated with bowel mucosal atrophy (80).

As Deitch et al. have shown, malnutrition can promote BT and sepsis (81). Mice on a diet completely free of protein for three weeks, however, did not develop BT, although their mortality was proportional to the duration of the malnutrition. Alverdy has reported that a TPN solution that contained amounts of amino acids and calories sufficient to support growth and weight gain can induce BT (82). Possible explanations for these discordant results are intrinsic species differences between mice and rats and the fact that the mice in Deitch's study had received some dietary fiber. Therefore, they had compared oral diets in Charles River rats with intravenous TPN and oral TPN, both of which contained 25% glucose and 4.5% amino acids but were free of fiber. BT occurred in 60% of the both TPN groups. The addition of corn-syrup solids, which contained 2.5 g cellulose per day, significantly reduced the BT but did not prevent cecal overgrowth of gram-negative bacilli, nor did it reduce mucosal mass. The cellulose appeared to diminish subepithelial edema.

In another study of BT in Sprague-Dawley rats, Illig et al. noted no great differences between oral and parenteral feeding although parenteral feeding led to gut atrophy, cecal bacterial overgrowth, and increased gut permeability to lactulose (83).

In an impromptu, nonrandomized retrospective controlled trial, Sedman et al. studied the effects of 10 days of TPN therapy immediately before laparotomy in 203 critically ill patients (84). Twenty-eight of these patients, who were considered unable to tolerate oral nutrition, were arbitrarily assigned to the control group. The other 175, who were thought to be unable to take an oral diet, were assigned to the oral-diet treatment group. The two groups were similar in demographic characteristics and in the disorders for which the laparotomies were performed. Three patients in the TPN group (11%) and 14 in the oral-diet group (8%) developed BT defined as a positive culture of MLN or serosal scrapings taken as soon as the abdomen had been opened. This difference is not statistically significant. The types of bacteria cultured, which were predominantly *E. coli* (81%), were similar in the two groups. Five of the 17 patients who developed BT (29%) subsequently developed postoperative infectious complications compared to only two of 186 patients who did not exhibit BT (1%) (p < 0.001). This investigation, which is the only one so far performed in human subjects suggests that short courses of TPN under such circumstances do not induce or prevent BT. The fact that BT occurs much less commonly in human studies than in animal models probably reflects the greater tendencies of experimental animals in such experiments to develop BT more frequently than humans.

Because of the suspected association of TPN and BT, Spaeth et al. compared three groups of rats: Group I received a normal oral diet; Group II received a TPN solution intravenously; and Group III received the same TPN solution, which contained 28% glucose, orally (85). BT occurred in both groups on TPN (85). The TPN solutions contained no fiber, and therefore two additional groups were studied to assess the role of fiber on BT (intravenous TPN and oral TPN plus cellulose powder [2.5 g per day]). The addition of cellulose prevented the occurrence of BT. The cellulose appeared to act by preventing the alterations in mucosal structure and function induced by the TPN.

Spaeth et al. also studied the effects of bulk-forming agents such as cellulose fiber, and kaolin but not citrus pectin (a fully fermentable, nonresidue fiber) reduced the incidence of BT in TPN-fed mice to control levels (86).

Nettelbladt et al. made similar observations in rats with brief starvation-induced BT (78a).

B.   Prevention of "Spontaneous" BT by Epidermal Growth Factor

Of the many causes of BT, the most surprising is the so-called spontaneous BT, which can be prevented by breast milk in newborn rabbits (87). Go found it only in formula-fed neonatal rabbits (87). Among many substances postulated to play the primary role in breast milk that prevents BT is epidermal growth factor (EGF). Secretory IgA, lactoformin, glutamine, specific enteric bacteria, and oligosaccharides have also been implicated. Okuyama et al. studied three groups: (a) breast-fed pups, (b) those given EGF (1.5 µg per g) subcutaneously three times daily, and (c) those not given EGF (88). All rats were sacrificed after seven days and the MLN, liver, and spleen were cultured. In the breast-fed animals there was no BT. In the EGF treated rabbits, 30–45% had BT whereas 30–80% of the control animals had BT ($p < 0.05$). The organisms in the cecum and ileum were similar in the EGF (+) animals and EGF (−) groups. Goblet cells were much fewer in the EGF (+) animals. The authors concluded that EGF decreases BT in formula-fed rabbits and induces an increase in the number of goblet cells in the small bowel mucosa. These findings suggest that EGF plays a role in maintaining gastrointestinal mucus barrier function. Furthermore, the implication that synthetic parenteral formula diets are less healthy than normal enteral nutrition is supported.

Protoglycan is a biological response modifier that appears to suppress BT. Nakasaki et al. administered TPN to rats and noted that up to 60% of them had positive MLN as well as a reduction in plasma cells and a decrease in secretory IgA production and secretion in gut-associated lymphoid tissue (GALT), bile, and portal venous blood (89). The oral ingestion of protoglycan (1000 mg per g per day) suppressed the TPN-induced BT and prevented degeneration of GALT.

The effects of the nutritional state on BT in experimental animals is a complex, contradictory, and controversial issue in which the results reported are quite diverse and overlapping. Both high- and low-protein dietary intake induce BT, as do a variety of TPN diets, whether these diets are taken parenterally or orally. These studies were designed to answer specific questions that differ from investigator to investigator, and the animals were subjected to a broad array of substances known to induce BT. Often multiple means of inducing BT were applied simultaneously. The measurements made and the methods of making them differ. The animals used vary in species, in type, and in immunological characteristics, and were often selected because of such differences. Central to this whole problem are the hepatic complications of TPN especially in children (90), one of which is BT.

Most of the bacterial infections are caused by organisms that are indigenous to the patient's gut and the bacterial source of the infection is never found even at autopsy. The process of BT may be promoted by the overgrowth of bacterial flora in the gut, by host immune defenses, or by physical defects in the mucosal barrier of the gut. Nutritional deficiencies are often associated with these conditions and therefore a complete in-depth dispassionate review of nutrition per se in relationship to BT is needed.

REFERENCES

1. Brook I, Ledney GD. Ofloxacin and penicillin G combination therapy in prevention of bacterial translocation and animal mortality after irradiation. Antimicrob Agents Chemother 35:1685–1787, 1991.
2. Goris RJA, van Bebber IPT, Mollen RMH, Koopman JP. Does selective decontamination of the gastrointestinal tract prevent multiple organ failure? Arch Surg 126:561–565, 1991.
3. Yao Y-M, Lu L-R, Yu Y, Liang H-P, Chen J-S, Shi Z-G, Zhou B-T, Sheng Z-Y. Influence of selective decontamination of the digestive tract on cell-mediated immune function and bacteria/endotoxin translocation in thermally injured rats. J Trauma 42:1073–1079, 1997.
4. Marotta F, Geng TC, Wu CC, Barbi G. Bacterial translocation in the course of acute pancreatitis: Beneficial role of nonabsorbable antibiotics and lactitol enemas. Digestion 57:446–452, 1996.
5. Privitera G, Rossi G, Conte E, Gatti S, Matinato C, Reggiani P. Parenteral fluoroquinolones prevent translocation of enterobacteria following combined liver-small bowel transplantation in pigs. Transplant Proc 28:2669–2670, 1996.
6. Runyon BA, Borzio M, Young S, Squier SU, Giarner C, Runyon MA. Effect of selective bowel decontamination with norfloxacin on spontaneous bacterial peritonitis, translocation, and survival in an animal model of cirrhosis. Hepatology 21:1719–1724, 1995.
7. Khardori N, Elting L, Wong E, Schable B, Bodey GP. Nosocomial infections due to *Xanthomonas maltophilia (Pseudomonas maltophilia)* in patients with cancer. Rev Infect Dis 12:943–1003, 1990.
8. Lingnau W, Berger J, Javorsky F, Lejeune P, Mutz N, Benzer H. Selective intestinal decontamination in multiple trauma patients: Prospective, controlled trial. J Trauma Injury and Crit Care 42:687–694, 1997.
9. Shannon FL, Moore EE, Moore FA, McCroskey BL. Value of distal colon wash-

out in civilian rectal trauma: reducing gut bacterial translocation. J Trauma 28: 989–994, 1988.

10. Deitch EA, Berg RD, Specien H. Endotoxin promotes the translocation of bacteria from the gut. Arch Surg 122:185–190, 1987.

11. Adjei AA, Yamauchi K, Nakasone Y, Konishi M, Yamamoto S. Arginine-supplemented diets inhibit endotoxin-induced bacterial translocation in mice. Nutrition 11:371–374, 1995.

12. Reynolds JV, Daly JM, Zhang S. Immunomodulatory mechanisms of arginine. Surg 194:141–145, 1988.

13. Gennari R, Alexander JW, Eaves-Pyles T. Effect of different combinations of dietary additives on bacterial translocation and survival in gut-derived sepsis. JPEN 19:319–325, 1995.

14. Gianotti L, Alexander JW, Pyles T, Fukushima R. Arginine-supplemented diets improve survival in gut-derived sepsis and peritonitis by modulating bacterial clearance. The role of nitric oxide. Ann Surg 217:644–654, 1993.

15. Deitch EA. Multiple organ failure. Ann Surg 216:117–134, 1992.

16. Mishima S, Yudioda T, Matsuda H, Shimazaki S. Mild hypotension and body burns synergistically increase bacterial translocation in rats consistent with a "two-hit phenomenon." J Burn Care Rehab 18:L22–26, 1997.

17. Gonce SJ, Peck MD, Alexander JW, Miskell PW. Arginine supplementation and its effect on established peritonitis in guinea pigs. JPEN 14:237–244, 1990.

18. Sorrels DL, Friend C, Koltuksuz U, Courcoulas A, Boyle P, Garrett M, Watkins S, Rowe MI, Ford HR. Inhibition of nitric oxide with aminoguanidine reduces bacterial translocation after endotoxin challenge in vivo. Arch Surg 131:1155–1163, 1996.

19. Rannekampff OH, Tenehaus M, Hansbrough J, Kiessig V, Zapata-Sirvent RL. Effects of recombinant, bactericidal, permeability-increasing protein on bacterial translocation and pulmonary neutrophil sequestration in burned mice. J Burn Care Rehabil 18:17–21, 1997.

20. Yao YM, Bahrami S, Leichtined G. Pathogenesis of hemorrhage-induced bacteria/endotoxin translocation in rats: effects of recombinant bacteriocidal/permeability-increasing protein. Ann Surg 221:398–405, 1995.

21. Walker RI, Porvaznik MJ. Disruption of the permeability barrier (zona occludens) between intestinal epithelial cells by lethal doses of endotoxin. Infect Immun 21:655–658, 1978.

22. Gennari R, Alexander JW. Effects of hyperoxia on bacterial translocation and mortality during gut-derived sepsis. Arch Surg 131:57–62, 1996.

23. Liehr H, Englisch G, Rasenack U. Lactulose: a drug with antiendotoxin effect. Hepatogastroenterology 27:356–360, 1980.

24. Greve JW, Gouma KJ, van Leeuwen PAM, Bauman WA. Lactulose inhibits endotoxin induced tumour necrosis factor production by monocytes. An in vitro study. Gut 31:198–203, 1990.

25. Mortensen PB, Holtug K, Bonnen H. The degradation of proteins and blood to short-chain fatty acids in colon is prevented by lactulose. Gastroenterology 98: 353–360, 1990.

26. Wesselius-De Casparis A, Braadbaart S, Bergh-Bohlken GE. Treatment of chronic constipation with lactulose syrup: results of a double-blind study. Gut 9:84–86, 1968.

27. Sander-Treske R, Czermak L. Lactulose in Salmonella enteritis–an alternative to antibiotic chemotherapy. Therapiewoche 26:740–745, 1976.

28. McCutcheon J, Fulton JD. Lowered prevalence of infection with lactulose therapy in patients win long-term hospital care. J Hosp Infect 13:81–86, 1989.

29. Thornton JR, Heaton KW. Do colonic bacteria contribute to cholesterol gallstone formation: Effects of lactulose on bile. Br Med J 282:1018–1020, 1981.

30. Roncucci L, Di Donato P, Carati L. Antioxidant vitamins or lactulose for the prevention of the recurrence of colorectal adenomas. Dis Colon Rectum 67:227–234, 1993.

31. de Groote GH, Schalm SW, Batavier P. Incidence of endotoxaemia in pigs with eschaemic hepatic necrosis treated by haemodialysis. Prevention of endotoxaemia with lactulose. Hepatogastroenterology 30:240–242, 1983.

32. Pain JA, Cahill CJ, Gilbert JM. Prevention of postoperative renal dysfunction in patients with obstructive jaundice: a multicentre study of bile salts and lactulose. Br J Surg 78:467–469, 1991.

33. Guzman-Stein G, Bonsack M, Liberty J. Intestinal handling facilitates enteric bacterial translocation. Surg Forum 38:75–76, 1987.

34. Deitch EA, Bridges RM. Effects of stress and trauma on bacterial translocation from the gut. J Surg Res 42:536–542, 1987.

35. Salman FT, Buyruk MN, Gürler Çelik A. The effect of surgical trauma on the bacterial translocation from the gut. J Pediatr Surg 27:802–804, 1992.

36. Özçelik MF, Eroğlu C, Pekmezci S, Öztürk R, Paksoy M. The role of lactulose in the prevention of bacteria in surgical trauma. Acta Chir Belg 96:44–48, 1996.

37. Sakata T, Yaima T. Influence of SCFAs on the epithelial cell division of the gastrointestinal tract. Q J Exp Physiol, 68:639–641, 1994.

38. Mao Y, Kasravi B, Nobaek S, Wang LQ, Adawi D, Roos G, Stenram U, Molin G, Bengmark S, Jeppsson B. Pectin-supplemented enteral diet reduces the severity of methotrexate-induced enterocolitis in rats. Scand J Gastroenterol, in press.

39. Fernandes CF, Shahami KM, Amer MA. Therapeutic role of dietary lactobacilli and lactobacilli fermented dairy products. FEMS Microbiol Rev 46:343–356, 1987.

40. Fabia R, Ar'Rajab A, Johansson ML, Willen R, Andersson R, Molin G, Bengmark S. The effect of exogenous administration of Lactobacillus reuteri R2LC and oat fiber on acetic acid-induced colitis in the rat. Scand J Gastroenterol 28: 155–162, 1993.

41. Johansson M-L, Molin G, Jeppsson B, Nobaek S, Ahrne S, Bengmark S. Administration of different Lactobacillus strains in fermented oatmeal soup: in vivo colonization of human intestinal mucosa and effect on the indigenous flora. Appl Environ Microbiol 59:15–20, 1993.

42. Mao Y, Nobaek W, Kasravi B, Adawi D, Stenram U, Molin G, Jeppsson B. The

effect of *Lactobacillus* strains and oat fiber on methotrexate-induced enterocolitis in rats. Gastroenterology 111:334–344, 1996.
43. Wang XD, Guo W, Wang Q, Andersson R, Soltesz V, Bengmark S. The association between enteric bacterial overgrowth and gastrointestinal motility after subtotal liver resection or portal vein obstruction in rats. Eur J Surg 160:153–160, 1994.
44. Wang XD, Soltesz V, Axelson J, Andersson R. Cholecystokinin increases small intestinal motility and reduces enteric bacterial overgrowth and translocation in rats with surgically induced acute liver failure. Digestion 57:67–72, 1996.
45. Wang XD, Soltesz V, Andersson R. Cisapride prevents enteric bacterial overgrowth and translocation by improvement of intestinal motility in rats with acute liver failure. Eur Surg Res 28:402–412, 1996.
46. Tokyay R, Zeigler ST, Loick HM, Heggers FP, De la Garza P, Traber DL, Herndon DN. Mesenteric lymphadenectomy prevents postburn systemic spread of translocated bacteria. Arch Surg 127:384–388, 1992.
47. Spaeth G, Specien RD, Berg RD, Deitch EA. Splenectomy influences endotoxin-induced bacterial translocation. J Trauma 30:1267–1272, 1990.
48. Silva RM, Keller R, Montero IJS, Silva MHG, Goldenberg S, Koh IHJ. Role of Peyer's patch in bacterial translocation. Transplantation Proc 28:2672, 1996.
49. Gennari R, Alexander JW. Arginine, glutamine, and dehydroepiandrosterone reverse the immunosuppressive effect of prednisone during gut-derived sepsis. Crit Care Med 25:1110–1111, 1997.
50. Schimpl G, Pesendorfer P, Steinwender G, Feierl G, Ratschek M, Höllwarth ME. Allopurinol reduces bacterial translocation, intestinal mucosal lipid peroxidation, and neutrophil-derived myeloperoxidase activity in chronic portal hypertensive and common bile duct-ligated growing rats. Ped Res 40:422–428, 1996.
51. Schimpl G. The effect of vitamin C and vitamin E supplementation of bacterial translocation in chronic portal hypertensive and common-bile-duct-ligated rats. Eur Surg Res 29:187–194, 1997.
52. Wang XD, Andersson R, Soltesz V, Wang WQ, Ar'rajab A, Bengmark S. Phospholipids prevent enteric bacterial translocation in the early state of experimental acute liver failure in the rat. Scan J Gastroenterol 29:1117–1121, 1994.
53. Wang S, Andersson R, Soltesz V, Guo W, Bengmark S. Water-soluble ethylhydroxyethyl cellulose prevents bacterial translocation induced by major liver resection in the rat. Ann Surg 217:155–167, 1993.
54. Lipkin M, Newmark H. Calcium and the prevention of colon cancer. J Cell Biochem 22:65–73, 1995.
55. Bovee-Oudenhoven IMJ, Termont DSML, Weerkamp AH, Faassen-Peters MAW, Van Der Meer R. Dietary calcium inhibits the intestinal colonization and translocation of Salmonella in rats. Gastroenterology 113:550–557, 1997.
56. Hartcroft WS. Experimental reproduction of human hepatic disease. In: *Progress in Liver Diseases*, Vol. 1, J Popper and F Schaffner, eds., New York: Grune and Stratton, pp. 68–85.
57. Conn HO. Dietary management of portal-systemic encephalopathy. In: *Hepatic*

Encephalopathy: Syndromes and Therapies, HO Conn and J Bircher, eds., East Lansing, MI: Medi-Ed Press, 1994, pp. 331–350.

58. Owens WE, Berg RD. Bacterial translocation from the gastrointestinal tracts of thymectomized mice. Current Microbiol 7:169–174, 1982.

59. Wells CL, Balish E. Immune response modulation by colonization of GF rats with *Propionibacterium acnes*. Infect Immun 26:473–479, 1979.

60. Fuller DG, Berg RD. Inhibition of bacterial translocation from the gastrointestinal tract by nonspecific immunostimulation. In: *Germfree Research: Microflora Control and Its Application to the Biomedical Sciences*, New York: Alan R. Liss Inc., 1985, pp. 195–198.

61. Fauve RM. Stimulating effect of *Corynebacterium parvum* extract on the macrophage activities against *Salmonella typhimurium* and *Listeria monocytogenes*. In: *Corynebacterium parvum: Applications in Experimental and Clinical Oncology.* Halpern, ed., New York: Plenum Press, 1975, p. 77.

62. Wang XO, Sun ZW, Soltesz V, Deng XM, Andersson R. The role of intravenous administration of *dextran 70* in enteric bacterial translocation after partial hepatectomy in rats. Eur J Clin Inv 27:936–942, 1997.

63. Armstrong CP, Dixon K, Taylor TV, et al. Surgical experience of deeply jaundiced patients with bile duct obstruction. Br J Surg 71:234–238, 1984.

64. Deitch EA, Sittig K, Ma L, et al. Obstructive jaundice promotes bacterial translocation from the gut. Am J Surg 159:79–84, 1990.

65. Ding JW, Andersson R, Norgren I, Stenram U, Bengmark S. The influence of biliary obstruction and sepsis on reticuloendothelial function. Eur J Surg 158:157–164, 1992.

66. Drivas G, James O, Wardle N. Study of reticuloendothelial phagocytic capacity in patients with cholestasis. Br Med J 1:1568–1569, 1976.

67. Cakmakci M, Tirnaksiz B, Hayran M, Belek S, Gürbüz, Sayek I. Effects of obstructive jaundice and external biliary diversion on bacterial translocation in rats. Eur J Surg 162:567–571, 1996.

68. Deitch EA, Ma L, Ma LW, et al. Inhibition of endotoxin-induced bacterial translocation in mice. J Clin Invest 84:36–42, 1989.

69. Kocsar LT, Bertok L, Varteresz V. Effect of bile acids on the intestinal absorption of endotoxin in rats. J Bacteriol 100:220–223, 1969.

70. Gouma DJ, Goelho JCU, Fisher JD. Endotoxemia after relief of biliary obstruction by internal-external drainage in rats. Int J Surg Sci 15:111–115, 1985.

71. Slocum MM, Sittig KM, Specian RD, Deitch EA. Absence of intestinal bile promotes bacterial translocation. Am Surg 58:305–310, 1993.

72. Ding JW, Andersson R, Soltesz V, Bengmark S. The role of bile and bile acids in bacterial translocation in obstructive jaundice in rats. Eur Surg Res 25:11–19, 1993.

73. Ding JW, Nässberger L, Andersson R, Bengmark S. Macrophage phagocytic dysfunction and reduced metabolic response in experimental obstructive jaundice. Eur J Surg 160:437–442, 1994.

74. Ding JW, Andersson R, Soltesz VL, Pärsson H, Johansson K, Wang W, Beng-mark S. Inhibition of bacterial translocation in obstructive jaundice by muramyl tripeptide phosphatidylethanolamine in the rat. J Hepatol 20:720–728, 1994.

75. Ding JW, Andersson R, Stenram U, Lundquist A, Bengmark S. The effect of biliary decompression on reticuloendothelial function in jaundiced rats. Br J Surg 79:648–652, 1992.

76. Parks RW, Clements WDB, Smye MG, Pope C, Rowlands BJ, Diamond T. Intes-tinal barrier dysfunction in clinical and experimental obstructive jaundice and its reversal by internal biliary drainage. Br J Surg 83:1345–1349, 1996.

77. Karsten TM, van Gulik TM, Spanjaard L, Bosma A, van der Bergh Weerman MA, Dingemans KP, Dankert J, Gouma DJ. Bacterial translocation from the biliary tract to blood and lymph in rats with obstructive jaundice. J Surg Res 74:125–130, 1998.

78. Casafont F, Sanchez E, Martin L, Aguero J, Romero FP. Influence of malnutri-tion on the prevalence of bacterial translocation and spontaneous bacterial perito-nitis in experimental cirrhosis in rats. Hepatology 25:1334–1337, 1997.

78a. Nettelbladt, C-G, Katouli M, Bark T. Bulking fibre prevents translocation to mes-enteric lymph nodes of an efficiently translocating *Escherichia coli* strain in rats. Clin Nutri 17:185–190, 1988.

79. Nelson JL, Alexander JW, Gianotti L, Chalk CL, Pyles T. High protein diets are associated with increased bacterial translocation in septic guinea pigs. Nutri-tion 12:195–199, 1996.

80. Barber AE, Jones WG, Minei JP, Fahey TJ, Moldawer LL, Rayburn JL, Fischer E, Keogh CV, Shires T, Lowry SF. Glutamine or fiber supplementation of a defined formula diet: impact on bacterial translocation, tissue composition, and response to endotoxin. JPEN 14:335–343, 1990.

81. Deitch EA, Ma W-J, Ma L, Berg RD, Specian RD. Protein malnutrition predis-poses to inflammatory-induced gut-origin septic states. Ann Surg 211:560–568, 1990.

82. Alverdy JC, Aoys E, Moss GS. Total parenteral nutrition promotes bacterial translocation from the gut. Surgery 104:185–190, 1988.

83. Illig KA, Ryan CK, Hardy DJ, Rhodes J, Locke W, Sax HC. Total parenteral nutrition-induced changes in gut mucosal function: atrophy alone is not the issue. Surg 112:631–637, 1992.

84. Sedman PC, MacFie J, Palmer MD, Mitchell CJ, Sagar PM. Preoperative total parenteral nutrition is not associated with mucosal atrophy or bacterial tansloca-tion in humans. Br J Surg 82:1663–1667, 1995.

85. Spaeth G, Berg RD, Specian RD, Deitch EA. Food without fiber promotes bacte-rial translocation from the gut. Surg 108:240–247, 1990.

86. Spaeth G, Specian RD, Berg RR, Deitch EA. Bulk prevents bacterial transloca-tion induced by the oral administration of total parenteral nutrition solution. JPEN 14:442–447, 1990.

87. Go LL, Albanese CT, Watkins SC. Breast milk protects the neonate from bacte-rial translocation. J Pediatr Surg 29:1059–1064, 1994.

88. Okuyama H, Urao M, Lee D, Drongowski RA, Coran AG. The effect of epidermal growth factor on bacterial translocation in newborn rabbits. J Ped Surg 33: 225–228, 1998.
89. Nakasaki H, Mitomi T, Tajima T, Ohnishi N, Fujii K. Gut bacterial translocation during total parenteral nutrition in experimental rats and its countermeasure. Am J Surg 175:38–43, 1998.
90. Kelly DA. Liver complications of pediatric parenteral nutrition—epidemiology. Nutrition 14:153–157, 1998.

9
Prognosis of Spontaneous Bacterial Peritonitis

Xavier Aldeguer, Roser Vega, Josep Maria Llovet, and Ramon Planas
Hospital Universitari Germans Trias i Pujol, Badalona, Spain

I. INTRODUCTION

Spontaneous bacterial peritonitis (SBP), defined as an infection of ascitic fluid that occurs in the absence of any obvious intraabdominal source, is a frequent complication of cirrhosis. Although SBP was first reported in France around the turn of this century, over the next 70 years only sporadic reports appeared in the medical literature. After the landmark series of Conn and Fessel (1) in 1971, a large number of studies have helped to characterize further the spectrum of this complication. In prospective series encompassing cirrhosis of different etiologies, the *prevalence of SBP* on admission to hospital ranged from 4% to 20% (2–7). Increased awareness of SBP and the performance of almost routine paracentesis explains, in part, the increasing prevalence of this complication of cirrhosis.

This chapter deals with the evolution of the *prognosis* of SBP during the last three decades and the reasons for the improvement in prognosis. In addition, current knowledge of the prognostic predictors, the resolution, and survival of SBP will also be discussed.

II. EVOLUTION OF PROGNOSIS IN RECENT DECADES

The prognosis of SBP has varied to a great extent since its clinical description in 1971. In the 78 episodes of SBP analyzed in the study by Conn and Fessel, the hospital mortality rate was approximately 95% (1). *Survival rates* and resolution of infection rates improved dramatically in the 1980s to 50–85% and 37–77%, respectively (8–17). This trend has been confirmed in the reports of the current decade with corresponding figures of 83–92% and 74–83%, respectively (8,18–20).

This improvement in the prognosis of the SBP was attributed to several factors: (a) the recognition in the 1970s and early 1980s of SBP as a frequent and life-threatening complication of ascitic cirrhosis that led to the use of systematic paracentesis not only when suspecting SBP, but also whenever the overall condition of a cirrhotic patient with ascites deteriorates, as occurs with the appearance of hepatic encephalopathy, fever, or gastrointestinal bleeding ; (b) the lowering of the threshold in polymorphonuclear (PMN) count for the diagnosis of SBP from 500 to 250 cells/mm^3 (8,9), which allows the treatment of patients in an earlier, less severe stage of the infection with the resultant improvement in the survival rate; and (c) the progress in antibiotic treatment, with the usage of very effective, well-tolerated, non-nephrotoxic antibiotic agents, such as third-generation cephalosporins (15,16), the combination of amoxicillin and clavulanic acid, or oral quinolones, such as pefloxacin or ofloxacin, in patients with noncomplicated SBP (21).

In addition to these factors, others may also account for the improved hospital survival in cirrhotic patients with SBP. Shortened courses of antibiotics, such as the withdrawal of antibiotics two days after disappearance of all clinical signs and symptoms of the infection and normalization of ascitic fluid leucocyte count, have proved to be as effective as the longer therapy regimes (17,19). Such changes might contribute to the decrease in duration of hospitalization and thus for the occurrence of new, nosocomial complications. Finally, recent advances in the management of variceal bleeding and ascites also contribute to improved hospital survival (22).

III. CAUSES OF DEATH

At present, antibiotic treatment in SBP achieves the resolution of the infection in approximately 90% of cases. Despite this high resolution rate, 20–40% of the patients die during the hospitalization period, probably because the infection triggers progressive impairment of liver and renal function. Although it is difficult to establish the primary cause of death precisely in patients with as many complications as those who suffer from SBP, presently only those patients with more severe and advanced SBP, usually with shock and renal failure, die as a consequence of the infection itself (3,14,23–26). In cases of

SBP resolution as well as in nonadvanced SBP patients, other complications of the underlying liver disease, such as gastrointestinal bleeding, liver failure, or hepatorenal syndrome, are responsible for death (8,9,26,27). It has been estimated that the frequency of death during the period of hospitalization is five to six times higher in infected cirrhotic patients than in noninfected patients (28).

Even though the resolution of the infection and survival have improved in recent years, the occurrence of an episode of SBP implies a poor prognosis. In fact, the 1-year probability of survival after the first episode of SBP is approximately 30–40%, which is much lower than the survival rates observed in patients with noninfected ascites (57–64%). Relapse of the infection, gastrointestinal bleeding, and hepatic failure are the main causes of death (14,29). Currently, a history of resolved SBP in a patient with advanced cirrhosis is considered per se to be a clinical indication for liver transplantation.

IV. PROGNOSTIC FACTORS

In recent years, several clinical and laboratory findings obtained prior to or during the course of SBP have been considered to be predictors of the failure of the resolution of infection or of the development of renal impairment and death. The identification of these risk factors allows treatment of SBP patients at especially high risk with specific measures to prevent renal impairment and, perhaps, to increase survival. On the other hand, SBP patients in relatively good clinical condition and with indicators of high resolution rates of infection and the absence of SBP-associated complications may be treated with oral antibiotic agents. Such patients might well complete their treatment as outpatients, thus reducing the cost and improving the quality of life of these patients.

The most important prognostic factors identified as independent predictors of the resolution of infection and hospital survival in cirrhotic patients with SBP in most of the studies are (a) the absence of renal impairment; (b) the degree of liver failure; and (c) the severity of the infection itself.

A. Renal Impairment

Renal impairment in cirrhotic patients with ascites, the so-called hepatorenal syndrome (HRS), has been widely assessed. Though the hepatorenal syndrome was described originally in patients with a rapidly progressive impairment in renal function that led to death within few days or weeks, later studies have showed the existance of a subset of patients with renal failure and all the characteristics of HRS except for a stable, less-severe impairment in renal function and longer survival. Based on these observations, two different types of HRS, which probably represent distinct expressions of the same pathogenic mechanism, have been defined recently by the latest Consensus of the International Ascites Club (30): (a) Type I HRS, which is characterized by rapidly progressive reduction of renal function, as defined by a doubling of the initial serum creatinine concentration to a level higher than 2.5 mg/dl, or a 50% reduction of the initial 24-h creatinine clearance to a level lower than 20 ml/min in less than two weeks; and (b) Type II HRS, in which the renal failure is not characterized by a rapidly progressive course. The overall risk of developing this severe complication in a cirrhotic patient with ascites is approximately 18% in the first year and 39% within five years after the development of ascites. The prognosis of the Type I HRS is poor, with a median survival time of less than two weeks after the onset of the renal impairment, regardless of the therapeutic approach used. Type II HRS has a better prognosis, with survivals of 54% and 39%, after three and 12 months, respectively (31,32), but worse than that of cirrhotic patients with ascites but without HRS.

Taking into account the importance of renal impairment in the prognosis of cirrhotic patients with ascites, it is not surprising that the previous existence and/or the development of renal impairment during an episode of SBP plays an important prognostic role. This assumption has been assessed in many studies (8,25,26,29,33). In a retrospective study of 213 consecutive episodes of SBP empirically treated with cefotaxime in 185 cirrhotic patients, Toledo et al. (26) found that renal function, assessed by blood urea nitrogen (BUN) levels at the time of the diagnosis of SBP, was the most significant independent predictor of the resolution of infection and of patient survival (Table 9.1). Similarly, Llovet et al. (18), in an assessment of short-term prognosis of 64 patients with SBP, found that certain parameters of renal insufficiency, such as serum creatinine and serum sodium concentration, were independently associated with hospital mortality in addition to other variables such as the polymorphonuclear count in the ascites, prothrombin time, and serum cholesterol.

A recent study reported by Follo et al. (20) must be mentioned because of its definitive conclusions. This study was the first directed at investigating the incidence, predictive factors, and prognosis of renal impairment (RI) in 252 consecutive episodes of SBP in 197 cirrhotic patients. Clinical and laboratory data were obtained before and after the episode of SBP and considered as possible predictors of RI and hospital mortality. The results of this study clearly indicate that renal impairment is an important event in the clinical course of SBP in patients with cirrhosis. In fact, the incidence of renal impairment induced by an episode of SBP (SBP-RI) was 33%. In this study, SBP-

Table 9.1 Independent Prognostic Factors in the Resolution of Infection and Survival in 185 Cirrhotic Patients with Spontaneous Bacterial Peritonitis Treated with Cefotaxime

	p value
SBP resolution	
Band neutrophils in WBC count/mm^3	<0.001
Site of SBP acquisition (community or hospital)	0.001
BUN level	0.004
Serum AST level	0.041
Hospital survival	
BUN level	<0.001
Serum ALT level	<0.001
Site of SBP acquisition (community or hospital)	0.001
Age	0.002
Child-Pugh score	0.008
Ileus	0.012

Source: Ref. 26.

RI was defined as an increase in BUN or serum creatinine levels to greater than 30 mg/dL or 1.5 mg/dL, respectively, in patients who had had normal baseline values, or as a 50% increase in BUN or serum creatinine over baseline values in those patients with preexisting renal impairment (BUN > 30 mg/dL or creatinine > 1.5 mg/dL). According to the evolution of kidney function, renal impairment was divided into three categories: (a) *progressive,* which is characterized by a progressive increase in BUN and serum creatinine during hospitalization, i.e., is identical to Type I HRS; (b) *static,* when the initial impairment in renal function stabilized during hospitalization; and (c) *transient,* when serum creatinine levels and BUN remained constant or returned to normal values during hospital admission after resolution of the infection. The episodes of SBP comprised 42%, 33%, and 25% of types a, b, and c, respectively (Fig. 9.1).

Llovet et al. (34), in a recently published study performed in 229 episodes of SBP, found a slightly higher incidence of SBP-RI (46.4%), which was transient in 26% of the episodes, static in 35%, and progressive in the remaining 38% of cases. In both studies (20,34), SBP-RI occurred in the setting of arterial hypotension and was characterized by oliguria, low urinary sodium concentration, and high urinary osmolality. These features are identical to those observed in cirrhotic patients with ascites in whom functional kidney failure spontaneously develops as a consequence of intense renal arteri-

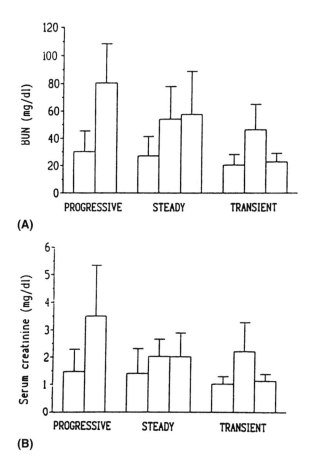

Figure 9.1 Evolution of (A) BUN and (B) serum creatinine levels in the three types of SBP-RI. The first and second bars in progressive SBP-RI represent baseline and peak levels. In steady SBP-RI, levels obtained in basal conditions (first bars), at the time of detection of SBP-RI (second bars), and at the end of hospitalization (third bars) are represented. The first, second, and third bars in transient SBP represent baseline, peak, and recovery levels, respectively. (From Ref. 20.)

olar vasoconstriction. These data suggest that SBP-RI represents a functional renal impairment induced by the infection. However, unlike HRS, which is rarely transient, SBP-RI may be reversible in 25% of the cases.

   The leukocyte count in blood at the time of diagnosis, which probably reflects the severity of the infection, the BUN (or serum creatinine concentration, in hospital-acquired episodes of SBP), and the serum bilirubin level before the onset of SBP were the only independent predictors of the development of SBP-RI in the study by Follo et al. (20). These findings indicate that cirrhotic patients with ascites and severely impaired liver or kidney function are especially predisposed to develop SBP-RI. The exact mechanisms that induce SBP-RI are not completely understood. However, it is possible that several different mechanisms may simultaneously operate to produce SBP-RI in cirrhotic patients with ascites and SBP. These mechanisms may represent: (a) an impairment of liver function related to the infection; (b) the deterioration of circulatory function caused by the endothelial vasodilator substances, which can induce renal vasoconstriction by a baroreceptor-mediated stimulation of the renin-angiotensin-catecholamine-vasopressin systems; or (c) a direct stimulation of renal vasoconstrictors by endotoxin, which is a normal constituent of the bacterial cell wall.

The most outstanding finding of the study by Follo et al. (20) was the observation that renal impairment is the strongest independent predictor factor of hospital mortality in the whole series of patients with SBP and in the subgroup of patients with hospital-acquired SBP. In fact, more than half (54%) of the patients who developed renal impairment during an episode of SBP died during the hospitalization, as compared to only 9% of episodes of SBP in the absence of RI. Although the contribution of kidney dysfunction to the high mortality rate in SBP episodes associated with SBP-RI is difficult to ascertain, the observation that the mortality rate correlated directly with the degree of impairment of kidney function is compatible with a cause-and-effect relationship (Table 9.2).

The major role of RI in the prognosis of hospital mortality in cirrhotic

Table 9.2 Hospital Mortality According to the Evolution of Kidney Function in 231 SBP Episodes that Responded to Treatment

SBI-RI status	Number	Deaths
Episodes without SBP-IR	166	12 (7%)
Episodes with SBI-IR	65	27 (42%)*
Transient SBP-RI	21	1 (5%)
Steady SBP-RI	26	8 (31%)*
Progressive SBP-RI	181	8 (100%)*

*p = 0.001 vs. episodes without SBP-IR.
Source: Ref. 20.

patients with SBP has been confirmed in two recent studies by Navasa et al. (21,35). The first study (21) was a multicenter, randomized trial comparing the efficacy of intravenous cefotaxime vs. oral ofloxacin in 123 cirrhotic patients with SBP without shock, gastrointestinal hemorrhage, ileus, severe renal failure, or grade II–IV hepatic encephalopathy. Oral ofloxacin was as effective as intravenous cefotaxime in uncomplicated SBP. In this study, the BUN at the time of diagnosis was again the strongest predictor of hospital survival. In fact, none of the 36 nonazotemic patients with community-acquired SBP and without hepatic encephalopathy developed complications during hospitalization, and all were alive at time of discharge. In the second study (35), performed in 52 cirrhotic patients with SBP in the absence of shock or gastrointestinal bleeding, the only independent predictive factor of hospital mortality identified in the multivariate analysis was renal failure at the time of the diagnosis of SBP. Renal failure, interleukin-6 ascitic levels, a measure of the inflammatory response to infection in ascitic fluid, and mean arterial pressure were the three independent predictors of SBP-RI at the time of the diagnosis of SBP in this study.

In summary, these data indicate that renal impairment is a frequent event in cirrhotic patients with SBP, and that SBP-RI is the most important predictor of hospital mortality in patients with SBP. The prevention of renal failure may, therefore, improve short-term survival in patients with SBP. Unfortunately, at present, effective methods of preventing SBP-RI have not been clearly established.

B. Degree of Liver Failure

The degree of liver failure, which may be assessed by different parameters, such as Child-Pugh score, prothrombin activity, and serum bilirubin or albumin concentrations, has been related to the short-term prognosis of the SBP. The association of liver failure with mortality in SBP is not surprising, since SBP occurs usually in patients with advanced cirrhosis, and the prognostic value of these measurements of liver failure is well documented (7,8,25).

In early series of SBP, the degree of liver failure was associated not only with hospital survival, but also with the resolution of SBP. In 1978, Weinstein et al. (24) found that hepatic encephalopathy, total serum bilirubin levels greater than 8 mg/dL, and albumin levels lower than 2.5 g/dL, respectively, were associated with poor prognosis in the group of 28 episodes of SBP in 25 cirrhotic patients studied. These findings suggest that the worse the liver function, the worse the prognosis of SBP. A few years later, Hoefs et al. (8), in a review of 43 cirrhotic patients with SBP, noted similar prognostic indices. In addition, they identified two different prognostic groups according to their hepatic function. The first group (serum bilirubin > 8 mg/dL and/ or serum creatinine > 2.1 mg/dL) had acute liver injury, which is usually superimposed on chronic liver disease, whereas the second group was characterized by advanced relatively inactive chronic liver disease. The majority of patients in the first group died (75%) within the first seven days of the onset of SBP, whereas 90% of the patients in the second group survived the initial episode of SBP, and 50% survived the hospitalization. These criteria described by Hoefs et al. (8) have become less accurate in the last decade. In 1993, we performed a multivariate study in order to identify the predictive factors of hospital mortality in 64 cirrhotic patients with SBP (18). Eleven patients (17%) died while in hospital, six of them before the infection was considered cured. The prothrombin rate and serum cholesterol concentration, two indices of liver failure, were identified as independent prognostic factors of hospital mortality. Moreover, when a discriminant function in a randomly selected sample of the patients (60%) was analyzed, it correctly predicted the outcome in 36/39 cases (92.3%), with a 87.5% sensitivity and a 93.5% specificity for death. When the prediction was made using the criteria described by Hoefs at al. (8), the number of cases classsified with the predicted outcome were only 30/36 (77%), with lower sensitivity and specificity for death (50% and 83.8%, respectively).

In the last decade, some studies including large numbers of patients have clarified the role of the severity of liver failure in the resolution of infection and hospital survival in cirrhotic patients with an episode of SBP. In the study by Toledo et al. (26), the Child-Pugh score did not predict correctly the resolution of SBP, although it was one of the six variables that were independently correlated with survival at the end of hospitalization. Serum bilirubin, one of the components of Child-Pugh score, was also found to be an independent prognostic factor with mortality during hospitalization in the study by Follo et al. (20).

Finally, among the 45 clinical and laboratory features analyzed as possible prognostic factors in the study by Navasa et al. (21), only the BUN and the presence of grade I hepatic encephalopathy at the time of the diagnosis of SBP independently correlated with survival. As shown in Table 9.3, BUN and grade I hepatic encephalopathy closely correlated with both the clinical course and the hospital mortality in patients with community- and hospital-acquired SBP.

C. Severity of Infection

The severity of the infection has also been considered as an important prognostic factor in most of the studies carried out so far. Many clinical symptoms

Table 9.3 Clinical Course of Cirrhotic Patients with Community- and Hospital-Acquired SBP Classified According to the Presence or Absence of Grade I Hepatic Encephalopathy and BUN Values at the Time of Diagnosis of SBP

	Patients with treatment failure and/or developing complications during hospitalization[a]	Deaths
Community-acquired SBP		
BUN of <25 mg/dL and no HE (n = 36) (%)	0 (0)	0 (0)
BUN of >25 mg/dL and/or HE (n = 52) (%)	20 (38)	14 (27)
P value	<0.001	0.002
Hospital-acquired SBP		
BUN of <25 mg/dL and no HE (n = 16) (%)	3 (19)	1 (6)
BUN of >25 mg/dL and/or HE (n = 19) (%)	13 (68)	8 (42)
p value	0.009	0.042

HE, grade I hepatic encephalopathy.
[a] Gastrointestinal bleeding, development or worsening of HE, or bacterial infections other than SBP or hepatorenal syndrome.
Source: Ref. 21.

and analytical or microbiological variables which reflect directly or indirectly the severity of the infection have been assessed. As early as 1978, Weinstein et al. (24) analyzed some of these parameters in their review of 28 cases documented over a five-year period. They found that both clinical signs, such as increasing hepatic encephalopathy, and an analytical variable indicative of the severity of the infection, such as the percentage of granulocytic leukocytes greater than 85% in the peripheral blood, were associated with an adverse prognosis, whereas no differences were observed among patients with bacteremia and with sterile blood cultures. Three other clinical variables, hepatic encephalopathy, ileus, and septic shock have also achieved statistical significance for prognostic value in some studies (7,21,25,26). Fortunately, the presence of septic shock, which is associated with a deleterious prognosis, is now very infrequent because of the earlier diagnosis of SBP.

Other analytical variables obtained from blood or ascitic fluid such as the total leukocytosis, the polymorphonuclear cell count in blood, the absolute polymorphonuclear count or the percentage of PMNs in the ascitic fluid, and the ascitic fluid lactate concentration and pH have been defined as indendendent prognostic variables in some studies (17,18,26,29,36). Regular monitoring of the PMN count in the ascitic fluid during antibiotic therapy (usually every 48 h) provides important information for establishing the endpoint for antibiotic therapy and for predicting the outcome of the patient's hospital course. This assumption was confirmed in a study by Fong et al. (17) that was performed in 33 cirrhotic patients with an episode of SBP. Among the 30 patients with an initial PMN cell count in the ascitic fluid >500/mm^3, the percentage change of PMN cell count after 48 h of therapy correlated with survival. The survivors had a mean decrease of 92% compared to 67% for nonsurvivors. These data suggest that patients who show a rapid drop in the ascitic PMN count at 48 h have a better prognosis than those who exhibit a smaller decrement. This effect may reflect a better bactericidal response by the host in patients with less severe underlying liver disease.

It is well known that infection causes the release of multiple endogenous mediators such as cytokines and interleukins, which are responsible for the inflammatory response. Although the aim of this response is to suppress the infection, it may be associated with adverse hemodynamic and metabolic consequences. Cytokines, particularly tumor necrosis factor alpha (TNFα), interleukin-1beta (IL-1β), and interleukin-6 (IL-6), are probably the most important mediators of sepsis. It has been established that patients with chronic liver disease respond to sepsis with a greater and longer-lasting increase in the circulating levels of IL-6 and TNFα than patients without cirrhosis (37). Furthermore, the intraperitoneal release of IL-6 is greatly increased in cirrhotic patients with ascites and SBP (38). All these data suggest that the inflammatory response to infection, as reflected by the levels of cytokines in plasma or ascitic fluid, is greater in cirrhotic patients than in noncirrhotic patients, and that cytokines may be of prognostic significance in patients with liver failure. The possible relationship between the degree of the inflammatory response triggered by the intra-abdominal infection, development of SBP-RI, and hospital mortality has recently been assessed in a series of 52 cirrhotic patients with SBP in the absence of shock or gastrointestinal bleeding (35). In addition to confirming the results of previous studies, they suggest that plasma and ascitic fluid levels of cytokines are greatly increased in these patients, that renal impairment is a frequent complication during the course of SBP. Furthermore, renal failure at the time of diagnosis or the development of SBP-RI are important negative predictors of survival during hospitalization. The most dramatic findings in this study were as follows: First, a rapid decrease in the concentration of cytokines in ascitic fluid and in plasma following antibiotic treatment occurred, as shown by the fact that 48 h after cefotaxime treatment a sharp fall in cytokine levels was observed in all patients who responded to treatment. Second, cirrhotic patients with SBP do not constitute a homogeneous population in terms of intra-abdominal cytokine production. The ascitic fluid concentration of TNFα, IL-6, and PMN were significantly higher in patients with culture-positive SBP than in those with culture-negative SBP. Among patients with culture-positive SBP, those with gram-negative isolates showed higher cytokine levels in plasma and ascitic fluid and PMN concentrations in ascites, suggesting that the intra-abdominal inflammatory response in SBP depends on the concentration and the type of infecting organisms. Third, there was a relationship between the degree of inflammatory response at the time of the diagnosis of the infection and the development of SBP-RI. Patients developing SBP-RI showed significantly higher ascitic fluid PMN concentration and plasma and ascitic fluid levels of cytokines at diagnosis than those without deterioration in renal function. In summary, the results of this study suggest that the degree of the inflammatory response at the time of diagnosis may be important in the pathogenesis of SBP-RI. The numbers and types of organisms in ascitic fluid are important predictors of the development of renal impairment and of the prognosis in cirrhotic patients with SBP.

1. Culture Positive vs. Culture Negative

The positivity of ascitic fluid cultures in cirrhotic patients with SBP suggests the existence of a higher concentration of bacteria in ascitic fluid than in culture-negative SBP, the so-called culture-negative neutrocytic ascites (CNNA), as a consequence of a greater entry of microorganisms into the ascitic fluid and/or a lower bactericidal capacity of ascitic fluid. Data about the prognostic role of positive-culture SBP are controversial: culture-positive SBP was found to be a prognostic factor of survival in some studies (11,17,20), but not in others (8,26,29,39). Some studies have reported that CNNA is a less severe variant of SBP (11,40). However, other studies have not confirmed these data, and short-term mortality of patients with CNNA seems to be the same or only slightly lower than that of patients with SBP (39). Therefore, CNNA should be considered to be a true infection of ascitic fluid, which must be treated with appropriate antibiotics.

The presence of highly virulent bacteria may be associated with the development of invasive infections, such as neonatal meningitis, bacteremia, and pyelonephritis. *Escherichia coli* is the most frequent bacterium isolated in SBP, and encapsulated *Escherichia coli* are more frequently associated with invasive infections than nonencapsulated strains. Recently, Soriano et al. (41) studied the capsular serotypes of the *Escherichia coli* that cause SBP and their possible role in prognosis of cirrhotic patients with SBP. Two-thirds of the episodes of SBP were caused by encapsulated *Escherichia coli*. Patients with

Table 9.4 Morbidity and Mortality of Patients According to the Presence or Absence of Capsular Polysaccharide of *Escherichia coli*

	Group I (n = 27)	Group 2 (n = 10)	P
Patients with complications[a]	25 (92.5)	5 (50)	<0.01
Complications per patient[b]	1.9 ± 1.1	0.8 ± 1.0	<0.01
Septic shock	8 (29.6)	1 (10)	NS
Gastrointestinal hemorrhage	8 (29.6)	0	NS
Encephalopathy	20 (74.1)	4 (40)	NS
Renal failure	17 (62.9)	3 (30)	NS
Mortality	12 (44.4)	2 (20)	NS

Note: Group 1, patients with encapsulated *E coli;* group 2, patients with nonencapsulated *E coli.* The numbers in parentheses refer to percentages.
[a] Number of patients who developed one or more complications.
[b] Number of complications per patient (mean ± SD). The other numbers in the table refer to number of patients.
Source: Ref. 41.

encapsulated *Escherichia coli* SBP showed a higher incidence of severe complications, such as shock, gastrointestinal bleeding, and renal failure, and a trend to a higher mortality rate than patients with SBP induced by nonencapsulated *Escherichia coli* (Table 9.4). These observations suggest that virulence factors of bacteria may play a role in the prognosis of cirrhotics with SBP.

2. Hospital- vs. Community-Acquired SBP

The site of SBP acquisition may also be an important predictor of the resolution of the infection and of patient survival. In fact, in the study by Toledo et al. (26), SBP resolved in 89% and 68% of community-acquired and hospital-acquired episodes, respectively. On the other hand, 73% of patients with community-acquired SBP and only 50% of those with hospital-acquired SBP were discharged alive from hospital. It is not surprising, therefore, that the site of SBP acquisition was found to be an independent prognostic factor for both SBP resolution and hospital survival in that study. As mentioned above, in the study by Navasa et al. (21) hospital mortality was also higher in hospital-acquired than in community-acquired SBP, especially when associated with renal impairment and/or hepatic encephalopathy (Table 9.3). As hospital-acquired SBP appeared in patients previously admitted to hospital because of problems other than infection, the most logical explanation for these findings is that patients in whom SBP developed during hospitalization had more severe disease than those with community-acquired SBP. However, other studies did not demonstrate that the site of SBP acquisition has prognostic value (8,18,20,25).

V. OTHER PROGNOSTIC FACTORS

There are other variables associated with survival in cirrhotic patients with SBP. Age has been identified as one such prognostic factor in some studies (20,26). The existence of a recent upper gastrointestinal hemorrhage was shown to be a poor prognostic sign for survival in the study by Llovet et al. (18). Although gastrointestinal bleeding itself is a severe complication of cirrhosis, the detrimental effects of gastrointestinal bleeding on the immune response in cirrhosis could also account for its negative prognostic value in SBP. This observation is a further argument for using selective intestinal de-contamination in cirrhotic patients with gastrointestinal hemorrhage. Finally, the existence of a hepatocarcinoma at the time of diagnosis of SBP has been found to be associated with a very poor prognosis (29).

REFERENCES

1. Conn HO, Fessel JM. Spontaneous bacterial peritonitis in cirrhosis: variation on a theme. Medicine 1971; 50:161–197.
2. Bar-Meir S, Lerner E, Conn HO. Analysis of ascitic fluid in cirrhosis. Am J Dig Dis 1979; 24:136–144.
3. Correiz JP, Conn HO. Spontaneous bacterial peritonitis in cirrhosis: endemic or epidemic. Med Clin North Am 1975; 59:963–981.
4. Kline MM, McCallum RW, Guth PH. The clinical value of ascitic fluid culture and leukocyte count in alcoholic cirrhosis. Gastroenterology 1976; 70:408–412.
5. Planas R, Arroyo V. Spontaneous bacterial peritonitis. Acta Gastroenterol Belg 1995; 58:297–310.
6. Garcia-Tsao G. Spontaneous bacterial peritonitis. Gastroenterol Clin North Am 1992; 21:257–275.
7. Almdal TP, Skinhoj P. Spontaneous bacterial peritonitis in cirrhosis: incidence, diagnosis, and prognosis. Scand J Gastroenterol 1987; 22:295–300.
8. Hoefs JC, Canawati HN, Sapico FL, Hopkins RR, Weiner J, Montgomerie JZ. Spontaneous bacterial peritonitis. Hepatology 1982; 2:339–407.
9. Pinzello G, Simonetti RG, Craxi A, DiPiazza S, Spano C, Pagliaro L. Spontane-ous bacterial peritonitis: a prospective investigation in predominantly non-alco-holic cirrhotic patients. Hepatology 1983; 3:545–549.

10. Carey WD, Boayke A, Leatherman J. Spontaneous bacterial peritonitis: clinical and laboratory features with reference to hospital-acquired cases. Am J Gastroenterol 1986; 81: 1156–1161.

11. Pelletier G, Salmon D, Ink O, Attali P, Buffet C, Etienne JP. Culture-negative neutrocytic ascites: a less severe variant of spontaneous bacterial peritonitis. J Hepatol 1990; 10:327–331.

12. Akriviadis EA, Runyon BA. Utility of an algorithm in differentiating spontaneous from secondary bacterial peritonitis. Gastroenterology 1990; 98:127–133.

13. Rimola A, Bory F, Terés J, Pérez-Ayuso RM, Arroyo V, Rodés J. Oral, nonabsorbable antibiotics prevent infection in cirrhotics with gastrointestinal hemorrhage. Hepatology 1985; 5:463–467.

14. Titó Ll, Rimola A, Ginès P, Llach J, Arroyo V, Rodés J. Recurrence of spontaneous bacterial peritonitis in cirrhosis: frequency and predictive factors. Hepatology 1988; 8:27–31.

15. Felisart J, Rimola A, Arroyo V, Pérez-Ayuso RM, Quintero E, Ginès P, Rodés J. Cefotaxime is more effective than ampicillin-tobramycin in cirrhotics with severe infections. Hepatology 1985; 5:457–462.

16. Ariza J, Xiol X, Esteve M, Fernández-Bañares F, Liñares J, ALonso T, Gudiol F. Aztreonam vs cefotaxime in the treatment of gram-negative spontaneous bacterial peritonitis in cirrhotic patients. Hepatology 1991; 14:91–98.

17. Fong T, Akriviadis E, Runyon BA, Reynolds TB. Polymorphonuclear cell count response and duration of antibiotic therapy in spontaneous bacterial peritonitis. Hepatology 1989; 9:423–426.

18. Llovet JM, Planas R, Morillas R, Quer JC, Cabré E, Boix J, Humbert P, Guilera M, Doménech E, Bertrán X, Gassull MA. Short-term prognosis of cirrhotics with spontaneous bacterial peritonitis: multivariate study. Am J Gastroenterol 1993; 88:388–392.

19. Runyon BA, McHutchinson JC, Antillon MR, Akriviadis E, Montano A. Short-course versus long course antibiotic treatment of spontaneous bacterial peritontis. A randomized controlled study of 100 patients. Gastroenterology 1991; 100: 1737–1742.

20. Follo A, Llovet JM, Navasa M, Planas R, Forns X, Francitorra A, Rimola A, Gassull MA, Arroyo V, Rodés J. Renal impairment following spontaneous bacterial peritonitis in cirrhosis. Incidence, clinical course, predicitive factors and prognosis. Hepatology 1994; 20:1495–1501.

21. Navasa M, Follo A, Llovet JM, Clemente G, Vargas V, Rimola A, Marco F, Guarner C, Forné M, Planas R, Bañares R, Castells L, Jiménez de Anta MT, Arroyo V, Rodés J. Randomized comparative study of oral ofloxacin versus intravenous cefotaxime in spontaneous bacterial peritonitis. Gastroenterology 1996; 111:1011–1017.

22. Arroyo V, Ginès P, Planas R. Treatment of ascites in cirrhosis. Gastroenterol Clin North Am 1992; 21:237–256.

23. Wyke RJ. Problems of bacterial infection in patients with liver disease. Gut 1987; 28:623–641.

24. Weinstein MP, Iannini PB, Stratton CW, Eickhoff TC. Spontaneous bacterial peritonitis: a review of 28 cases with emphasis on improved survival and factors influencing prognosis. Am J Med 1978; 64:592–598.
25. Ariza J, Fernández J, Garau J, Rufi G, Casanova A, Gudiol F. Peritonitis espontánea del cirrótico. Consideraciones sobre su patogénesis y factores pronósticos. A propósito de 59 casos. Med Clin (Bar) 1982; 79:305–310.
26. Toledo C, Salmerón JM, Rimola A, Navasa M, Arroyo V, Llach J, Ginès A, Ginès P, Rodés J. Spontaneous bacterial peritonitis in cirrhosis: predictive factors of infection resolution and survival in patients treated with cefotaxime. Hepatology 1993; 17:251–257.
27. Wilcox M, Dismukes W. Spontaneous bacterial peritonitis. A review of pathogenesis, diagnosis and treatment. Medicine 1987; 66:447–456.
28. Caly WR, Strauss E. A prospective study of bacterial infections in patients with cirrhosis. J Hepatol 1993; 18:271–272.
29. Ink O, Pelletier G, Salmon D, Attali P, Pessione F, Hannoun S, Buffet C, Etienne JP. Pronostic de l'infection spontaneé de l'ascite chez le cirrhotique. Gastroenterol Clin Biol 1989; 13:556–561.
30. Arroyo V, Ginès P, Gerbes AL, Dudley FJ, Gentilini P, Laffi G, Reynolds TB, Ring-Larsen H, Schölmerich J. Definition and diagnostic criteria of refractory ascites and hepatorenal syndrome in cirrhosis. Hepatology 1996; 23:164–176.
31. Ginès A, Escorsell A, Ginès P, Saló J, Jiménez W, Inglada L, Navasa M, Rimola A, Arroyo V, Rodés J. Incidence, predictive factors, and prognosis of the Hepatorenal Syndrome in cirrhosis with ascites. Gastroenterology 1993; 105:229–236.
32. Llach J, Ginès P, Arroyo V, Rimola A, Titó Ll, Badalamenti S, Jiménez W, Gayá J, Rivera F, Rodés J. Prognostic value of arterial pressure, endogenous vasoactive systems and renal function in cirrhotic patients admitted to the hospital for the treatment of ascites. Gastroenterology 1988; 94:482–487.
33. Mihas AA, Toussaint J, Hsu HS, Dostherow P, Achord JL. Spontaneous bacterial peritonitis in cirrhosis. Clinical and laboratory features, survival and prognostic factors. Hepato Gastroenterol 1992; 39:520–522.
34. Llovet JM, Rodríguez-Iglesias MP, Moitinho E, Planas R, Bataller R, Navasa M, Menacho M, Pardo A, Castells A, Cabré E, Arroyo V, Gassull MA, Rodés J. Spontaneous bacterial peritonitis in patients with cirrhosis undergoing selective intestinal decontamination. A retrospective study of 229 spontaneous bacterial peritonitis episodes. J Hepatol 1997; 26:88–95.
35. Navasa M, Follo A, Filella X, Jiménez W, Francitorra A, Planas R, Ruiz del Arbol L, Rimola A, Arroyo V, Rodés J. Tumor necrosis factor and interleukin-6 in spontaneous bacterial peritonitis in cirrhosis. Renal impairment and mortality. Hepatology 1998; 27:1227–1232.
36. Attali P, Turne K, Pelletier G, Ink O, Etienne JP. PH of ascitic fluid. Diagnostic and prognostic value in cirrhotic and non-cirrhotic patients. Gastroenterology 1986; 90:1255–1260.
37. Byl B, Roucloux I, Crusiaux A, Dupont E, Devière J. Tumor necrosis factor

alpha and interleukin 6 plasma levels in infected cirrhotic patients. Gastroenterology 1993; 104:1492–1497.

38. Propst T, Propst A, Herold M, Schauer G, Judnaier G, Braunsteiner H, Stöffler G, Vogel W. Spontaneous bacterial peritonitis is associated with high levels of interleukin-6 and its secondary mediator in ascitic fluid. Eur J Clin Invest 1993; 23:832–836.

39. Runyon BA, Hoefs JC. Culture-negative neutrocytic ascites: a variant of spontaneous bacterial ascites. Hepatology 1984; 4:1209–1211.

40. al Amri SM, Allam AR, al Mofleh IA. Spontaneous bacterial peritonitis and culture-negative neutrocytic ascites in patients with non-alcoholic liver cirrhosis. J Gastroenterol Hepatol 1994; 9:433–436.

41. Soriano G, Coll P, Guarner C, Such J, Sánchez F, Prats G, Vilardell F. *Escherichia coli* capsular polysaccharide and spontaneous bacterial peritonitis in cirrhosis. Hepatology 1995; 21:668–673.

10
General Management of Patients with Spontaneous Bacterial Peritonitis

Joan M. Salmerón, Miguel Navasa, and Juan Rodés
Hospital Clínic i Provincial de Barcelona, University of Barcelona, Barcelona, Spain

Patients with advanced cirrhosis frequently develop bacterial infections. The incidence of infectious complications in hospitalized cirrhotic patients is very high, with different studies showing that 30–50% of such patients have bacterial infections at admission or develop these complications during hospitalization (1–4). The incidence of different types of bacterial infections are detailed in Table 10.1. As shown in this table, spontaneous bacterial peritonitis (SBP) is, after urinary tract infections, the second most frequent infectious complication in cirrhotic patients with ascites.

SBP characteristically occurs in patients with advanced cirrhosis with the Child-Pugh class of these patients being C in 75% of the cases and B in the remaining 25% (5). In this setting, the development of clinical complications such as ascites, hepatic encephalopathy, renal failure, or gastrointestinal bleeding and the derangement of liver function in the course of SBP is not surprising. Therefore, the general management of patients with SBP must take the following factors into consideration: (a) the treatment of the infection and (b) the treatment and prevention of complications.

In the last 15 years, a number of different antibiotic regimens have demonstrated both their efficacy, in terms of sensitivity of the microorganisms isolated in episodes of SBP (>90%), and the resolution of infection (80%), as well as their safety in terms of low rates of superinfection (<2%) and other

Table 10.1   Bacterial Infections in Liver Cirrhosis:
Incidence

Infection	Percentage (%)	
	Limits	Average
Total incidence	33–46	39
Types of infection:		
Urinary tract infection	18–29	21
Spontaneous bacterial peritonitis	7–23	15
Respiratory infection	6–10	8
Bacteremia	4–10	7
Other infections	3–6	5

From Refs. 1–4.

adverse effects such as renal failure ($<1\%$) (5–11). It is clear that further improvement of this figure can only be achieved by careful management of these patients including the prevention, early recognition, and treatment of complications related to SBP and chronic liver disease as well as the use of new therapeutic strategies in the treatment of SBP.

I.   EVALUATION OF SEVERITY OF INFECTION

The clinical presentations of SBP have been described in detail in different studies including large series of patients with this complication (5,12–18). The clinical manifestations at the time of diagnosis of SBP in different historical series of patients treated at the Hospital Clinic in Barcelona may be seen in Table 10.2. As shown in this table, the clinical signs at diagnosis and the in-hospital prognosis of this complication vary over time. Two phenomena may explain the differences observed: the time of diagnosis of SBP, which is earlier in recent series; and the availability of highly effective, safe antibiotic agents to treat SBP since the 1980s with the introduction of third-generation cephalosporins, mainly cefotaxime (5–7,10).

Fever and abdominal pain, with or without rebound tenderness, are the most frequent clinical signs identified in patients with SBP. Hepatic encephalopathy, gastrointestinal dysfunction (nausea, vomiting, diarrhea, or ileus), oliguria, and gastrointestinal hemorrhage may be present at diagnosis and/or during the course of SBP. The presence of septic shock carries a very poor

Table 10.2 Clinical Manifestations and Complications at Time of Diagnosis of Spontaneous Bacterial Peritonitis and Survival at End of Hospitalization in Two Historical Series of Patients Treated in the Hospital Clinic of Barcelona

	1971–1979 (n = 91)	1981–1989 (n = 294)
Abdominal pain	73 (80%)	205 (70%)
Fever	61 (67%)	183 (62%)
Ileus[a]	39 (43%)	14 (5%)
Hepatic encephalopathy[a]	60 (66%)	124 (42%)
Gastrointestinal bleeding[a]	20 (22%)	29 (10%)
Septic shock[a]	38 (42%)	25 (8%)
Renal failure[a]	78 (86%)	116 (39%)
Survival[a]	15 (16%)	185 (63%)

[a] Statistically significant differences, <0.5.
From Refs. 5, 6, 19–22.

prognosis. Death occurs within a few hours or days regardless of adequate therapy, with the expected mortality in these cases being more than 70% (5,6,10). Generalized hemorrhage, as a consequence of disseminated intravascular coagulation, metabolic acidosis, derangement of mental status, acute respiratory insufficiency, and oliguria due to acute renal failure are usually present in the setting of septic shock. Septic shock and its associated abnormalities are directly related to the time of diagnosis and to the initiation of empiric therapy. The later SBP is suspected and antibiotic treatment initiated, the more severe the clinical signs of infection.

Patients with SBP almost always present hematological changes suggestive of severe infection. Most patients show increased white blood cell (WBC) counts, but normal or decreased WBC counts may be seen in up to 30% of the cases. The appearance of leukocyte band forms is the most frequent abnormality observed in patients with SBP (20). Other analytical disturbances in cases of severe SBP are lactic metabolic acidosis, hypoxemia, hypoglycemia (23), and derangement of clotting factor levels and the detection of circulating fibrinogen degradation products.

Mortality in episodes of SBP may be related to the lactate concentration and pH in ascitic fluid at the time of diagnosis of SBP. It has been suggested that the lower the pH, the higher the lactate concentrations in ascitic fluid and the poorer the prognosis of SBP (24), but these measurements have been abandoned in clinical practice. It seems that SBP caused by bacteria of enteric origin or culture-positive episodes of SBP are associated with a higher mortality than non-enteric and culture-negative episodes (17,21,25,26). Other reports, however, do not agree with these results (5,10,18). Finally, the initial response to antibiotic therapy as estimated by the percentage decrease in the polymorphonuclear count in ascitic fluid appears to be directly related to survival (25).

The results of a retrospective analysis including 213 consecutive episodes of SBP treated with cefotaxime have recently been published (5). Of 51 clinical and laboratory parameters assessed in this study (other than antibiotic therapy), nine variables were identified as predictors of the resolution of infection on univariate analysis. These variables were a lower total WBC count, the percentage of neutrophils and band neutrophils in the WBC count, serum aspartate transaminase (AST) levels, blood urea nitrogen (BUN) and serum creatinine concentrations, and the grade of hepatic encephalopathy, as well as the absence of shock and community-acquired SBP. On multivariate analysis only four parameters were seen to be independent predictors of the resolution of SBP: band neutrophils in WBC counts, community-acquired SBP, and BUN and serum AST activity.

In the same series, 82 patients (38%) died during hospitalization, and 46 died shortly before the resolution of SBP. The main causes of death were liver failure in 23 patients (associated with unresolved infection in nine cases and hepatorenal syndrome in three), gastrointestinal hemorrhage in 13, and septic shock in 10. Thirty-six patients died after the resolution of SBP with the cause of death being liver failure in 22 (associated with hepatorenal syndrome in four and with hepatocellular carcinoma in two), severe infections acquired after the resolution of SBP in eight (five cases of bacteremia, two new SBP episodes, and one case of pneumonia), gastrointestinal hemorrhage in five, and brain hemorrhage in the remaining case. On multivariate analysis only six variables independently correlated with better survival at the end of hospitalization: lower age, BUN, serum AST activity, and the Child-Pugh score as well as community-acquired SBP and the absence of ileus.

II. COMPLICATIONS: PREVALENCE AND TREATMENT OR PROPHYLAXIS

As indicated, the development of SBP may follow a worsening of the clinical condition of the patient. The clinical data in 213 episodes of SBP are shown in Table 10.3; More than 50% of cirrhotic patients with SBP exhibit hepatic encephalopathy, renal failure, gastrointestinal bleeding, ileus, or septic shock.

Table 10.3 Clinical Data at Time of
Diagnosis of Spontaneous Bacterial Peritonitis

	Number of cases (%)
Episodes of SBP	213
Abdominal pain	137 (64)
Fever	131 (62)
Vomiting	17 (8)
Diarrhea	15 (7)
Ileus	10 (5)
Gastrointestinal bleeding	21 (10)
Hepatic encephalopathy	93 (44)
Shock	16 (8)
Serum bilirubin (mg/dl)[a]	6.3 ± 6.6
Serum albumin (gm/dl)[a]	2.7 ± 0.6
Prothrombin activity (%)[a]	49 ± 16
Child-Pugh classification[b]	
Grade A	1 (1)
Grade B	47 (22)
Grade C	157 (74)

[a] Mean ± SD.
[b] Available in 205 cases.
From Ref. 5.

It is obvious that the early diagnosis and early application of antibiotic therapy may reduce the incidence of these complications.

A. Renal Impairment

Renal impairment is a very frequent event both at the time of diagnosis and during the clinical course of SBP, being observed in nearly 40% of the cases (5,10,11,26).

Recently the results of a retrospective study aimed at investigating the incidence, clinical course, predictive factors, and prognosis of renal impairment in cirrhotic patients with SBP have been reported (26). Two hundred fifty-two consecutive episodes of SBP in 197 patients were analyzed. Renal impairment (hepatorenal syndrome) occurred in 83 episodes (33%). In 45 cases (18%) renal failure was present before the development of SBP. Renal impairment was progressive in 35 episodes (42%), steady in 27 (33%), and transient in 21 (25%). BUN and serum sodium concentrations before SBP and the band neutrophil count at diagnosis were independent predictors of the development of renal impairment. Renal failure was the strongest independent predictor of mortality during hospitalization (42% mortality in patients with renal impairment versus 7% in those without; p < 0.001), almost exclusively related to progressive or persistent renal failure but not in the transient type (100%, 31%, and 5% mortality rates, respectively). In addition, there were other independent prognostic factors, such as the BUN concentration before SBP, age, positive ascitic fluid culture, and the serum bilirubin level.

The mechanisms leading to renal impairment in cirrhotic patients with SBP have rarely been studied. In a recent study in patients with SBP it has been shown that the development of renal impairment (RI) was related to the degree of inflammatory response at the time of diagnosis (27). Patients developing SBP-RI showed significantly higher ascitic fluid polymorphonuclear cell concentrations and plasma and ascitic fluid levels of cytokines at the time of diagnosis than those without changes in renal function during the course of the infection (Fig. 10.1). Similarly, plasma and ascitic fluid levels of cytokines were found to be significantly higher in patients with SBP who died than in those who did not (Fig. 10.2). On the other hand, the ascitic fluid levels of interleukin-6 (IL-6) were the only independent predictors of the development of SBP-RI in association with the presence of renal failure and mean arterial pressure at the time of diagnosis. An important part of this study was the observed changes in plasma renin activity, a good indicator of effective plasma volume, and the evolution of renal function. Whereas plasma renin activity significantly decreased following resolution of infection in cases without SBP-RI, it increased markedly in patients developing SBP-RI despite the resolution of the infection, suggesting that the mechanism of SBP-RI is related to a deterioration of systemic hemodynamics throughout the course of the infection. Renal dysfunction that occurs spontaneously in patients with cirrhosis with ascites is currently considered to be related to arteriolar vasodilation, which takes place predominantly in the splanchnic circulation and leads to arterial vascular underfilling (28). The hepatorenal syndrome is the most extreme expression of this circulatory dysfunction. Nitric oxide (NO) is thought to play a major role in the pathogenesis of this abnormality. Since cytokines stimulate the vascular production of NO, SBP-RI could be the consequence of an activation of vascular inducible-NO synthase, and perhaps of other cytokine-induced vasodilatory mediators, and therefore this may produce an accentuation of the arteriolar vasodilation already present prior to the infection (29–32).

The observation that SBP-RI develops in many cases despite the resolu-

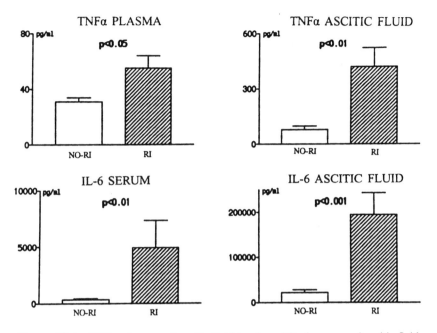

Figure 10.1   TNFα plasma and ascitic fluid levels and IL-6 serum and ascitic fluid levels in cirrhotic patients with SBP who developed or did not develop renal impairment.

tion of infection and a rapid decrease of the initial cytokine levels toward values observed in noninfected cirrhotic patients with ascites does not argue against this hypothesis. Investigations of changes in effective arterial blood volume following therapeutic paracentesis in decompensated cirrhosis indicate that circulatory function is extraordinarily unstable in these patients and that events that would be expected to have only a transitory circulatory effect may induce an irreversible deterioration of systemic hemodynamics. Therefore, the initial increase in cytokine levels may lead to a series of events that, in turn, may produce a deterioration of circulatory and renal function that is not reversed by the resolution of infection (33–37).

In addition to early diagnosis and therapy, the high prevalence of renal failure either before or at the time of diagnosis of SBP makes prevention of renal impairment during SBP very difficult. Theoretically, minimization of both derangements of liver function during infection and deterioration of circulatory disturbances should offer some degree of protection against SBP-in-

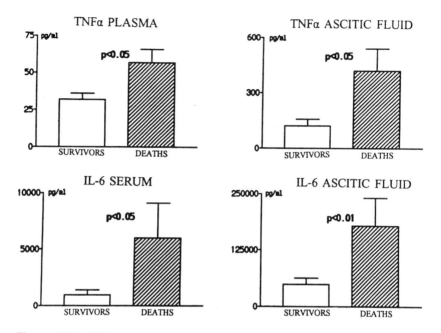

Figure 10.2 TNFα plasma and ascitic fluid levels and IL-6 serum and ascitic fluid levels in cirrhotic patients with SBP who died and did not die.

duced renal impairment. Correction of shock when present and of patient hydration by both parenteral fluid replacement and discontinuation of diuretic drugs are mandatory. Administration of potentially nephrotoxic drugs such as nonsteroidal anti-inflammatory drugs (NSAIDs) and aminoglycoside antibiotic agents must be avoided or limited as much as possible. The same measures should be applied in the case of the development of renal impairment. Although not proven in patients with SBP, plasma expansion with human albumin, alone or combined with systemic vasoconstrictors, which have reversed a number of cases of hepatorenal syndrome in cirrhotic patients (38), may be useful in preventing and/or treating renal impairment during episodes of SBP.

B. Hepatic Encephalopathy

Bacterial infection is a well-known precipitating factor for hepatic encephalopathy (HE) in cirrhotic patients. HE generally complicates SBP in approximately 40% of patients at the time of diagnosis (5,10). Mild to moderate HE (grades I and II) may be seen in most cases, although 25% of the patients exhibit severe HE. Despite the appearance or worsening of HE, which are common events during SBP, no study has specifically investigated this point up to now. It is well established that in approximately 10% of patients without HE or with only grade I HE at diagnosis of SBP the mental status worsens during the evolution of the infection (26).

The precise mechanisms leading to HE during SBP are not completely understood. Different studies have proposed an important role for endotoxin and cytokines in the pathogenesis of hepatic encephalopathy (39). Duchini (40) proposed that central nervous system endothelial cells are directly or indirectly responsible for injury to the brain in hepatic encephalopathy, and that this damage to the central nervous system is mediated by specific cytokines and nitric oxide, which activate endothelial cells and thereby cell function. Interactions between these cytokines and endothelial cells of the central nervous system may trigger a cascade of events including enhanced permeability of the blood–brain barrier, brain edema, alterations in astrocytes, and gliosis. Cytokine-induced production of nitrogen reactive molecules by endothelial cells may also lead to further cellular damage and neuronal dysfunction. Since SBP is characterized by very high circulating levels of tumor necrosis factor (TNFα) and IL-6 (27), a pathogenic role could easily be attributed to these cytokines in hepatic encephalopathy. In addition, these substances may have potential therapeutic implications. However, as mentioned above, patients with higher circulating levels of cytokines also have a higher incidence of renal failure and more severe infection, and probably other conditions such as dehydration, electrolyte disturbances, gastrointestinal bleeding, and derangements of liver function, which have been recognized as precipitating factors of hepatic encephalopathy (41). There are no effective measures for the prevention and treatment of hepatic encephalopathy in patients with SBP. As in other cirrhotic patients with hepatic encephalopathy, treatment includes correction of electrolyte disturbances and other precipitating factors and the administration of oral and/or rectal lactulose or lactitol.

C. Gastrointestinal Bleeding

More than 10% of the patients present with gastrointestinal hemorrhage at the time of the diagnosis of SBP (5,10,26). This prevalence rate increases to nearly 25% when considering bleeding episodes that occur during the week prior to the diagnosis of SBP (5). Moreover, gastrointestinal hemorrhage is the cause of death in up to 28% of the patients with SBP who die before the infection is resolved and 14% of those who die after the resolution of infection during the same hospitalization. Overall, gastrointestinal bleeding accounts for 22% of the deaths of patients with SBP (5).

The relationship between gastrointestinal bleeding and SBP has been clearly established. On one hand, cirrhotic patients with gastrointestinal bleeding are prone to develop bacterial infections, predominantly caused by bacteria of intestinal origin (42–45). It seems clear that acute hypovolemia and splanchnic vasoconstrictor drugs that are commonly used during bleeding episodes favor disturbances in barrier mechanisms of the intestinal wall and potentiate the depression of the reticuloendothelial system present in advanced cirrhosis. As a result, bacterial translocation and persistent bacteremia may be more frequent during hemorrhagic episodes. In this setting, colonization of ascitic fluid by circulating bacteria is a frequent event, particularly in those cirrhotic patients with decreased antimicrobial activity of their ascitic fluid (46,47). On the other hand, it is well known that severe bacterial infection predisposes to gastrointestinal bleeding, with this event being significantly more frequent in cirrhotic than in noncirrhotic patients (48). Endotoxin and cytokines may cause disturbances in blood perfusion of the gastrointestinal mucosa leading to ischemia and the appearance of acute ulcers. Moreover, circulatory disturbances associated with the infection may also induce deterioration of splanchnic hemodynamics, leading to variceal rupture by increasing the portal pressure. This phenomenon, together with the impairment of different clotting factors by the infection, may explain why cirrhotic patients with bacterial infections are more prone to show variceal bleeding. It is not surprising that acute episodes of gastrointestinal bleeding of any origin have a worse outcome and response to treatment in cirrhotic patients with, than in those without, bacterial infection (49).

There are no studies to date demonstrating any beneficial effect of antisecretory drugs in the prevention of gastrointestinal bleeding in patients with SBP. In cases with gastrointestinal bleeding of any origin (esophageal and gastric varices, hypertensive gastropathy, erosive and ulcerative lesions), treatment does not differ from that used in hemorrhagic episodes in noninfected cirrhotic patients (48). However, special attention should be paid to the correction of infection-related disturbances that may interfere with hemostatic mechanisms such as lactic acidosis and coagulopathy.

D. Ileus

Clinically significant disturbances of gastrointestinal motility may be seen in up to 20% of the patients at the time of diagnosis of SBP (5,10). Among these abnormalities, vomiting and diarrhea are the most frequently observed. Ileus, which may be observed in more than 5% of these patients, has prognostic significance (5,10), and its presence is associated with a higher mortality (5).

There is no specific treatment for ileus secondary to SBP. Usually, intestinal motility becomes normal in response to antibiotic therapy. However, persistent ileus may be seen in a number of cases. Electrolyte disturbances, mainly hypokalemia, and the administration of opiates in an attempt to ameliorate abdominal pain may be responsible for persistent ileus. The presence of ileus makes the administration of intravenous fluid solutions and a close monitoring and correction of electrolyte and metabolic disturbances mandatory. In cases of persistent vomiting, especially in patients with hepatic encephalopathy, the placement of a nasogastric tube and continuous aspiration of the gastric content is indicated. This measure may prevent the occurrence of tracheal aspiration of gastric contents and aspiration pneumonia. Prokinetic drugs (metroclopramide, cisapride, domperidone) have not been shown to be useful in resolving ileus associated with SBP.

It should be emphasized that the general management of cirrhotic patients with SBP requires a very active attitude by the physician. The diagnosis of SBP requires a high degree of suspicion and must be made as soon as possible. Initiation of antibiotic therapy must not be delayed. Associated complications must be detected and treated rapidly. Renal impairment is a frequent complication and carries a poor prognosis. Prevention of renal impairment should be an important goal in the treatment of SBP. Finally, it should be kept in mind that whereas SBP in the past was considered to be one of the terminal events in the course of cirrhotic patients, SBP is now considered a formal indication for liver transplantation and therefore all the measures aimed at helping these patients achieve liver transplant should be applied.

REFERENCES

1. Rimola A. Infecciones bacterianas en la cirrosis hepática. In: Actualidades en Gastroenterología y Hepatología. Rodés J, Chantar C, eds., Barcelona: J.R. Prous, 1988, 149–189.
2. Suárez C, Pajares JM. Epidemiología de las infecciones en la cirrosis hepática. Rev Clin Esp 1981; 160:299–303.
3. Andreu M, Barrufet P, Force L, Sol R, Verdaguer A, Panadés A, Arán R. Fiebre en el enfermo con cirrosis hepática: estudio prospectivo durante seis meses. Med Clín (Barcelona) 1985; 433–436.
4. Clemente-Ricote G, Barajas JM, Serrano MI, Perez de Ayala MV, Menchén P, Senent MC, Castellanos D, Loeches N, Velo JL, Alcalá-Santaella R. Infecciones bacterianas en la cirrosis hepática. Gastroenterol Hepatol 1986; 9:285–290.
5. Toledo C, Salmerón JM, Rimola A, Navasa M, Arroyo V, Llach J, Ginès A, Ginès P, Rodés J. Spontaneous bacterial peritonitis in cirrhosis: predictive factors

of infection resolution and survival in patients treated with cefotaxime. Hepatology 1993; 17:251–257.

6. Felisart J, Rimola A, Arroyo V, Pérez-Ayuso RM, Quintero E, Ginès P, Rodés J. Cefotaxime is more effective than is ampicillin-tobramycin in cirrhotics with severe infections. Hepatology 1985; 5:457–462.

7. Rimola A, Tító Ll, Llach J, Salmerón JM, Marqués F, Badalamenti S, Rodés J. Efficacy of ceftizoxime in the treatment of severe bacterial infections in patients with cirrhosis. Drug Invest 1992; 4(suppl. 1):35–37.

8. Ariza J, Xiol X, Esteve M, Fernández-Bañares F, Linares J, Alonso T, Gudiol F. Aztreonam vs. cefotaxime in the treatment of gram-negative spontaneous peritonitis in cirrhotic patients. Hepatology 1991; 14:91–98.

9. Grange JD, Amiot X, Grange V, Gutmann L, Biour M, Bodin F, Poupon R. Amoxicillin-clavulanic acid therapy of spontaneous bacterial peritonitis: a prospective study of twenty-seven cases in cirrhotic patients. Hepatology 1990; 11: 360–364.

10. Rimola A, Salmerón JM, Clemente G, Rodrigo L, Obrador A, Miranda, ML, Guarner C, Planas R, Solà R, Vargas V, Casafont F, Marco F, Navasa M, Bañares R, Arroyo V, Rodés J. Two different dosages of cefotaxime in the treatmemt of spontaneous bacterial peritonitis in cirrhosis: results of a prospective, randomized, multicenter study. Hepatology 1995; 21:674–679.

11. Navasa M, Follo A, Llovet JM, Clemente G, Vargas V, Rimola A, Marco F, Guarner C, Forné M, Planas R, Bañares R, Castells L, Jiménez de Anta MT, Arroyo V, Rodés J. Randomized, comparative study of oral ofloxacin versus intravenous cefotaxime in spontaneous bacterial peritonitis. Gastroenterology 1996; 111:1011–1017.

12. Pinzello G, Simonetti RG, Craxi A, DiPiazza S, Spano C, Pagliaro L. Spontaneous bacterial peritonitis. A prospective investigation in predominantly nonalcoholic cirrhotic patients. Hepatology 1983; 3:545–549.

13. Hoefs JC, Runyon BA. Spontaneous bacterial peritonitis. Disease-a-Month 1985; 31:1–48.

14. Correia JP, Conn HO. Spontaneous bacterial peritonitis: endemic or epidemic? Med Clin N Am 1975; 59:963–981.

15. Hoefs JC, Canawati HN, Sapico FL, Hopkins RR, Weiner J, Montgomerie JZ. Spontaneous bacterial peritonitis. Hepatology 1982; 2:399–407.

16. Mihas AA, Toussaint J, Hsu HS, Dotherow P, Achord JL. Spontaneous bacterial peritonitis in cirrhosis: clinical and laboratory features, survival and prognostic indicators. Hepatogastroenterology 1992; 39:520–522.

17. Pelletier G, Salmon D, Ink O, Hannoun S, Attali P, Buffet C, Etienne JP. Culture-negative neutrocytic ascites: a less severe variant of spontaneous bacterial peritonitis. J Hepatol 1990; 10:327–331.

18. Terg R, Levi D, López P, Rafaelli C, Rojter S, Abecasis R, Villamil F, Aziz H, Podesta A. Analysis of clinical course and prognosis of culture-positive spontaneous bacterial peritonitis and neutrocytic ascites. Dig Dis Sci 1992; 37:1.499–1.504.

19. Sánchez-Tapias JM, Rodés J, Arroyo V, Bruguera M, Terés J, Bordas JM, Gasull MA, Revert L. Infección peritoneal en la cirrosis hepática con ascitis. Rev Clín Esp 1971; 123:375–380.

20. Sánchez-Tapias JM, Terés J, Arroyo V, Bosch J, Bruguera M, Rodés J. Infección peritoneal en la cirrosis hepática con ascitis. Cinco años de experiencia. Gastroenterol Hepatol 1978; 1:15–21.

21. Rimola A, Felisart J, Terés J, Gatell JM, Jiménez de Anta MT, Rodés J. Estudio controlado de la eficacia terapéutica de dos pautas antibióticas en la peritonitis bacteriana espontánea de la cirrosis. Valor pronóstico de los datos bacteriológicos. Gastroenterol Hepatol 1984; 7:235–241.

22. Planas R, Rimola A, Sánchez-Tapias JM, Terés J, Bruguera M, Rodés J. Antibióticos orales no absorbibles en el tratamiento de la peritonitis bacteriana espontánea en la cirrosis hepática. Gastroenterol Hepatol 1981; 4:499–503.

23. Nouel O, Bernuau J, Rueff B, Benhamou JP. Hypoglycemia. A common complication of septicemia in cirrhosis. Arch Intern Med 1981; 141:1.477–1.478.

24. Navasa M, Caballería J, Elena M, Ballesta AM, Ginès P, Rodés J. Valor pronóstico del pH y del lactato en ascitis en la peritonitis bacteriana espontánea de la cirrosis hepática. Gastroenterol Hepatol 1985; 8:455–460.

25. Fong TL, Akriviadis EA, Runyon BA, Reynolds TB. Polymorphonuclear cell count response and duration of antibiotic therapy in spontaneous bacterial peritonitis. Hepatology 1989; 9:423–426.

26. Follo A, Llovet JM, Navasa M, Planas R, Forns X, Francitorra A, Rimola A, Gassull MA, Arroyo V, Rodés J. Renal impairment after spontaneous bacterial peritonitis in cirrhosis: incidence, clinical course, predictive factors and prognosis. Hepatology 1994; 20:1495–1501.

27. Navasa M, Follo A, Filella X, Jiménez W, Francitorra A, Planas R, Rimola A, Arroyo V, Rodés J. Tumor necrosis factor and interleukin-6 in spontaneous bacterial peritonitis in cirrhosis. Relationship with the development of renal impairment and mortality. Hepatology 1998; 27:1227–1232.

28. Schrier RW, Arroyo V, Bernardi M, Rodés J. Peripheral arterial vasodilation hypothesis: a proposal for the initiation of renal sodium and water retention in cirrhosis. Hepatology 1988; 8:1151–1157.

29. Moncada S. The L-arginine: nitric oxide pathway. Acta Physiol Scand 1992; 145:201–227.

30. Stoclet JC, Fleming I, Gray G, Julou- Schaeffer G, Schneider F, Schott C, Schott C. Nitric oxide and endotoxemia. Circulation 1993; 87(suppl. V):V77–V80.

31. Henrich WL, Hamasaki Y, Said SI, Campbell WB, Cronin RE. Dissociation of systemic and renal effects in endotoxemia. J Clin Invest 1982; 69:691–699.

32. Ball HA, Cook JA, Wise WC, Halushka PV. Role of thromboxane, prostaglandins and leukotrienes in endotoxic and septic shock. Intensive Care Med 1986; 12:116–126.

33. Sugiura M, Inagami T, Kon V. Endotoxin stimulates endothelin release in vivo and in vitro as determined by radioimmunoassay. Biochem Biophys Res Commun 1989; 161:1220–1227.

34. Badr KF, Kelley VE, Rennke HG, Brenner BM. Roles for thromboxane A2 and leukotrienes in endotoxin-induced acute renal failure. Kidney Int 1986; 30:474–480.
35. Bremm KD, Konig W, Spur B, Crea A, Galanos C. Generation of slow reacting substance (leukotrienes) by endotoxin and lipid A from human polymorphonuclear granulocytes. Immunology 1984; 53:299–305.
36. Llach J, Ginès P, Arroyo V, Salmerón JM, Ginès A, Jiménez W, Gaya J. Effect of dipyridamole on kidney function in cirrhosis. Hepatology 1993; 17:59–64.
37. Osswald H. The role of adenosine in the regulation of glomerular filtration rate and renin secretion. Trends Pharmacol Sci 1984; 5:94–97.
38. Guevara M, Ginès P, Fernández-Esparrach G, Sort P, Salmerón JM, Jiménez W, Arroyo V, Rodés J. Reversibility of hepatorenal syndrome by prolonged administration of ornipressin and plasma volume expansion. Hepatology 1998; 27:35–41.
39. Odeh M. Endotoxin and tumor necrosis factor-alpha in the pathogenesis of hepatic encephalopathy. J Clin Gastroenterol 1994; 19:146–153.
40. Duchini A. The role of central nervous system endothelial cell activation in the pathogenesis of hepatic encephalopathy. Med Hypotheses 1991; 46:239–244.
41. Ferenci P. Hepatic encephalopathy. In: McIntyre N, Benhamou JP, Bircher J, Rizzetto M, Rodés J. Oxford Textbook of Clinical Hepatology. New York: Oxford University Press, 1991, 471–483.
42. Rimola A, Bory F, Terés J, Pérez-Ayuso R.M, Arroyo V, Rodés J. Oral nonabsorbable antibiotics prevent infection in cirrhotics with gastrointestinal hemorrhage. Hepatology 1985; 5:463–467.
43. Conn HO, Ramsby GR, Storer EN. Selective intraarterial vasopressin in the treatment of upper gastrointestinal hemorrhage. Gastroenterology 1972; 63:634–645.
44. Davis GB, Broodstein J, Hagan PI. The relative effects of selective intra-arterial and intravenous vasopressin infusion. Radiology 1976; 120:537–538.
45. Mallory A, Schaefer JW, Cohen JR, Holt SA, Norton LW. Selective intraarterial vasopressin infusion for upper gastrointestinal tract hemorrhage. Arch Surg 1980; 115:30–32.
46. Rimola A, Soto R, Bory F, Arroyo V, Piera C, Rodés J. Reticuloendothelial system phagocytic activity in cirrhosis and its relation to bacterial infections and prognosis. Hepatology 1984; 4:53–58.
47. Runyon BA. Patients with deficient ascitic fluid opsonic activity are predisposed to spontaneous bacterial peritonitis. Hepatology 1988; 8:632–635.
48. Burroughs AK, Bosch J. Clinical manifestations and management of bleeding episodes in cirrhotics. In: McIntyre N, Benhamou JP, Bircher J, Rizzetto M, Rodés J. Oxford Textbook of Clinical Hepatology. New York: Oxford University Press, 1991, 408–425.
49. Bernard B, Cadranel JF, Valla D, Escolano S, Jarlier V, Opolon P. Prognostic significance of bacterial infection in bleeding cirrhotic patients: a prospective study. Gastroenterology 1995; 108:1828–1834.

11
Antibiotic Therapy of Spontaneous Bacterial Peritonitis

Miguel Navasa and Juan Rodés
Hospital Clínic i Provincial de Barcelona, University of Barcelona, Barcelona, Spain

I. INTRODUCTION

Spontaneous bacterial peritonitis (SBP), the most characteristic infectious complication of cirrhotic patients, is defined as the infection of a previously sterile ascitic fluid with no apparent intra-abdominal source of infection. The incidence of SBP in cirrhotic patients admitted to the hospital with ascites has been estimated to range between 7% and 23% (1–4). Antibiotic therapy in SBP must be started as soon as the diagnosis is established. The diagnosis is established on the basis of clinical signs and symptoms and/or a polymorphonuclear cell count in ascitic fluid higher than 250 cells/mm³ (4). This diagnosis is confirmed by a positive culture in approximately 70% of the cases. The remaining 30% are considered culture-negative SBP but are empirically treated because bacteremia, severe peritonitis, and death may follow if these patients do not receive antibiotic therapy (3). Early diagnosis, routine use of diagnostic paracentesis in patients admitted to the hospital with ascites, and the use of effective antibiotics are the most important tools for the treatment of SBP. Table 11.1 shows the most common organisms isolated in patients with SBP. They include gram-negative and gram-positive aerobic bacteria. Empirical treatment should inhibit all these organisms without causing adverse effects. Because combinations of antibiotics including aminoglycoside agents are often associated with renal failure, such combinations have been abandoned and third-generation cephalosporins are considered the antibiotic agents

219

Table 11.1 Microorganisms Isolated
in Spontaneous Bacterial Peritonitis in
Cirrhosis

Culture-positive SBP	82(67%)
Gram-negative bacilli	61
Escherichia coli	45
Klebsiella spp.	7
Other	9
Gram-positive cocci	21
Streptococcus pneumoniae	12
Other *streptococci*	8
Staphylococcus aureus	1
Culture-negative SBP	41(33%)

From Ref. 29.

of choice in the treatment of SBP. However, other antibiotic drugs are also effective in the treatment of this infectious complication. In this chapter we will discuss the antibacterial activity, pharmacokinetic properties, and clinical efficacy of the antibiotic agents most commonly used in the treatment of SBP.

II. CEFOTAXIME

A. Antibacterial Activity

1. Gram-Negative Aerobic Bacteria

A recent study showed that the activites of cefotaxime against 3882 consecutive Enterobacteriaceae isolated from intensive care and hematology and oncology units in Europe were generally similar to those of both ceftazidime and ceftriaxone, with 93–96% of *E. coli. K. oxytoca, P. mirabilis*, and *P. vulgaris* susceptible to cefotaxime (5). In addition, around 85% of the tested strains of *K. pneumoniae, M. morgagni*, and *S. marcescens* were susceptible to cefotaxime. Other Enterobacteriaceae susceptible to cefotaxime include *Salmonella* spp., *Shigella* spp., and *Yersinia enterocolitica. Citrobacter freundii, Enterobacter aerogenes*, and *E. cloacae* are considered generally resistant to cefotaxime (5–11).

   Pseudomonas aeruginosa and *Stenotrophomonas (Xanthomonas) maltophilia* are also resistant to cefotaxime (6). Other gram-negative aerobic bacteria are usually susceptible to cefotaxime, including *Haemophilus influenzae, Moraxella catarrhalis, Neisseria gonorrhoeae, Aeromonas hydrophila, N.*

meningitidis, and *Acinetobacter wolffi*, whereas *A. johnsoni* and *A. caloaceti-cus* are generally resistant (11). Less commonly isolated gram-negative bacteria susceptible to cefotaxime include *Aeromonas sobria*, *Bordetella paraper-tussis*, *Campylobacter yeyuni*, *Haemophilus ducrei*, and *Pasteurella multocida* (5–8).

2. Gram-Positive Aerobic Bacteria

Cefotaxime is usually active against methicillin-susceptible *Staphylococcus aureus*, *Streptococcus pneumoniae*, *Streptococcus pyogenes*, and *S. viridans*. For *Staphylococcus epidermidis* the MIC_{90} is around 7 mg/L and has suboptimal or little activity against methicillin-resistant *S. aureus* and *enterococci* (5–7).

B. Pharmacokinetic Properties

The intravenous bolus administration of 1 g of cefotaxime causes a mean peak plasma concentration (C_{max} that ranges between 81 and 102 mg/L, whereas a single bolus dose of 2 g produces C_{max} values between 175 and 215 mg/L (12). Mean plasma concentrations of cefotaxime and desacetyl-cefotaxime, the active metabolite of cefotaxime, 8 h after the administration of cefotaxime range from 0.5 to 1.0 mg/L, although higher trough values have been reported in elderly patients (12–14). The apparent volume of distribution of cefotaxime is about 20–30 L/1.73 m^2, and in vitro protein binding is about 25–40%. Cefotaxime efficiently penetrates into the ascitic fluid and high concentrations are achieved in patients with cirrhosis and bacterial peritonitis (15–16). In addition, cefotaxime adequately penetrates wound, burn blister, and interstitial fluid, as well as cardiac, gynecological, and prostatic tissue. Approximately 50% of cefotaxime is excreted renally and 50% is converted in the liver to the antimicrobially active metabolite desacetyl-cefotaxime. Desacetyl-cefotaxime is partly excreted renally and is partly further converted into active metabolites that are eliminated in the urine. The plasma elimination half-life ($t_{1/2}$ β) ranges from 0.8 to 1.4 h for cefotaxime and is about 2 h for desacetyl-cefotaxime.

The disposition of cefotaxime is minimally affected in patients with impaired liver function. Although the total clearance is decreased and the apparent $t_{1/2}$ β increased in cirrhotic patients with ascites (16), concomitant renal impairment is probably the most important event responsible for the changes in the elimination of cefotaxime in these patients. Actually, doses of cefotaxime in cirrhotic patients with SBP are only slightly modified by abnormalities in renal function.

C. Therapeutic Efficacy

The efficacy of cefotaxime in patients with SBP has been evaluated in different studies (17–19). The first investigation consisted in a randomized controlled trial comparing cefotaxime (2 g every 4 h in patients without renal failure) versus the combination of ampicillin plus tobramycin in a large series of cirrhotic patients with SBP or other severe bacterial infections (17) (Table 11.2). Cefotaxime was more effective in achieving the resolution of SBP than ampicillin plus tobramycin, and, whereas no patient treated with cefotaxime developed nephrotoxicity or superinfections, these two complications occurred in more than 10% of the patients treated with ampicillin plus tobramycin. Following this study, cefotaxime has been considered to be the antibiotic of choice in the empiric treatment of SBP in cirrhotic patients.

Table 11.2 Comparison of Different Antibiotics in Treatment of Spontaneous Bacterial Peritonitis

	Resolution of infection	Nephrotoxicity	Superinfection	Hospital survival
Tobramycin + ampicillin	56%	7%	16%	61%
Cefotaxime				
2 g/4 h	85%	0%	0%	73%
2 g/6 h	77%	0%	1%	69%
2 g/8 h				
5-day therapy	93%	0%	0%	67%
10-day therapy	91%	0%	0%	58%
2g/12 h	79%	0%	1%	79%
Other cephalosporins				
Ceftriaxone	94%	0%	0%	63%
Ceftizoxime	88%	0%	0%	84%
Cefonicid	94%	0%	0%	70%
Aztreonam[a]	71%	0%	14%	57%
Amoxicillin-clavulanic acid	85%	0%	7%	63%
Oral pefloxacin + other antibiotics	87%	0%	7%	60%
Oral ofloxacin[b]	84%	0%	1%	81%

[a] The study included only spontaneous bacterial peritonitis caused by gram-negative organisms.
[b] The study included only uncomplicated spontaneous bacterial peritonitis, i.e., without septic shock, profound hepatic encephalopathy, gastrointestinal hemorrhage, ileus, or severe renal failure.

Two randomized controlled trials assessing the optimal duration of therapy and dosage of cefotaxime in cirrhotic patients with SBP have been reported. Runyon et al. (18) randomized 90 patients with SBP to receive cefotaxime (2 g intravenously [IV] every 8 h) for 10 days (43 patients) or for 5 days (47 patients). Resolution of the infection (93.1% vs. 91.2%), recurrence of SBP during hospitalization (11.6% vs. 12.8%), and hospital mortality (32.6% vs. 42.5%) were all comparable in the two groups (Table 11.2). Short-course treatment with cefotaxime is, therefore, as efficacious as long-course therapy in cirrhotic patients with SBP. Rimola et al. (19) reported the results of a randomized, multicenter controlled trial in 143 patients with SBP treated with cefotaxime in which two different dosages were compared: 2 g every 6 h (71 cases) vs. 2 g every 12 h (72 cases). The rate of resolution of SBP (77% vs. 79%) and patient survival (69% vs. 79%) were similar in both groups (Table 11.2). The results of this study suggest that doses of cefotaxime lower than those usually recommended are effective in SBP and may represent a significant reduction in the cost of the antibiotic therapy.

In 1998 Rodès et al. predicted that plasma expansion with intravenous albumin would enhance the efficacy of cefotaxime, and in 1999 they proved this prediction. They randomly assigned 126 fresh patients with cirrhosis and SBP, 63 to receive cefotaxime and 63 to receive cefotaxime plus plasma expansion with intravenous albumin (19a). The cefotaxime dosage varied depending on the serum creatinine concentration, and the albumin was given in a dosage of 1.5 g per kg on the day of randomization. The two groups were virtually identical in clinical and laboratory features. The infections resolved in more than 90% of both groups. One-fourth of the cefotaxime-treated patients died compared to one-tenth of those who received albumin, usually of renal impairment.

In an accompanying editorial (19b), Bass pointed out that albumin infusions are expensive ($1000 to $4000) and not always available and suggested ways of reducing the cost.

III. OTHER PARENTERAL ANTIBIOTICS

Several investigations have been carried out to assess the efficacy of other antibiotic regimes in these patients (Table 11.2).

A. Ceftriaxone and Cefonicid

Ceftriaxone is a third-generation cephalosporin that possesses antibacterial activity similar to that of cefotaxime and ceftizoxime. Ceftriaxone, however, has truly unique pharmacokinetics: it is 90% protein-bound, is excreted through both the biliary and urinary tracts, and has a serum half-life of 8 h. As a consequence, most serious infections can be treated with once-daily dosing (20). The presence of renal or hepatic dysfunction does not require dose adjustment. Cefonicid, which is structurally and biologically similar to cefamandole (a second-generation cephalosporin), is unique because it is 98% serum protein-bound and has a serum half-life of 4.4 h (21). Although it has been used effectively as single-daily dosing for infection caused by susceptible organisms, failures have been noted in more serious infections, including *S. aureus* bacteremia (20).

Mercader et al. (22) reported that ceftriaxone 2 g/day was effective in achieving the resolution of 83% of 18 episodes of SBP in cirrhotic patients. Three patients developed superinfections (*Candida* in two and *Enterococcus* in one). More recently, ceftriaxone (2 g/24 h) and cefonicid (2 g/12 h.) were compared in an unblinded randomized trial (23). Both antibiotics showed similar efficacy in the treatment of SBP, with a resolution rate of 100% for ceftriaxone and 94% for cefonicid. Despite this high efficacy, the hospital mortality rates were 30% and 37%, respectively. Three patients treated with ceftriaxone and two patients treated with cefonicid developed superinfection with *Enterococcus faecalis* or *Candida albicans*.

B. Aztreonam

Aztreonam is monocyclic β-lactam that binds primarily to penicillin-binding proteins (PBP 3) in Enterobacteriaceae, *Pseudomonas*, and other gram-negative aerobic organisms. In contrast, it does not bind to PBPs in gram-positive or anaerobic bacteria and this is why aztreonam has no appreciable antibacterial activity against these microorganisms (24). Aztreonam is not absorbed from the gastrointestinal tract. After the intravenous administration, the C_{max} is achieved immediately after completion of the infusion. The serum half-life of aztreonam ranges from 1.3 to 2.2 h and it is removed from the body by glomerular filtration and/or tubular secretion. No active metabolites have been found in the serum or urine. Aztreonam is widely distributed into body tissues and fluids. Therapeutic levels are present in many tissues and in peritoneal, pleural, and synovial fluids (25). The efficacy of aztreonam was evaluated in 16 episodes of SBP caused by Enterobacteria by Ariza et al. (26). Overall mortality during hospitalization was 62%. Superinfections due to resistant organisms were detected in three cases (19%). These results, together with the fact that aztreonam is only capable of inhibiting approximately 75% of the potential organisms causing SBP, suggest that this antibiotic is probably not optimal for the empirical treatment of cirrhotic patients with SBP.

C. Amoxicillin Plus Clavulanic Acid

The combination of amoxicillin plus clavulanic acid suppresses most of the bacteria responsible for SBP. Combining clavulanate with amoxicillin does not significantly alter the pharmacological parameter of either drug. Both drugs have good penetration into peritoneal fluid. Diarrhea and superinfections, particularly by *Candida albicans*, are not uncommon. The administration of 1 g per 6 h of amoxicillin associated with 200 mg of clavulanic acid was found to be effective in 85% of 27 episodes of SBP. Only one patient developed superinfection (27).

Although some of these studies evaluating the efficacy of other antibiotics in the treatment of SBP include a small number of patients, are not randomized, or do not determine the rate of complications, it is clear that the resolution rate of infection is similar to that obtained with cefotaxime. These other parenteral antibiotic agents, with the exception of aztreonam, can be used in the empiric treatment of SBP.

IV. ORAL ANTIBIOTICS

In most instances, patients with SBP are in relatively good clinical condition and can be treated with oral antibiotic agents. Two studies have been reported assessing the effectiveness of oral antibiotics in SBP (28,29). Both studies used broad spectrum quinolones, which are almost completely absorbed after oral administration, and which rapidly diffuse into the ascitic fluid.

A. Antibacterial Activity of Fluoroquinolones

1. Gram-Negative Bacteria

Most strains of Enterobacteriaceae are susceptible to fluoroquinolones. *Escherichia coli*, *Citrobacter diversus*, *Salmonella*, *Shigella*, and *Klebsiella* species, *Morgagnella morgagni*, *Serratia marcescens*, *Proteus mirabilis*, *Providencia stuarti*, and *Yersinia enterocholitica* are inhibited in 90% of the cases at fluoroquinolone concentrations of 1 mg/L or less (30). The inhibitory activity of fluoroquinolones against *Enterobacter* species, in particular *Enterobacter cloacae* and *E. aerogenes*, and *Citrobacter freundii* varies widely among different studies. *Neisseriaceae* and *Haemophilus* species are susceptible to fluoroquinolones. As a group, the fluoroquinolones are generally less active against *Pseudomonas aeruginosa* than they are against the Enterobacteriaceae and other gram-negative microorganisms, with ciprofloxacin the most active quinolone against *Pseudomonas* species. Among other gram-negative organisms, fluoroquinolones are active against *Aeromonas hydrophila* and *A. shigelloides*, *Plesiomonas* species, *Campylobacter jejuni*, and *Moraxella* species (30).

2. Gram-Positive Bacteria

Sparfloxacin and tosufloxacin are the most potent quinolone inhibitors of *Staphylococcus aureus*. The inhibitory activity of these newly developed compounds against staphylococci is substantially greater than that of ciprofloxacin. Ciprofloxacin is also active against other staphylococci, including *S. epidermidis*. However, *S. saprophyticus* and *S. haemolyticus* are resistant to ciprofloxacin and pefloxacin. The susceptibility of streptococci to quinolones is variable (30).

B. Pharmacokinetic Properties

With the exception of norfloxacin, which is only 30–40% bioavailable by the oral route, the 4-quinolones are 80–100% bioavailable, and absorption occurs between 1 and 3 h. Food has little influence on the absorption of quinolones. The newer quinolones are widely distributed throughout the body, with distribution volumes exceeding 1.5 L/kg. None of these newly developed fluoroquinolones are significantly bound to plasma proteins (10–37%). With this low degree of plasma protein binding, penetration into fluids and tissues is high and, in contrast to what occurs with many other antibiotics, fluoroquinolone tissue concentrations decline approximately in parallel with serum concentrations. The fluoroquinolones differ widely in the degree to which they are eliminated by metabolic transformation in the liver. Ofloxacin and sparfloxacin are minimally metabolized and are almost entirely eliminated unchanged in the urine. Pefloxacin, by contrast, is extensively converted to metabolic derivatives with reduced microbiological activity. Ciprofloxacin, enoxacin, fleroxacin, lomefloxacin, and norfloxacin are eliminated partly by metabolism and partly by renal excretion. Fluoroquinolones predominantly excreted by either renal or hepatic metabolism generally have longer serum half-lives than those agents that share both elimination pathways. The $t_{1/2}$ for ciprofloxacin is 3–5 h, for ofloxacin about 8 h, and for sparfloxacin approximately 20 h.

Plasma and ascitic fluid concentrations of ofloxacin were determined in 12 cirrhotic patients and in 12 healthy volunteers after a single dose and repeated 200-mg oral doses by Silvain et al. (31). The mean plasma elimination half-life was 11.6 h in cirrhotic patients and 7.0 h in control subjects. Mean total clearance was 2.3 times lower in patients than in controls due to a significant decrease of renal clearance of the drug. Ascitic fluid penetration of ofloxacin after the first oral dose was 80%, and ascitic fluid concentrations equaled corresponding plasma concentrations after 10 h, without pronounced accumulation of ofloxacin in ascites. Because of its broad spectrum of activity and its great ascitic fluid penetration after oral administration, these authors proposed that this antibiotic represents a new therapeutic approach for severe bacterial infections in cirrhotic patients, in particular SBP.

C. Mechanisms of Acquired Bacterial Resistance

Development of bacterial resistance among pathogens during the clinical use of quinolones has been predicted to occur, possibly reflecting the selective pressures of extensive use, particularly in cirrhotic patients undergoing prolonged selective intestinal decontamination. Bacteria acquire resistance to quinolones by spontaneously occurring mutation in chromosomal genes that alter either the target enzyme deoxynucleic acid (DNA) gyrase or drug permeation across the bacterial cell membranes (33,34). Alterations in the A subunit of DNA gyrase that cause quinolone resistance are clustered between amino acids 67 and 106 in the amino terminus of the A protein near the active site of the enzyme. Changes in serine-83 (to leucine or tryptophan) are most common and cause the largest increment in resistance as well as reduced binding of drug to the gyrase–DNA complex. The routes of quinolone across the bacterial cell membranes are not fully defined, but it appears that quinolones can diffuse across the gram-negative bacterial membrane through porin channels. Mutations in genes that affect expression of outer membrane proteins may cause a reduction in the amounts of porin protein in the outer membrane and contribute to quinolone resistance.

D. Therapeutic Efficacy

1. Introduction

Silvain et al. (28) reported the effectiveness of oral pefloxacin alone (1 case) and in combination with other oral antibiotics (cotrimoxazole, 9 cases; amoxicillin, 3 cases; cefadroxil, 1 case; and cotrimoxazole plus metronidazole, 1 case) in 15 episodes of SBP. The rates of resolution of infection was 87%, two patients developed superinfections, and the survival at the end of hospitalization was 60%. Navasa et al. (29) have recently reported the results of a randomized controlled trial in patients with SBP without septic shock, ileus, or serum creatinine >3 mg/dL comparing oral ofloxacin (400 mg every 12 h) vs. intravenous cefotaxime (2 g every 6 h). The rates of resolution of infection and patient survival were similar in the two groups. In addition, the incidence of superinfections and the duration of antibiotic treatment were also similar in both groups, suggesting that oral ofloxacin is as effective as intravenous cefotaxime in the treatment of nonseverely complicated SBP. The investigators also suggested that a small subgroup may be effectively treated as outpatients, i.e., those with uncomplicated, community-acquired SBP who have not received antibiotics in the previous two weeks and who have a blood urea nitrogen level <25 mg/dL, who have no encephalopathy, and who, after three days of therapy, show clinical improvement and a significant decrease ($\geq$59%) in the polymorphonuclear cell count in the ascitic fluid. Such patients could be safely discharged while still receiving oral ofloxacin. Although this idea carries great potential, many more such patients need to be studied before a general recommendation concerning outpatient management of SBP can be made (35).

2. Treatment of SBP in Patients Receiving Prophylaxis with Quinolones

The expected changes in the fecal flora and in the microorganisms responsible for the infections that occur in patients undergoing selective intestinal decontamination (SID) with quinolones, usually norfloxacin p.o. 400 mg/day, led to changes in the empiric treatment of SBP in these patients. On the basis of a theoretical increased risk of infections due to the *Enterococcus*, the association of ampicillin plus cefotaxime has been proposed as an empiric treatment of recurrent SBP. Llovet et al. (36) have shown that the frequency of SBP-caused by gram-negative bacilli is greater in 229 patients without SID than in 36 patients with SID (67% vs. 14%, respectively; p < 0.002). In this study, gram-positive cocci were isolated in 79% of culture-positive episodes of SBP that occurred in patients with SID, and in only 30% of the SBP episodes developing in patients not receiving SID. However, SBP in patients with and without prophylaxis with norfloxacin did not differ in clinical features or in response to treatment and prognosis. Almost all the organisms isolated from patients receiving norfloxacin were susceptible to cefotaxime in vitro. More recently, Novella et al. (37) have shown that the bacteria most frequently isolated from the infections of patients receiving norfloxacin for the prevention of the first episode of SBP was *Escherichia coli*. None of the *E. coli* isolated from these patients was resistant to cefotaxime. These two studies together (36,37) indicate that cefotaxime is effective against most of the gram-positive and gram-negative microorganisms that causes SBP in patients undergoing SID with quinolones. Therefore, it may be used alone as empiric treatment of recurrent SBP in such patients. It is important to note that in the latter study (37), *E. coli* was resistant to norfloxacin in 90% of the cases isolated from infections from patients undergoing SID with this antibiotic agent. Although other studies of long-term prophylaxis with norfloxacin (38,39), ciprofloxacin

(40), or trimethoprime-sulfamethoxazole (41) did not show resistance to these antibiotics by gram-negative bacilli, the emergence of infections caused by quinolone-resistant bacteria in cirrhotic patients undergoing SID may be expected (42–44), as occurs in the general population and in neutropenic patients (45). This phenomenon is thought to result from the current widespread use of quinolones and the possible mechanisms that have been previously considered. Nevertheless, the appearance of an increasing number of quinolone-resistant bacteria indicates that patients undergoing SID must be carefully selected.

Third-generation cephalosporins now may be considered the gold standard for the treatment of SBP. The efficacy of cefotaxime in SBP has been evaluated in large series of patients, at different doses and on different dosage schedules. Cefotaxime is probably the antibiotic agent of choice. However, other antibiotic agents, including other cephalosporins, the combination of amoxicillin plus clavulanic acid, and quinolones, are also effective in the treatment of SBP. Recent studies suggest that selected patients with SBP can be treated with oral antibiotic drugs. Cefotaxime can be used alone in the treatment of recurrent SBP in patients undergoing SID with norfloxacin. The addition of ampicillin does not seem necessary. In these patients, quinolones should not be used as empiric antibiotic treatment of recurrent SBP because the high-risk quinolone-resistant bacteria may be responsible for the infections.

REFERENCES

1. Rimola A, Navasa M. Infections in liver disease. In: *Oxford Textbook of Clinical Hepatology*, 2nd ed. McIntyre N, Benhamou JP, Bircher J, Rizzetto M, Rodés J, eds. Oxford: Oxford Medical Press, 1999, 1861–1874.
2. Caly WR, Strauss E. A prospective study of bacterial infections in patients with cirrhosis. J Hepatol 1993; 18:353–358.
3. Runyon BA, Hoefs JC. Culture-negative neutrocytic ascites: a variant of spontaneous bacterial peritonitis. Hepatology 1984; 4:1209–1211.
4. Navasa M. Treatment of spontaneous bacterial peritonitis and other severe bacterial infections in the setting of cirrhosis. In: *Treatments in Hepatology*, Arroyo V, Bosch J, Rodes J, eds. Barcelona: Masson, 1995, 109–115.
5. Verbist L. Epidemiology and sensitivity of 8625 ICU and hematology/oncology bacterial isolates in Europe. Scand J Infec Dis 1993; suppl. 91:14–24
6. Amyes SGB, Baird DR, Crook DW, Gillespie SH, Howard AJ, Oppenheim BA, Pedler SJ, Paull A, Tompkins DS, Lawrie SA. A multicentre study of the in-vitro activity of cefotaxime, cefuroxime, ceftazidime, ofloxacin and ciprofloxacin against blood and urinary pathogens. J Antimicrob Chemother 1994; 34:639–648.
7. Martínez-Beltran J, Cantón R, Liñares J, García de Lomas J, Gimeno C, Tubau

F, Baquero F. Multicentre comparative study of the antibacterial activity of FK-037, a new parenteral cephalosporin. Eur J Clin Microbiol Infect Dis 1995; 14: 244–252.

8. Gu JW, Neu HC. In vitro activity of Ro 23-9424, a dual action cephalosporin, compared with activities of other antibiotics. Antimicrob Agents Chemother 1990; 34:189–195.

9. Murphy SP, Erwin ME, Jones RN. Cefquinome (HR 111V): In vitro evaluation of a broad-spectrum cephalosporin indicated for infection in animals. Diagn Microbiol Infect Dis 1994; 20:49–55.

10. Bauernfeind A, Schweighart S, Eberlein E, Jungwirth R. In vitro activity and stability against novel beta-lactamases of investigational beta-lactams (cefepime, cefpirome, flomoxef, SCE 2787 and piperacillin plus tazobactam) in comparison with established compounds (cefotaxime, latamoxef and piperacillin). Infection 1991; 19(suppl. 5):S264–275.

11. Cormican MG, Jones RN. Antimicrobial activity of cefotaxime tested against infrequently isolated species (unusual pathogens). Diagn Microbiol Infect Dis 1995; 22:43–48.

12. Brogden RN, Spencer CM. Cefotaxime: A reappraisal of its antibacterial activity and pharmacokinetic properties, and a review of its therapeutic efficacy when administered twice daily for the treatment of mild to moderate infections. Drugs 1997; 53:483–510.

13. Lüthy R, Blaser J, Bonetti A, Simmen H, Wise R, Siegenthaler W. Human pharmacokinetics of ceftazidime in comparison to moxalactam and cefotaxime. J Antimicrob Chemother 1981; 8(suppl. B):273–276.

14. Lüthy R, Blaser J, Bonetti A, Simmen H, Wise R, Siegenthaler W. Comparative multi-dose pharmacokinetics of cefotaxime, moxalactam and ceftazidime. Antimicrob Agents Chemother 1981; 20:567–575.

15. Ings RMJ, Fillastre J-P, Godin M, Leroy G, Humbert G. The pharmacokinetics of cefotaxime and its metabolites in subjects with normal and impaired renal function. Rev Infect Dis 1982; 4:379–391.

16. Ko RJ, Sattler FR, Nichols S, Akriviadis E, Runyon B, Appleman M, Cohen JL, Koda RT. Pharmacokinetics of cefotaxime and desacetylcefotaxime in patients with liver disease. Antimicrob Agents Chemother 1991; 35:1376–1380.

17. Felisart J, Rimola A, Arroyo V, Perez-Ayuso RM, Quintero E, Ginès P, Rodés J. Cefotaxime is more effective than is ampicillin-tobramycin in cirrhotics with severe infections. Hepatology 1985; 5:457–462.

18. Runyon BA, McHutchison JG, Antillon MR, Akriviadis EA, Montano AA. Short-course versus long-course antibiotic treatment of spontaneous bacterial peritonitis: A randomized controlled study of 100 patients. Gastroenterology 1991; 100:1737–1742.

19. Rimola A, Salmeron JM, Clemente G, Rodrigo L, Obrador A, Miranda ML, Guarner C, Planas R, Solá R, Vargas V, Casafont F, Marco F, Navasa M, Bañares R, Arroyo V, Rodés J. Two different dosages of cefotaxime in the treatment of spontaneous bacterial peritonitis in cirrhosis: results of a prospective, randomized, multicenter study. Hepatology 1995; 21:674–679.

19a. Sort P, Navasa M, Arroyo V, Aldeguer X, Planas R, Rui-del-Arbol L, Castells L, Vargas V, Soriano G, Guevara M, Ginès P, Rodès J. Effect of intravenous albumin on renal impairment and mortality in patients with cirrhosis and spontaneous bacterial peritonitis. N Engl J Med 341:403–409, 1999.

19b. Bass NM. Intravenous albumin for spontaneous bacterial peritonitis in patients with cirrhosis. N Engl J Med 341:443–444, 1999.

20. Karchmer AW. Cephalosporins. In: *Principles and Practice of Infectious Diseases*, 4th Ed., Mandell GL, Bennet JE, Dolin R, eds., New York: Churchill Livingstone, 1995, 247–264

21. Actor P. In vitro experience with cefonicid. Rev Infect Dis 1984; suppl. 4:S783–790.

22. Mercader J, Gómez J, Ruiz J, Garre MC, Valdés M. Use of ceftriaxone in the treatment of bacterial infections in cirrhotic patients. Chemotherapy 1989; 35(suppl. 2):23–26.

23. Gómez-Jimenez J, Ribera E, Gasser I, Artaza MA, Del Valle O, Pamissa A, Martínez-Vázquez JM. Randomized trial comparing ceftriaxone with cefonicid for treatment of spontaneous bacterial peritonitis in cirrhotic patients. Antimicrob Agents Chemother 1993; 37:1587–1592.

24. Chambers HF, Neu HC. Other β-lactam antibiotics. In: *Principles and Practice of Infectious Diseases*, 4th Ed., Mandell GL, Bennet JE, Dolin R, eds., New York: Churchill Livingstone, 1995, 264–272.

25. Stutman HR, Marks MI, Swabb EA. Single-dose pharmacokinetics of aztreonam in pediatric patients. Antimicrob Agents Chemother 1984; 26:196–199.

26. Ariza J, Xiol X, Esteve M, Fernández Bañares F, Liñares J, Alonso T, Gudiol F. Aztreonam vs. cefotaxime in the treatment of gram-negative spontaneous peritonitis in cirrhotic patients. Hepatology 1991; 14:91–98.

27. Grange JD, Amiot X, Grange V, Gutmann L, Biour F, Poupon R. Amoxicillin-clavulanic acid therapy of spontaneous bacterial peritonitis: a prospective study of twenty-seven cases in cirrhotic patients. Hepatology 1990; 11:360–364.

28. Silvain C, Breux JP, Grollier G, Rouffineau J, Becq-Giraudon B, Beauchant M. Les septicémies et les infections du liquide d'ascite du cirrhotique peuvent-elles être traitées exclusivement par voie orale? Gastroenterol Clin Biol 1989; 13:335–339.

29. Navasa M, Follo A, Llovet JM, Clemente G, Vargas V, Rimola A, Marco F, Guarner C, Forné M, Planas R, Bañares R, Castells L, Jiménez de Anta MT, Arroyo V, Rodés J. Randomized, comparative study of oral ofloxacin versus intravenous cefotaxime in spontaneous bacterial peritonitis. Gastroenterology 1996; 111:1011–1017.

30. Rosenstiel N, Adam D. Quinolone antibacterials. An update of their pharmacology and therapeutic use. Drugs 1994; 47:872–901.

31. Silvain C, Bouquet S, Breux JP, Becq-Giraudon B, Beauchant M. Oral pharmacokinetics and ascitic fluid penetration of ofloxacin in cirrhosis. Eur J Clin Pharmacol 1989; 37:261–265.

32. Masecar BI, Celesk RA, Robillard HJ. Analysis of acquired ciprofloxacin resistance in a clinical strain of *Pseudomonas aeruginosa*. Antimicrob Agents Chemother 1990; 34:281–286.

33. Vila J, Ruiz J, Goni P, De Anta MT. Detection of mutations in parC in quinolone-resistant clinical isolates of *Escherichia coli*. Antimicrob Agents Chemother 1996; 40:491–493.

34. Hooper DC. Quinolones. In: *Principles and Practice of Infectious Diseases*, 4th Ed., Mandell GL, Bennet JE, Dolin R, eds., New York: Churchill Livingstone, 1995, 364–376.

35. García-Tsao G. Treatment of spontaneous bacterial peritonitis with oral ofloxacin: inpatient or outpatient therapy? Gastroenterology 1996; 111:1147–1150.

36. Llovet JM, Rodríguez-lglesias P, Moitinho E, Planas R, Bataller R, Navasa M, Menacho M, Pardo A, Castells A, Cabré E, Arroyo V, Gassull MA, Rodés J. Spontaneous bacterial peritonitis in patients with cirrhosis undergoing selective intestinal decontamination. J Hepatol 1997; 26:88–95.

37. Novella M, Sola R, Soriano G. Continuous versus inpatient prophylaxis of the first episode of spontaneous bacterial peritonitis with norfloxacin. Hepatology 1997; 25:532–536.

38. Ginès P, Rimola A, Planas R, Vargas V, Marco F, Almela M, Forné M, Miranda ML, Llach J, Salmerón JM, Esteve M, Marqués JM, Jiménez de Anta MT, Arroyo V, Rodés J. Norfloxacin prevents spontaneous bacterial peritonitis recurrence in cirrhosis: results of a double-blind, placebo-controlled trial. Hepatology 1990; 12:716–724.

39. Soriano G, Guarner C, Teixidó M, Such J, Barrios J, Enriquez J, Vilardell F. Selective intestinal decontamination prevents spontaneous bacterial peritonitis. Gastroenterology 1991; 100:477–481.

40. Rolanchon A, Cordier L, Bacq Y, Nousbaum JB, Franza A, Paris JC, Fratte S, Bohn B, Kitmacher P, Stahl JP, Zarski JP. Ciprofloxacin and long-term prevention of spontaneous bacterial peritonitis: results of a prospective controlled trial. Hepatology 1995; 22:1171–1174.

41. Singh N, Gayowski T, Yu VL, Wagener MM. Trimethoprim-sulfamethoxazole for the prevention of spontaneous bacterial peritonitis in cirrhosis: a randomized trial. Ann Intern Med 1995; 122:595–598.

42. Dupeyron C, Mangeney N, Sedrati L, Campillo B, Fouet P, Leluan G. Rapid emergence of quinolone resistance in cirrhotic patients treated with norfloxacin to prevent spontaneous bacterial peritonitis. Antimicrob Agents Chemother 1994; 38:340–344.

43. Muder RR, Brennen C, Goetz AM, Wagener MM, Rihs JD. Association with prior fluoroquinolone therapy of widespread ciprofloxacin resistance among gram-negative isolates in a Veterans Affairs Medical Center. Antimicrob Agents Chemother 1991; 35:356–358.

44. Peña C, Albareda JM, Parrarés R, Pujol M, Tubau F, Ariza J. Relationship between quinolone use and emergence of ciprofloxacin-resistant *Escherichia coli* in bloodstream infections. Antimicrob Agents Chemother 1995; 39:520–524.

45. Cometta A, Calandra T, Bille J, Glauser MP. *Escherichia coli* resistant to fluoro-quinolones in patients with cancer and neutropenia. N Engl J Med 1994; 330: 1240–1241.

12

Risk Factors for Spontaneous Bacterial Peritonitis in Cirrhosis: Efficacy of Norfloxacin in Preventing Recurrence of SBP

Pere Ginès, Pau Sort, and Vicente Arroyo
Hospital Clínic i Provincial de Barcelona, University of Barcelona, Barcelona, Spain

In recent years, much progress has been made in the field of pathogenesis and management of spontaneous bacterial peritonitis (SBP) in cirrhosis (1–5). Several predictive factors about the occurrence of SBP have been identified. Some of these factors are related to the bactericidal activity of ascitic fluid whereas others depend on the activity of systemic defense mechanisms against infection. Moreover, a better awareness of the infection and the use of potent and safe antibiotics has increased markedly the resolution and survival rates of cirrhotic patients with SBP (1–6). This improved prognosis has unveiled that SBP is a recurrent process. Patients who recover from the first episode of SBP are at very high risk for SBP recurrence (7). Long-term survival of these patients is poor, and recurrent SBP is a frequent cause of death. These data have prompted the use of prophylactic methods to prevent SBP in patients with cirrhosis (1–5). This chapter describes the conditions that are known to be associated with an increased risk of SBP in patients with cirrhosis and the use of antibiotics in the prophylaxis of the recurrence of SBP.

I. CONDITIONS ASSOCIATED WITH AN INCREASED RISK OF DEVELOPING SPONTANEOUS BACTERIAL PERITONITIS

A. Past History of SBP

Patients who have recovered from the first episode of SBP constitute the group of cirrhotic patients with the greatest risk of developing SBP. The demonstration and characterization of SBP as a highly recurrent disorder was made by Titó et al. in 1988 (7). These authors analyzed the long-term course of 75 consecutive patients with cirrhosis who recovered from their initial episode of SBP. No patient was excluded from the analysis and no prophylactic measures were attempted to prevent recurrence. Half of the patients developed one or more episodes of SBP during a mean follow-up period of 10 months (range 0.1–56 months). SBP recurred once in 22 patients, twice in 10, and three times or more in six patients. The cumulative probability of SBP recurrence was 43% at 6 months, 69% at one year, and 74% at two years of follow-up (Fig. 12.1). In addition to the highlighting of this high recurrence rate, four additional important clinical observations were made. First, gram-negative bacteria of enteric origin were the most common organisms that caused both the first and recurrent episode of SBP. Second, no relationship was found

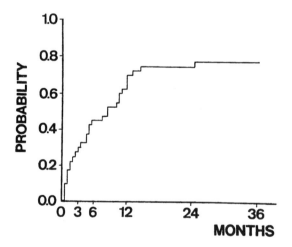

Figure 12.1 Cumulative probability of spontaneous bacterial peritonitis recurrence after a first episode of spontaneous bacterial peritonitis. (From Ref. 7.)

between the type of bacteria isolated in the first episode and in subsequent episodes of SBP. Third, liver function tests and the protein concentration of the ascitic fluid correlated with the recurrence of SBP. Patients with markedly impaired liver function, as indicated by elevated serum bilirubin levels and prolonged prothrombin times or low protein concentrations in the ascitic fluid (≤10 g/L) had an extremely high risk of SBP recurrence (a one-year probability between 80% and 90%). However, even patients with less severely impaired liver function tests had a high probability of recurrence (between 50% and 60% within one year). The only subset of patients with relatively low SBP recurrence rates was that of patients with high protein concentrations in the ascitic fluid (>10g/L) (Fig. 12.2). Finally, the last important clinical observation of this study was that cirrhotic patients who recovered from the first episode of SBP had an extremely poor overall outcome. The majority of patients died during the follow-up period, and death from the recurrence of SBP was the second most common cause of death after liver failure. The probability of survival was 38% at one year, 27% at two years, and 16% at three years, a much poorer outcome than that observed after other complications of cirrhosis such as ascites or gastrointestinal bleeding (Fig. 12.3). The high recurrence rate of SBP and the poor outcome of patients with cirrhosis with a past history of SBP were confirmed in subsequent studies (8–10) and stimulated the use of antibiotic prophylaxis in this setting (11,12).

B. Gastrointestinal Bleeding

Gastrointestinal bleeding is a major risk factor that precedes the development of bacterial infections in cirrhosis; approximately one-third of patients develop infections in close temporal relationship to an episode of bleeding (13–19). Bacterial infections show a bimodal distribution, with an early peak of incidence that corresponds to infections documented at admission or within the first 48 h after bleeding, and a second peak between 5 and 10 days after the index hemorrhage (18). Infections that develop in cirrhotic patients after gastrointestinal bleeding are particularly severe, the most common of which are SBP, bacteremia, and pneumonia. In the whole population of bleeding cirrhotic patients, the prevalence of SBP is relatively low, ranging from 7% to 15% in different studies. However, when only bleeding patients with ascites are considered the incidence of SBP is very high, ranging from 29% to 50% (Table 12.1).

Several factors may account for this high incidence of bacterial infections in patients with cirrhosis and gastrointestinal bleeding. Because cirrhotic

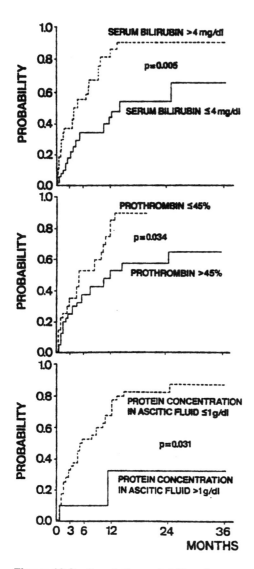

Figure 12.2 Cumulative probability of spontaneous bacterial peritonitis recurrence in patients who recovered from the first episode of spontaneous bacterial peritonitis classified according to serum bilirubin, prothrombin index, and protein concentration in ascitic fluid. (From Ref. 7.)

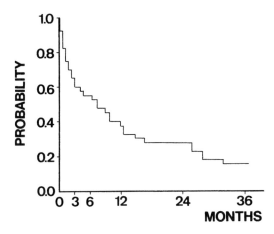

Figure 12.3 Cumulative probability of survival in patients who recovered from the first episode of spontaneous bacterial peritonitis. (From Ref. 7.)

patients are frequently submitted to aggressive diagnostic and therapeutic interventions, it is possible that some bacterial infections are related to the increased risk of infection associated with these invasive procedures. This fact may explain some episodes of urinary tract infection in patients with urinary catheters, of pneumonia in patients with tracheal intubation, and of gram-positive bacteremia in patients with central venous catheters. However, it is un-

Table 12.1 Incidence of Bacterial Infections and Spontaneous Bacterial Peritonitis (SBP) in Different Series of Cirrhotic Patients with Gastrointestinal Bleeding

Reference	Number of patients	Proven infections (% patients)	SBP (%)	SBP in patients with ascites (%)
Rimola et al. (13)	72	35	21[a]	—
Bleichner et al. (14)	149	22	14	—
Soriano et al. (16)	59	37	7[a]	29
Blaise et al. (17)	45	67	15	41
Bernard et al. (18)	64	36	14	30
Pauwels et al. (19)	89	27	12	52

[a] SBP and/or bacteriemia.

likely that medical interventions alone account for the high incidence of infections caused by gram-negative bacteria of intestinal origin, particularly SBP and bacteremia, because other observations suggest that these infections are in part the consequence of changes in the host defense mechanisms induced by the hemorrhage. In this regard, it is well known from studies in normal animals with hemorrhagic shock that hemorrhage temporarily impairs some of the systemic defense mechanisms, particularly the activity of the reticuloendothelial system (RES) (20,21). To our knowledge, no studies have been performed to assess the effects of hemorrhage on the activity of the RES in experimental or human cirrhosis. Nevertheless, it is likely that hemorrhage causes a further impairment of the already decreased activity of the RES in patients with cirrhosis (22,23). Moreover, hemorrhage also increases the permeability of intestinal mucosa to bacteria and causes bacterial translocation to the mesenteric lymph nodes, which is considered to be an important step in the development of SBP in cirrhosis (24–29). Moreover, pretreatment of animals with norfloxacin to induce selective intestinal decontamination almost completely prevents translocation of gram-negative bacteria to mesenteric lymph nodes (29). This observation provides a pathophysiological explanation for the efficacy of norfloxacin in the prevention of infections caused by gram-negative bacteria in cirrhotic patients with gastrointestinal bleeding (16).

Bacterial infections in patients with gastrointestinal bleeding have a suppressive influence on survival, because infected patients have a higher mortality than noninfected patients (14,18). However, this negative impact of bacterial infections is probably due to the fact that infections are more common in patients with severe liver disease, who are less likely to survive the bleeding episode. In fact, when prognostic factors are analyzed by multivariate analysis the risk of death correlates more closely with liver dysfunction than with bacterial infections (18). An intriguing observation in cirrhotic patients with overt gastrointestinal bleeding is that the presence of a bacterial infection is associated with an increased risk of rebleeding (18,30). This association between bacterial infections and rebleeding is worthy of study and provides a further reason for the use of prophylactic antibiotics to prevent infections in patients with gastrointestinal bleeding.

C. Reduced Protein Concentration and Opsonic Activity in Ascitic Fluid

It is now clearly established that impairment in local defense mechanisms against infection plays an important role in the pathogenesis of SBP in cirrhosis (3–5). First, it was demonstrated that the antimicrobial activity of ascitic fluid, as assessed by measuring opsonic activity, is more greatly reduced in ascites of cirrhosis compared to the ascites of other etiologies (such as malignant ascites and cardiac ascites) or with normal peritoneal fluid (31–33). Opsonization is a prerequisite for the elimination of bacteria by phagocytic cells and requires that bacteria be coated with immunoglobulin G and/or components of complement. By comparing ascitic fluids of different etiologies with a variety of protein concentrations, Runyon et al. showed that the opsonic activity of ascitic fluid correlated directly with total protein and C_3 and C_4 concentrations in ascitic fluid (33). The opsonic activity of ascitic fluid is almost nonexistent when ascitic fluid total protein concentration is decreased below 10 g/L or C_3 and C_4 concentrations in ascitic fluid are decreased to below 10 mg/dL and 2.5 mg/dL, respectively. Because patients with cirrhosis frequently have low total protein and C_3 and C_4 concentrations in ascitic fluid, it is likely that deficiencies in proteins with antimicrobial properties, particularly complement, are responsible for the reduced opsonic activity of ascitic fluid (33).

Patients with cirrhosis constitute a heterogeneous population with respect to the antimicrobial activity of ascites. The ascitic fluid opsonic activity is normal in some patients, whereas it is markedly reduced in others (34–36). Moreover, it was demonstrated that patients with reduced ascitic fluid opsonic activity were more likely to develop episodes of SBP during follow-up compared to patients with normal ascitic fluid opsonic activity (34–36). Given the close correlation between the ascitic fluid opsonic activity and total protein and C_3 and C_4 concentrations in ascitic fluid, the relationships between total protein or complement concentrations in ascitic fluid, which can be measured more easily than opsonic activity, and the risk of SBP were established in subsequent investigations. Not surprisingly, it was found that both low total protein or low complement concentrations in ascitic fluid are associated with an increased probability of developing SBP. In one study that included 107 patients with cirrhotic and noncirrhotic ascites, 15% of patients with ascitic fluid protein concentration ≤10 g/L developed SBP during their hospitalization compared with only 2% of patients with ascitic fluid protein concentration >10g/L (37) ($p < 0.01$). The relationship between total protein concentration in ascitic fluid and long-term probability of developing SBP has also been assessed in two investigations. In both studies, it was found that total protein concentration in ascitic fluid was the most important predictor of the occurrence of the first episode of SBP in ascitic cirrhotic patients (36–38). A reduced C_3 concentration in ascitic fluid is also associated with an increased risk of SBP development (35,36,39).

D. Impaired Reticuloendothelial System Phagocytic Activity

In addition to the altered local defensive mechanisms against infection in the peritoneal fluid, cirrhotic patients frequently have impaired activity of systemic defense mechanisms against infection (4,5). Dysfunction of neutrophils and monocytes, which affect phagocytosis and intracellular killing of bacteria and impair chemotaxis, is commonly seen in patients with cirrhosis (40–43). However, to our knowledge, the relationship between such abnormalities and the risk of developing bacterial infections, including SBP, has not yet been assessed. Advanced cirrhosis is usually associated with low serum complement levels, as some components of complement, especially C_3, are synthesized in the liver (44–46). This hypocomplementemia may be responsible, at least in part, for the reduced serum opsonic activity (47). Reduced serum C_3 levels have been found to be associated with an increased risk of SBP in some investigations but not in others (36,39). Finally, a depression in the RES phagocytic activity is also common in advanced cirrhosis (22,23,48–51). The RES is a crucial defensive component against infection, particularly bacteremia, due to its efficiency by removing bacteria from the bloodstream (52–54). The hepatic RES constitutes the largest fraction of the total body RES and is mainly dependent on the activity of Kupffer cells. The impaired RES phagocytic activity present in cirrhosis is related, at least in part, to the existence of intrahepatic and/or extrahepatic shunting of blood (22,55). Only two studies have been reported that assess the relationship between the RES phagocytic activity and the likelihood of bacteremia and/or SBP in cirrhosis. In the first investigation, Rimola et al. (22) found that cirrhotic patients with reduced RES phagocytic activity, as assessed by the reduction in the rate constant of [99m]technetium–sulfur colloid, had a greater risk of developing bacteremia and/ or SBP during follow-up than did patients with normal RES phagocytic activity. Similarly, Bolognesi et al. (23) found that impaired RES phagocytic activity, as assessed by the maximum removal capacity of human albumin millimicrospheres tagged with [99m]technetium, was associated with an increased risk of the development of SBP during follow-up. In patients with depressed RES activity, the one-year probability of developing SBP was 52% compared to 0% in patients with normal RES activity. Although the results of these two studies clearly indicate that the RES phagocytic activity is a predictive factor for the development of SBP, it is important to point out that the number of patients included in these studies was relatively small (41 and 43 patients, respectively) and that only 23 patients in each study had ascites. Furthermore, other potential risk factors of SBP occurrence were not assessed.

II. PREVENTION OF RECURRENCE OF SPONTANEOUS BACTERIAL PERITONITIS

Patients with a recent episode of SBP and those suffering from gastrointestinal bleeding were the high-risk groups of patients in whom prophylactic measures to prevent SBP were first investigated (13,16,56). Because most episodes of SBP are caused by gram-negative bacteria, prophylaxis of SBP has been based on the oral administration of antibiotics that produce a selective decontamination of the gastrointestinal tract, i.e., elimination of aerobic gram-negative bacteria without affecting aerobic gram-positive and anaerobic bacteria (57–60). Quinolones are the most suitable antibiotics for this purpose (61,62). Because norfloxacin is the only antibiotic that has been used in the prevention of the recurrence SBP, the information discussed below refers to this antibiotic, although other quinolones may also be effective.

A. Antibacterial Spectrum and Pharmacokinetics of Norfloxacin

Norfloxacin and other fluoroquinolones (ciprofloxacin, ofloxacin, enoxacin, and pefloxacin) have very potent activity against gram-negative bacilli, including *Escherichia coli* and the *Enterobacter, Klebsiella, Salmonella, Shigella, Arizona, Proteus, Serratia*, and *Citrobacter species* (MIC$_{90}$ 0.06–0.25 µg/mL), although resistance is emerging in some regions (Table 12.2). The activity of norfloxacin against most of these gram-negative bacteria is comparable with that of cefotaxime. *Flavobacterium* and *Acinetobacter species* as well as *Burkholderia* (previously *Pseudomonas*) *maltophilia* and *pseudomallei* are usually resistant to most quinolones. However, these bacteria rarely cause SBP (5). Norfloxacin has only moderate activity against *Staphylococcus aureus* and *Staphylococcus epidermidis*, whereas both of these bacteria are usually susceptible to ciprofloxacin and ofloxacin. *Streptococcus pneumoniae, pyogenes*, and *viridans*, and *Enterococcus faecalis* and *faecium* are often resistant to norfloxacin and other fluoroquinolones (MIC$_{90}$ 4–16 µg/mL). All fluoroquinolones have little or no activity against most anaerobic bacteria, including *Bacteroides* and *Clostridium species*.

Norfloxacin is available only as an oral preparation, whereas ciprofloxacin and ofloxacin are available for both oral and intravenous administration. Norfloxacin is the fluoroquinolone with the lowest intestinal absorption. After oral administration, only 30–40% of the dose is absorbed, while the absorption of ciprofloxacin and ofloxacin reaches 60–80%. After a single norfloxacin

Table 12.2 In Vitro Susceptibility of Different
Bacteria to Norfloxacin

Type of bacteria	MIC_{90} (micrograms/ml)
Aerobic Gram-Negative Bacteria	
Escherichia coli	0.6–1.2
Klebsiella pneumoniae	0.25
Proteus mirabilis	0.06
Citrobacter freundii	0.25
Enterobacter cloacae	0.25
Salmonella spp.	0.06–0.25
Campylobacter jejuni	0.5–8
Aerobic Gram-Positive Bacteria	
Enterococcus faecalis	4–8
Enterococcus faecium	8–16
Streptococcus pneumoniae	4–16
Methicillin-sensitive	
Staphylococcus aureus	1–4
Methicillin-resistant	
Staphylococcus aureus	4–16
Anaerobic Bacteria	
Bacteroides fragilis	32
Peptostreptococcus spp.	16
Clostridium perfringens	2

dose of 400 mg, mean peak serum levels occur 1–2 h later and reach 1.6 µg/mL. The serum half-life of norfloxacin is approximately 4 h. There is no significant accumulation of norfloxacin after repeated doses in healthy subjects. The pharmacokinetics of norfloxacin do not appear to be altered in patients with liver disease (63). In patients with cirrhosis and ascites, the trough serum levels of norfloxacin after seven days of treatment with 400 mg/day are 0.5 ± 0.1 µg/mL (range 0.2–1.1 µg/mL) (12). The absorbed norfloxacin is either metabolized in the liver or excreted unchanged by the kidneys. Concentrations of norfloxacin in the urine are usually 100–300 times the simultaneous serum concentration and exceed the MIC_{90} of most urinary pathogens for 12–24 h. Due to its high kidney excretion, the pharmacokinetics of norfloxacin are markedly altered in the presence of renal failure. In healthy subjects, up to 50% of a single 400-mg oral dose may be recovered from the feces in the subsequent 48-h period. Peak concentrations in fecal specimens are in the range of 207–2715 µg/g at 24–36 h after dosing (64,65). Similar fecal concentrations have been found in patients with cirrhosis seven days after administration of norfloxacin 400 mg/day (12). Because of its marked activity against aerobic gram-negative bacteria, lack of efficacy against other bacteria, and high fecal concentrations after oral administration, norfloxacin is an excellent drug to induce a selective intestinal decontamination (61,66). Studies in patients with cirrhosis have confirmed that the administration of norfloxacin 400 mg/day for seven days is associated with selective intestinal decontamination (12).

In clinical practice, norfloxacin has been used almost exclusively in the treatment of urinary tract infections and enteric infections (61). For systemic infections, other fluoroquinolones, especially ciprofloxacin and ofloxacin, are preferred due to their higher intestinal absorption and better distribution and penetration in the tissues. Norfloxacin as well as ciprofloxacin have been shown to be effective in the prevention of infection in neutropenic patients (66). Adverse effects, most of them minor, are very uncommon during norfloxacin administration (61).

B. Efficacy of Norfloxacin in the Prevention of the Recurrence of SBP

Long-term norfloxacin administration has been shown to be effective in the prevention of the recurrence of SBP in patients with cirrhosis. In the only study published so far, patients received norfloxacin 400 mg/day or placebo, in a double-blind manner, for up to 19 months (mean treatment period six months) (56). The probability of the recurrence of SBP during one year of follow-up was only 20% in the norfloxacin group compared to 68% in the placebo group. This latter figure is similar to that reported in previous studies (7). This reduction was exclusively due to a decrease in the probability of developing a recurrence of SBP caused by gram-negative bacteria (3% vs. 60% at one year) (Fig. 12.4). Recurrent episodes of SBP in patients treated with norfloxacin were almost exclusively due to gram-positive bacteria or were culture-negative. When compared with the placebo group, it is evident that the probability of developing SBP caused by gram-positive bacteria was not increased by long-term norfloxacin administration (Fig. 12.4). The absence of differences in survival in this study among patients treated with norfloxacin and those treated with placebo has been used by some authors as an argument against the use of prophylaxis in patients who have recovered from the first episode of SBP (67,68). However, it must be pointed out that the only endpoint

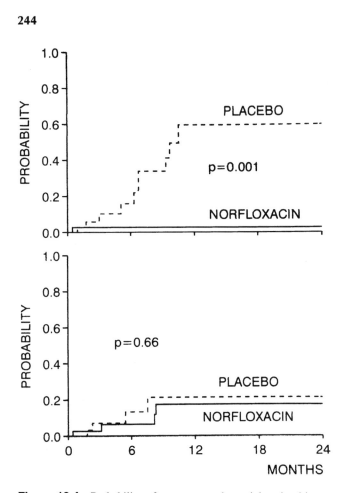

Figure 12.4 Probability of spontaneous bacterial peritonitis recurrence in patients receiving norfloxacin (400 mg/day) and patients treated with placebo after the first episode of spontaneous bacterial peritonitis. Top: episodes caused by gram-negative bacteria. Bottom: episodes caused by gram-positive bacteria or culture-negative. (Modified from Ref. 56.)

of the study was the recurrence of SBP and not survival. Accordingly, treatment with norfloxacin or placebo was definitively interrupted in patients developing a new episode of SBP. Further studies are required to evaluate the effect of continuous norfloxacin administration on survival. On the other hand, it has been demonstrated that the use of prophylactic antibiotics to decrease the incidence of SBP does reduce greatly the overall costs of management of SBP compared with the traditional "diagnose and treat" strategy (69,70).

The efficacy of norfloxacin administration in the prevention of the recurrence of SBP by gram-negative bacteria is probably related to its ability to cause a selective intestinal decontamination, which is maintained throughout the treatment period (56) (Fig. 12.5). Studies in experimental cirrhosis have shown that this effect is associated with a reduction of translocation of gram-negative bacteria to the mesenteric lymph nodes (71). Preliminary data in patients with cirrhosis investigated at the time of liver transplantation indicate that the frequency of bacterial translocation by gram-negative bacteria in patients treated with norfloxacin is markedly reduced compared with patients not receiving norfloxacin, suggesting that norfloxacin also prevents bacterial translocation to mesenteric lymph nodes in human cirrhosis (72). In experimental cirrhosis, norfloxacin administration was found to be associated with an increased risk of bacterial translocation and peritonitis caused by gram-positive bacteria (71). However, these findings appear to be exclusive of experimental cirrhosis because in human cirrhosis long-term norfloxacin administration neither increases bacterial translocation nor the risk of SBP or other infections by gram-positive bacteria (56,72,73). Besides its effect in preventing bacterial translocation, the existence of bactericidal levels of norfloxacin in serum and, presumably, ascitic fluid, for most gram-negative bacteria (12) could also contribute to the efficacy of norfloxacin in the prevention of the recurrence of SBP.

The duration of norfloxacin administration to prevent the recurrence of SBP has not been established. Because of the high risk of recurrence after the first episode of SBP, it seems advisable to maintain norfloxacin prophylaxis indefinitely. Nevertheless, norfloxacin may probably be discontinued in those few patients in whom ascites disappears during follow-up.

C. Side Effects of Norfloxacin: Development of Resistant Bacteria

The major concerns about continuous norfloxacin administration in the prevention of the recurrence of SBP have been the appearance of bacteria resistant to norfloxacin in the intestinal flora and the development of SBP caused by these resistant organisms (68,71).

The effects of continuous norfloxacin administration on fecal flora in patients with cirrhosis have been assessed carefully in two investigations (56,74). In the first study, which was performed in patients who were treated

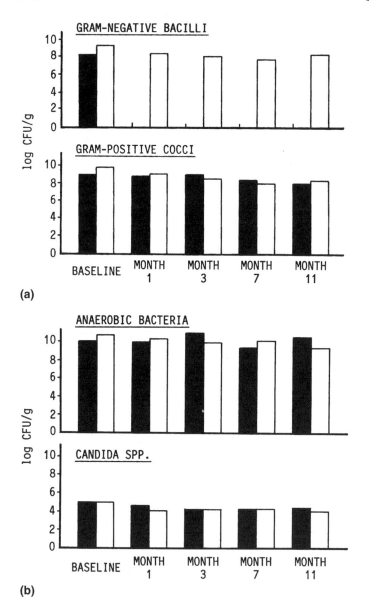

Figure 12.5 Changes in concentration of (a) gram-negative bacilli and gram-positive cocci and (b) anaerobic bacteria and *Candida* spp. in fecal flora during long-term administration of norfloxacin (black columns) or placebo (white columns). Results are expressed as logarithm colony-forming units per gram of feces.

with norfloxacin 400 mg/day for the prevention of the recurrence of SBP in whom quantitative analyses of fecal flora were performed bimonthly for up to 11 months, colonization of fecal flora by *Pseudomonas* species, *Aeromonas hydrophila*, or *Staphylococcus epidermidis* was found in some cases (56). However, in all cases low counts of resistant bacteria were found and colonization was transient. The second study was performed in a group of alcoholic cirrhotic patients treated with 400 mg/day of norfloxacin weekly for the first month and then every two weeks thereafter (74). In half of the patients, bacteria resistant to norfloxacin not present in baseline cultures were isolated from fecal flora at some time during a median follow-up of 25 days. Isolated bacteria were either gram-positive cocci (*Staphylococcus aureus*, coagulase-negative *Staphylococcus* species, and *Streptococcus* species), against which norfloxacin is poorly active, or fluoroquinolone-resistant gram-negative bacteria (*Citrobacter freundii*, *Enterobacter cloacae*, *Klebsiella oxytoca*, and *Proteus rettgen*). In contrast to the findings of the previous study, in this latter investigation most resistant isolates persisted until the end of follow-up. Differences between the two studies may be due, at least in part, to the fact that patients in the first study were outpatients, whereas the population of the second study consisted exclusively of hospitalized patients. Because a control group of patients was not included in the latter investigation, some instances of colonization, especially those due to gram-positive bacteria, may represent the acquisition of resistant bacteria in the hospital setting.

The concern about the possible appearance of SBP caused by fluoroquinolone-resistant gram-negative bacteria during continuous norfloxacin administration for prevention of SBP recurrence has been more theoretical than based on available evidence. In fact, among 229 episodes of SBP observed in two institutions during a six-year period (1988–1994), 193 episodes occurred in patients without norfloxacin prophylaxis and 36 in patients under norfloxacin prophylaxis. Only three episodes of SBP (0.1%) were caused by gram-negative bacteria resistant to fluoroquinolones, and all of them occurred in patients not receiving norfloxacin (75). In another study assessing the efficacy of norfloxacin in preventing the first episode of SBP, none of the 56 patients receiving continuous norfloxacin prophylaxis developed SBP caused by gram-negative bacteria (73). In this study, an increased incidence of mild urinary tract infections caused by gram-negative bacteria resistant to norfloxacin was observed.

Development of fungal infections is very uncommon during continuous norfloxacin prophylaxis in patients with cirrhosis. In the only published double-blind, placebo-controlled study, only one of 40 patients (2.5%) treated with norfloxacin developed oral and esophageal candidiasis, which resolved with oral nystatin therapy. In another study, oral candidiasis was observed in only one of the 109 patients included (0.9%) (73). These results are in keeping with the observation that administration of fluoroquinolones for prevention of gram-negative infections in neutropenic patients is not associated with an increased risk of fungal infections (76–78).

III. SUMMARY

In recent years we have learned a great deal about the natural history of cirrhosis with regard to the occurrence of SBP. Gastrointestinal bleeding has been identified as one of the major risk factors for the development of infections, including SBP, in patients with cirrhosis. It has also been shown that the likelihood of developing SBP in nonbleeding patients is closely related to the impairment of local defense mechanisms against infection in ascitic fluid. A reduced opsonic activity in ascitic fluid is associated with an increased risk of the occurrence of SBP. In clinical practice, the opsonic activity of ascitic fluid can be estimated by measuring total protein complement concentrations in ascitic fluid. Increased risk of the occurrence of SBP occurrence has been found in patients with protein concentrations in ascitic fluid below 15 g/L. Factors not related to the ascitic fluid that have been found to correlate with the risk of SBP occurrence are poor liver function and impaired activity of the reticuloendothelial system. However, the relationship between these two factors and the development of SBP deserves further investigation. Finally, SBP has been shown to be a recurrent process. Patients who have recovered from the first episode of SBP are at very high risk of recurrence of SBP. Long-term survival of these patients is poor and recurrent SBP accounts for a significant number of deaths among them.

The immediate clinical consequence of the identification of cirrhotic patients with a high risk of SBP occurrence has been the investigation of methods capable of preventing SBP in these patients. Because most episodes of infection are caused by aerobic gram-negative bacteria present in normal endogenous flora, the strategy used has been based on the administration of antibiotic agents that induce a selective decontamination of the intestinal tract. It has been shown that continuous administration of norfloxacin, a fluoroquinolone with potent effects against aerobic gram-negative bacteria and poor activity against aerobic gram-positive bacteria and anaerobes, reduces dramatically the risk of recurrence of SBP. Although colonization of intestinal flora by gram-negative bacteria resistant to norfloxacin or gram-positive cocci has been reported in some patients under norfloxacin prophylaxis, this finding is not associated with an increased risk of developing SBP caused by these organisms. Therefore, continuous norfloxacin administration appears to be very effective in the prevention of the recurrence of SBP by gram-negative bacteria and should be recommended in all cirrhotic patients recovering from their first episodes of SBP.

REFERENCES

1. Navasa M, Rodès J. Management of ascites in the patient with portal hypertension with emphasis on spontaneous bacterial peritonitis. Semin Gastrointest Dis 1997; 8:200–209.
2. Gaurner C, Soriano G. Spontaneous bacterial peritonitis. Semin Liver Dis 1997; 17:203–217.
3. Runyon BA. Bacterial translocation and spontaneous infections in liver disease. In: *Therapy in Liver Diseases: The Pathophysiological Basis of Therapy*, Arroyo V, Bosch J, Bruguera M, Rodés J, eds., Barcelona: Masson SA, 1997, 101–108.
4. Ginès P, Arroyo V, Rodés J. Pathophysiology, complications and treatment of ascites. In: *Portal Hypertension*, LaBrecque D, ed., Clin Liver Dis 1997; 1:129–155.
5. Rimola A, Navasa M. Infections in liver disease. In: *Oxford Textbook of Clinical Hepatology*, 2nd ed., McIntyre N, Benhamou JP, Bircher J, Rizetto M, Rodés J, eds., New York: Oxford University Press, 1999, 1861–1874.
6. Toledo C, Salmerón JM, Rimola A, Navasa M, Arroyo V, Llach J, Ginès A, Ginès P, Rodès J. Spontaneous bacterial peritonitis in cirrhosis: predictive factors of infection resolution and survival in patients treated with cefotaxime. Hepatology 1993; 17:251–257.
7. Titó L, Rimola A, Ginés P, Llach J, Arroyo V, Rodés J. Recurrence of spontaneous bacterial peritonitis in cirrhosis. Frequency and predictive factors. Hepatology 1988; 8:27–31.
8. Silvain C, Mannant PG, Ingrad P, Fort E, Besson I, Beauchant M. Récidive de l'infection spontanée du liquide d'ascite au cours de la cirrhose. Gastroenterol Clin Biol 1991; 15:106–109.
9. Altmann C, Grangé D, Amiot X, Pelletier G, Lacaine F, Bodin F, Etienne JP. Survival after a first episode of spontaneous bacterial peritonitis. Prognosis of potential candidates for orthotopic liver transplantation. J Gastroenterol Hepatol 1995; 10:47–50.
10. Terg R, Levi D, López P, Rafaelli C, Rojter S, Abecasis R, Villamil F, Aziz H, Podesta A. Analysis of clinical course and prognosis of culture-positive spontaneous bacterial peritonitis and neutrocytic ascites. Evidence of the same disease. Dig Dis Sci 1992; 37:1499–1504.
11. Ginès P, Rimola A, Salmerón JM, del Pino JI, Ginès A, Llach J, Arroyo V,

Rodés J. Utilidad de la administración oral de quinolonas en la profilaxis de la recidiva de la peritonitis bacteriana espontánea en la cirrosis hepática. Gastroenterol Hepatol 1990; 13:329–333.

12.   Ginès P, Rimola A, Marco A, Almela M, Marqués JM, Salmerón JM, Ginès A, Llach J, Jiménez de Anta MT, Arroyo V, Rodés J. Efecto de la administración de norfloxacina sobre la flora fecal en pacientes cirróticos. Gastroenterol Hepatol 1990; 13:325–328.

13.   Rimola A, Bory F, Terés J, Pérez-Ayuso R, Arroyo V, Rodés J. Oral non-absorbable antibiotics prevent infections in cirrhotic patients with gastrointestinal hemorrhage. Hepatology 1985; 5:463–467.

14.   Bleichner G, Boulanger R, Squara P, Sollet JP, Parent A. Frequency of infections in cirrhotic patients presenting with acute gastrointestinal haemorrhage. Br J Surg 1986; 73:724–726.

15.   Bercoff E, Chassagne P, Frébourg T, Manchon D, Bourreille J. Infections bactériennes et hémorragie digestive du cirrhotique. Gastroenterol Clin Biol 1990; 14: 34B–37B.

16.   Soriano G, Guarner C, Tomás A, Villanueva C, Torras X, González D, Sainz S, Anguera A, Cussó X, Balanzó J, Vllardell F. Norfloxacin prevents bacterial infection in cirrhotics with gastrointestinal hemorrhage. Gastroenterology 1992; 103:1267–1272.

17.   Blaise M, Pateron D, Trinchet JC, Levacher S, Beaugrand M, Pourriat JL. Systemic antibiotic therapy prevents bacterial infections in cirrhotic patients with gastrointestinal hemorrhage. Hepatology 1994; 20:34–38.

18.   Bernard B, Cadranel JF, Valla D, Escoland S, Jarlier V, Opolon P. Prognostic significance of bacterial infection in bleeding cirrhotic patients: a prospective study. Gastroenterology 1995; 108:1828–1834.

19.   Pauwels A, Mostefa-Kara N, Debenes B, Degoutte E, Lévy VG. Systemic antibiotic prophylaxis after gastrointestinal hemorrhage in cirrhotic patients with a high risk of infection. Hepatology 1996; 24:802–806.

20.   Altura BM, Hershey SG. Sequential changes in reticuloendothelial system function after acute hemorrhage. Proc Soc Exp Biol Med 1972; 139:935–939.

21.   Loegering DJ. Humoral factor depletion and reticuloendothelial depression during hemorrhagic shock. Am J Physiol 1977; 232:283–287.

22.   Rimola A, Soto R, Bory F, Arroyo V, Piera C, Rodés J. Reticuloendothelial system phagocytic activity in cirrhosis and its relation to bacterial infections and prognosis. Hepatology 1984; 4:53–58.

23.   Bolognesi M, Merkel C, Bianco S, Angeli P, Sacerdoti D, Amodio P, Gatta A. Clinical significance of the evaluation of hepatic reticuloendothelial removal capacity in patients with cirrhosis. Hepatology 1994; 19:628–634.

24.   Arden WA, Yacko M, Jay M, Beihn R, Debrin M, Gross D, Scwartz R. Scintigraphic evaluation of bacterial translocation during hemorragic shock. J Surg Res 1993; 54:102–106.

25.   Sorell W, Eamonn M, Quigley M, Gongliang JIN, Johnson T, Rikkers L. Bacterial translocation in the portal-hypertensive rat: studies in basal conditions

and on exposure to hemorragic shock. Gastroenterology 1993; 104:1722–1726.

26. Llovet JM, Bartoli R, Planas R, Cabré E, Jiménez M, Urban A, Ojanguren I, Arnal J, Gassull M. Bacterial translocation in cirrhotic rats. Its role in the development of spontaneous bacterial peritonitis. Gut 1994; 35:1648–1652.

27. Runyon B, Squier S, Borzio M. Translocation of gut bacteria in rats with cirrhosis to mesenteric lymph nodes partially explains the pathogenesis of spontaneous bacterial peritonitis. J Hepatol 1994; 21:792–796.

28. García-Tsao G, Lee FY, Barden G, Cartun R, West A. Bacterial translocation to mesenteric lymph nodes is increased in cirrhotic rats with ascites. Gastroenterology 1995; 108:1835–1841.

29. Llovet JM, Bartolí R, Planas R, Viñado B, Pérez J, Cabré E, Arnal J, Ojanguren I, Ausina V, Gassull MA. Selective intestinal decontamination with norfloxacin reduces bacterial translocation in ascitic cirrhotic rats exposed to hemorrhagic shock. Hepatology 1996; 23:781–787.

30. Goulis J, Armonis A, Patch D, Sabin C, Greensdale L, Burroughs AK. Bacterial infection is independently associated with failure to control bleeding in cirrhotic patients with gastrointestinal hemorrhage. Hepatology 1998; 27:1207–1212.

31. Simberkoff M, Moldover N, Weiss G. Bactericidal and opsonic activity of cirrhotic ascites and nonascitic peritoneal fluid. J Lab Clin Med 1978; 91:831–839.

32. Erdal Akalin H, Laleli Y, Telatar H. Bactericidal and opsonic activity of ascitic fluid from cirrhotic and non-cirrhotic patients. J Infect Dis 1983; 147:1011–1017.

33. Runyon BA, Morrissey RL, Hoefs JC, Wyle FA. Opsonic activity of human ascitic fluid: a potentially important protective mechanism against spontaneous bacterial peritonitis. Hepatology 1985; 5:634–637.

34. Runyon B. Patients with deficient ascitic fluid opsonic activity are predisposed to spontaneous bacterial peritonitis. Hepatology 1988; 8:632–635.

35. Mal F, Phan Huu T, Bendahou M, Trinchet J, Garnier M, Hakim J, Beaugrand M. Chemoattractant and opsonic activity in ascitic fluid. A study in 47 patients with cirrhosis and malignant peritonitis. J Hepatol 1991; 12:45–49.

36. Andreu M, Sola R, Sitges-Serra A, Alia C, Gallen M, Vila C, Coll S, Oliver MI. Risk factors for spontaneous bacterial peritonitis in cirrhotic patients with ascites. Gastroenterology 1993; 104:1133–1138.

37. Runyon B. Low-protein-concentration ascitic fluid is predisposed to spontaneous bacterial peritonitis. Gastroenterology 1986; 91:1343–1346.

38. Llach J, Rimola A, Navasa M, Ginès P, Salmerón JM, Ginès A, Arroyo V, Rodés P. Incidence and predictive factors of first episode of spontaneous bacterial peritonitis in cirrhosis with ascites: relevance of ascitic fluid protein concentration. Hepatology 1992; 16:724–727.

39. Such J, Guarner C, Enriquez J, Rodriguez JL, Seres I, Vilardell F. Low C3 in cirrhotic ascites predisposes to spontaneous bacterial peritonitis. J Hepatol 1988; 6:80–84.

40. Hassner A, Kletter Y, Shlag D, Yedvab M, Aronson M, Shibolet S. Impaired monocyte function in liver cirrhosis. Br Med J 1981; 16:481–489.

41. Rajkovic IA, Williams R. Abnormalities of neutrophil phagocytosis, intracellular killing and metabolic activity in alcoholic cirrhosis and hepatitis. Hepatology 1986; 6:252–262.
42. Feliu E, Gougerot MA, Hakim J, Cramer A, Auclair C, Rueff B, Boivin P. Blood polymorphonuclear dysfunction in patients with alcoholic cirrhosis. Eur J Clin Invest 1977; 7:571–577.
43. De Meo An, Andersen BR. Defective chemotaxis associated with a serum inhibitor in cirrhotic patients. N Engl J Med 1972; 286:735–740.
44. Potter BJ, Trueman AM, Jones EA. Serum complement in chronic liver disease. Gut 1971; 12:574–578.
45. Fox RA, Dudley FS, Sherlock S. The serum concentrations of the third component of complement in liver disease. Gut 1971; 12:574–578.
46. Kourilsky O, LeRoy R, Peltier AP. Complement and liver cell function in 53 patients with liver disease. Am J Med 1973; 55:783–790.
47. Erdal Akalin H, Laleli Y, Telatar H. Serum bactericidal and opsonic activities in patients with non-alcoholic cirrhosis. Q J Med 1985; 220:431–437.
48. Lahnborg F, Friman L, Berghem L. Reticuloendothelial function in patients with alcoholic liver cirrhosis. Scand J Gastroenterol 1981; 16:481–489.
49. Wardle N, Anderson A, James O. Kupffer cell phagocytosis in relation to BSP clearance in liver and inflammatory bowel diseases. Dig Dis Sci 1980; 25:414–419.
50. Halpern BN, Biozzi G, Pécquignot G. Mésure de la circulation sanguine du foie et de l'activité phagocytaire du système réticuloendothélial chez le sujet normal et le sujet cirrhotique. Path Biol 1959; 7:1537–1553.
51. Cooksley WGE, Powell LW, Halliday KW. Reticuloendothelial phagocytic function in human liver disease and its relationship to haemolysis. Br J Haematol 1973; 25:147–164.
52. Beeson PB, Brannon ES, Warren JV. Observations on the sites of removal of bacteria from the blood in patients with bacterial endocarditis. J Exp Med 1945; 81:9–23.
53. Rogers De. Host mechanisms which act to remove bacteria from the blood stream. Bact Rev 1960; 24:50–66.
54. Rutenburg AM, Sonnenblick E, Koven I. Comparative response of normal and cirrhotic rats to intravenously injected bacteria. Proc Soc Exp Biol Med 1959; 101:279–281.
55. Horisawa M, Goldstein G, Waxman A. The abnormal hepatic scan of chronic liver disease: its relationship to hepatic hemodynamics and colloid extraction. Gastroenterology 1976; 71:210–213.
56. Ginès P, Rimola A, Planas R, Vargas V, Marco F, Almela M, Forné M, Miranda ML, Llach J, Salmerón JM, Esteve M, Marqués J, Jiménez de Anta MT, Arroyo V, Rodés J. Norfloxacin prevents spontaneous bacterial peritonitis recurrence in cirrhosis: results of a double-blind, placebo controlled trial. Hepatology 1990; 12:716–724.
57. Van der Waaij D. Antibiotic choice: The importance of colonization of the diges-

tive tract: clinical consequences and implications. New York: Research Study Press, 1981, 300–310.

58. Van der Waaij D. Colonization resistance of the digestive tract: Clinical consequences and implications. Antimicrob Agents Chemother 1982; 10:263–270.

59. De Vries-Hospers HG, Sleijfer DT. Mulder NH, Van der Waaij D, Nieweg HO, Van Saene HKF. Bacteriological aspects of selective intestinal decontamination of the digestive tract as a method of infection prevention in the granulocytopenic patients. Antimicrob Agents Chemother 1981; 19:813–820.

60. Rogers C, Van Saene H, Suter P, Horner R, L'E Orme M. Infection control in critically ill patients: effects of selective decontamination of the digestive tract. Am J Hosp Pharm 1994; 51:631–648.

61. Kucres A, Crowe SM, Grayson ML, Hoy JF, eds. Norfloxacin, In: *The Use of Antibiotics. A Clinical Review of Antibacterial, Antifungal and Antiviral Drugs*, Oxford: Butterworth-Heinemann, 1997, 1061–1075.

62. Kucres A, Crowe SM, Grayson ML, Hoy JF, eds. Ciprofloxacin, In: *The Use of Antibiotics. A Clinical Review of Antibacterial, Antifungal and Antiviral Drugs*. Oxford: Butterworth-Heinemann, 1997, 981–1060.

63. Eandi M, Viano I, DiNola F, Leone L, Genazzani E. Pharmacokinetics of norfloxacin in healthy volunteers and patients with renal and hepatic damage. Eur J Clin Microbiol 1983; 2:253–259.

64. Cofsky RD, DuBouchet L, Landesman SH. Recovery of norfloxacin in feces after administration of a single oral dose to human volunteers. Antimicrob Agents Chemother 1984; 26:110–111.

65. Edlund C, Lidbeck A, Kager L, Nord CE. Comparative effects of enoxacin and norfloxacin on human colonic flora. Antimicrob Agents Chemother 1987; 31: 1846–1848.

66. Engels EA, Lau J, Barza M. Efficacy of quinolone prophylaxis in neutropenic cancer patients: A meta-analysis. J Clin Oncol 1998; 16:1179–1187.

67. Hoefs JC. Spontaneous bacterial peritonitis: prevention and therapy. Hepatology 1990; 12:776–781.

68. Schubert ML, Sanyal AJ, Wong ES. Antibiotic prophylaxis for prevention of spontaneous bacterial peritonitis? Gastroenterology 1991; 101:550–557.

69. Inadomi J, Sonnenberg A. Cost-analysis of prophylactic antibiotics in spontaneous bacterial peritonitis. Gastroenterology 1997; 114:1289–1294.

70. Younossi ZM, McHutchison JG, Ganiats TG. An economic analysis of norfloxacin prophylaxis against spontaneous bacterial peritonitis. J Hepatol 1997; 27: 295–298.

71. Runyon BA, Borzio M, Young S, Squier S, Guarner C, Runyon M. Effect of selective bowel decontamination with norfoxacin on spontaneous bacterial peritonitis, translocation, and survival in an animal model of cirrhosis. Hepatology 1995; 21:1719–1724.

72. Cirera I, Suárez MJ, Navasa M, Vila J, García-Valdecasas JC, Grande L, Taurá P, Rimola A, Rodés J. Bacterial translocation in patients with cirrhosis (abstract). J Hepatol 1997; 26:101A.

73. Novella M, Solà R, Soriano G, Andreu M, Gana J, Ortiz J, Coll S, Sàbat M, Vila MC, Guarner C, Vilardell F. Continuous versus inpatient prophylaxis of the first episode of spontaneous bacterial peritonitis with norfloxacin. Hepatology 1997; 25:532–536.

74. Dupeyron C, Mangeney N, Sedrati L, Campillo B, Fouet P, Leluan G. Rapid emergence of quinolone resistance in cirrhotic patients treated with norfloxacin to prevent spontaneous bacterial peritonitis. Antimicrob Agents Chemother 1994; 38:340–344.

75. Llovet JM, Rodríguez-Iglesias P, Moitinho E, Planas R, Bataller R, Navasa M, Menacho M, Pardo A, Castells A, Cabré E, Arroyo V, Gassull MA, Rodés J. Spontaneous bacterial peritonitis in patients with cirrhosis undergoing selective intestinal decontamination. J Hepatol 1997; 26:88–95.

76. Karp JE, Menz WG, Hendriksen C, Laughon B, Redden T, Bamberger BJ, Bartlett JG, Saral R, Burke PJ. Oral norfloxacin for prevention of gram-negative bacterial infections in patients with acute leukemia and granulocytopenia. A randomized double-blind placebo-controlled trial. Ann Intern Med 1986; 106:1–7.

77. Dekker AW, Rozenberg-Arska M, Verhoef J. Infection prophylaxis in acute leukemia; a comparison of ciprofloxacin with trimethoprim-sulphamethoxazole and colistin. Ann Intern Med 1987; 106:7–11.

78. Jansen J, Cromer M, Akard L, Black JR, Wheat LJ, Allen SD. Infection prevention in severely myelosuppressed patients: a comparison between ciprofloxacin and a regimen of selective antibiotic modulation of the intestinal flora. Amer J Med 1994; 96:335–341.

13

Primary Prophylaxis of Spontaneous Bacterial Peritonitis

Germán Soriano and Carlos Guarner
Hospital de la Santa Creu i Sant Pau, Universitat Autónoma de Barcelona, Barcelona, Spain

I. RATIONALE FOR PRIMARY PROPHYLAXIS OF SPONTANEOUS BACTERIAL PERITONITIS

Spontaneous bacterial peritonitis (SBP) is a frequent complication in cirrhotic patients with an incidence ranging between 8% and 27% during a single hospitalization (1–3). Considering patients with ascites and without previous SBP, the one-year probability of developing the first episode of SBP is 11–29% (4,5). These figures increase to 20–50% when considering high-risk groups defined by low ascitic fluid total protein (<10 g/L) or high serum bilirubin levels (>2.5 mg/dL) (4,5). Moreover, both short- and long-term prognosis are affected in cirrhotic patients who develop SBP or other severe bacterial infections. Actually, between 7% and 25% of deaths in cirrhotic patients are related to bacterial infections (1,6,7), and the frequency of death during hospitalization is 5–6 times higher in infected as compared to noninfected cirrhotic patients (1). It should be noted, however, that the short-term prognosis of patients with SBP has dramatically improved during the last decade (8–10), probably as a consequence of early diagnosis and treatment with non-nephrotoxic antibiotic agents (11). Although most patients survive the episode of SBP, 20–40% die during hospitalization in the most recent series, mainly as a consequence of other complications of cirrhosis, that are frequently triggered by the episode of SBP (9–12).

In fact, SBP frequently determines the occurrence of other complications of cirrhosis, such as gastrointestinal hemorrhage, hepatic encephalopathy, renal failure, and the hepatorenal syndrome (9–12). It has been observed that bacterial infections increase the risk of rebleeding during the early days of hospitalization in cirrhotic patients with gastrointestinal bleeding (13,14). On the other hand, 32–44% of patients show hepatic encephalopathy at the time of the diagnosis of SBP (9,10,12). Finally, the development of renal dysfunction occurs in one-third of patients with SBP and has been demonstrated to be the most important independent predictive factor of mortality during hospitalization in patients with SBP (10,15).

Both short-term and long-term prognoses are severely affected in cirrhotic patients by an episode of SBP. Between 40% and 70% of survivors of an episode of SBP will develop a new episode during the first year of follow-up (16,17). In addition, the one-year probability of survival after the first episode of SBP is approximately 30–40% (16,17), and is notably worse in those patients with more advanced liver insufficiency (Child-Pugh class C) (18).

II. CIRRHOTIC PATIENTS AT HIGH RISK OF THE FIRST EPISODE OF SPONTANEOUS BACTERIAL PERITIONITIS

During the last decade, several groups of cirrhotic patients at especially high risk of developing their initial episode of SBP have been identified (Table 13.1). Some of these patients are at high risk during hospitalization and are candidates for prophylaxis of SBP in the hospital, but other patients will remain at high risk indefinitely and are candidates for long-term (inpatient and outpatient) prophylaxis.

Table 13.1 Cirrhotic Patients at High Risk of the First Episode of Spontaneous Bacterial Peritonitis

I.   Short-term risk (during hospitalization)
Gastrointestinal hemorrhage
Ascites and low ascitic fluid total protein ($<$1–1.5 g/dL)
II. Long-term risk (during hospitalization and as outpatients)
Patients with ascites and low ascitic fluid total protein
($\leq$1 g/dL) and/or high serum bilirubin ($>$2.5 mg/dL)

The severity of liver insufficiency is probably the primary predisposing factor for developing SBP (19). More than 70% of episodes of SBP occur in patients who belong to Child-Pugh class C and the remainder are class B patients (4,9,10). It is extremely rare for a Child-Pugh class A patient to develop an episode of SBP. When SBP is suspected in such a patient, the possibility of secondary peritonitis should be kept in mind. This strong relationship between liver insufficiency and predisposition to SBP is probably related to the fact that most of the disturbances in the antimicrobial mechanisms observed in cirrhotic patients are closely correlated with liver function (20).

Impairment in the activity of the reticuloendothelial system seems to be one of the most relevant disturbances that explains the predisposition to develop bacterial infections and SBP in cirrhotic patients. Rimola et al. (21) demonstrated that cirrhotic patients with impaired reticuloendothelial activity show a higher incidence of bacteremia, both during and after hospitalization, than cirrhotic patients with normal reticuloendothelial activity. Recently, Bolognesi et al. (22) observed that cirrhotic patients with low maximal removal capacity by the hepatic reticuloendothelial system are more predisposed to develop SBP than those with higher capacity.

Ascites is a prerequisite for the development of SBP, but not all patients with ascites are at equal risk of developing SBP. Among other factors, it depends on the capacity of ascitic fluid to kill potentially infecting bacteria reaching ascites, mainly on the opsonic activity of the ascitic fluid (23). Ascitic fluid opsonic activity is directly correlated to the ascitic fluid protein concentration and C_3 levels in cirrhotic patients (24). Different studies have confirmed that low opsonic activity, total protein concentration, or C_3 levels in ascitic fluid predispose to the development of an episode of SBP (25–27). Among these parameters, the ascitic fluid total protein concentration is the easiest to perform in clinical practice, provides a surrogate index of ascitic fluid antimicrobial activity, and has become the most important marker of impending SBP in ascitic cirrhotic patients. Actually, Runyon (25) demonstrated that patients with ascitic fluid total protein levels ≤ 1 g/dL have a statistically significant higher risk of nosocomial SBP than those with higher levels (15% vs 1.5%).

Moreover, low ascitic fluid total protein levels not only predispose to SBP during hospitalization but also during long-term follow-up (4,5). Two multivariate analysis have identified predictive factors for the development of the first episode of SBP during long-term follow-up. Llach et al. (5) studied 127 cirrhotic patients without previous SBP and observed that the only independent predictive factor of the first episode of SBP was the total protein concentration of ascitic fluid. In this study, cirrhotic patients with total protein levels <1 g/dL in ascitic fluid showed a probability of developing their first episode of SBP of 24% within one year of follow-up. In the other study, Andreu et al. (4) prospectively analyzed 110 cirrhotic patients who had not previously had SBP, and demonstrated that the probability of developing SBP in patients with low ascitic fluid total protein (≤ 1 g/dL) or high serum bilirubin (>2.5 mg/dL) approached 50% during a one-year period of follow-up. It is of interest that 60% of the episodes of SBP were community-acquired.

Cirrhotic patients who have had gastrointestinal hemorrhage constitute another high-risk group for developing bacterial infections, including SBP (28,29). This predisposition appears to be related to several other dysfunctions of acute hemorrhage in the already impaired antimicrobial mechanisms of cirrhotic patients, such as a depression of reticuloendothelial activity and an increase in intestinal permeability and bacterial translocation due to hypovolemia (30,31). An enhanced incidence of bacterial translocation to mesenteric lymph nodes after hemorrhagic shock has recently been observed in rats with cirrhosis and shock compared to shocked noncirrhotic rats and to nonshocked cirrhotic rats (32,33). These observations suggest that both cirrhosis and hypovolemia are independent factors that favor bacterial translocation. As a consequence of these disturbances, 20% of cirrhotic patients admitted with gastrointestinal hemorrhage are already infected at the time of admission to the hospital (29), and 30–60% of them will develop a nosocomial bacterial infection, usually during the first three to four days of hospitalization (28,34–36). Therefore, up to 50% of cirrhotic patients present a bacterial infection during hospitalization for gastrointestinal bleeding.

Two studies have identified subgroups of cirrhotic patients with gastrointestinal bleeding at even higher risk of bacterial infection. In one study, the presence of a Child-Pugh's class C and/or rebleeding identified a subgroup with an especially high risk of nosocomial infection (37), who showed an incidence greater than 50% in a subsequent validating study (36). In the other study, the presence of ascites, encephalopathy, severe or recurrent hemorrhage, and serum albumin levels were independent predictive factors of bacterial infection in bleeding cirrhotic patients despite receiving prophylactic norfloxacin (38).

It had been suggested that endoscopic treatment of variceal hemorrhage could play a significant role in the predisposition to bacterial infections in the setting of acute hemorrhage (39,40). This predisposition, however, according to several recent studies, seems to be more related to the hemorrhage per se than to the endoscopic treatment. In one randomized study, Rolando et al. (41) prospectively evaluated the efficacy of two doses of an intravenous combination of antibiotic agents (imipenem/cilastatin) in the prevention of bacterial infections in cirrhotic patients who were treated with endoscopic sclerotherapy of esophageal varices. In this controlled study, the authors observed a low incidence of early postsclerotherapy bacteremia in both groups, and the incidence of bacterial infections during the first seven days after sclerotherapy was similar in both prophylactically treated patients (20%) and control subjects (23%), suggesting that this prophylactic antibiotic regimen may not be truly useful in the prevention of bacterial infections. Moreover, they observed that the infections were significantly more common after emergency sclerotherapy (34.8%) than after elective sclerotherapy (3.8%), thus confirming that the risk of bacterial infection in bleeding cirrhotic patients is related more to the hemorrhage than to its endoscopic therapy. Selby et al. (42) have recently confirmed these results in a randomized study that evaluated the efficacy of a single dose of prophylactic intravenous cefotaxime before emergency sclerotherapy. These authors performed routine blood and ascitic fluid cultures after sclerotherapy. Although the incidence of bacteremia was 31.6% in the control group and 5.3% in the treated group (p = 0.04), no clinical infection attributable to sclerotherapy developed in any patient in either of the two groups. Band ligation of esophageal varices appears to be more effective and safer than sclerotherapy (43,44), and the incidence of bacteremia and bacterial infections seems to be lower in patients treated with banding than in those treated with endoscopic sclerotherapy (45). According to these studies, endoscopic procedures with or without sclerotherapy or band ligation of esophageal varices do not seem to increase appreciably the risk of developing bacterial infections in cirrhotic patients. Therefore, short-course antibiotic prophylactic therapy for endoscopic treatment is not recommended.

Paracentesis is also an invasive procedure that has been considered in the past to be a predisposing factor for the development of SBP (46). However, diagnostic paracentesis appears to be an extremely safe procedure (47), since the diagnosis of SBP is almost always established by the first paracentesis (2,47). In addition, Runyon et al. (48) observed that the incidence of polymicrobial bacterascites as a consequence of a bowel puncture with the paracentesis needle was lower than 1%, and only one of the 10 such instances detected progressed to clinical peritonitis. Large-volume therapeutic paracentesis is currently the first-line treatment in cirrhotic patients with tense or refractory ascites (49,50). However, repeated paracentesis decreases ascitic fluid protein contents, including antimicrobial proteins such as C_3, in cirrhotic patients with or without previous SBP (51,52). A single large-volume paracentesis followed by diuretic administration decreased ascitic fluid C_3 in cirrhotic patients, but not in those patients treated with diuretic therapy alone (53). Therefore, just as patients with low total protein levels (25) and C_3 levels (26) in ascitic fluid are predisposed to develop SBP, repeated large-volume paracentesis may theoretically predispose to SBP. Solà et al. (54) compared prospectively the short and long-term incidence of SBP in cirrhotic patients with tense ascites treated with diuretics or with large-volume paracentesis. Although the short-term incidence of SBP was slightly higher in the diuretic-treated patients, the one-year probability of developing SBP was similar in both groups. This study suggests that large-volume paracentesis does not increase the risk of developing an episode of SBP. It should be noted, however, that only 40% of patients in the paracentesis group required more than one large-volume paracentesis during follow-up, which may have masked a potential deleterious effect of large-volume paracentesis on the incidence of SBP. Available data suggest that cirrhotic patients with ascites who undergo diagnostic or therapeutic paracentesis do not seem to constitute a group of patients at an especially high risk of developing SBP. Other invasive procedures such as intravenous and urinary catheters could predispose to bacterial infections in cirrhotic patients (3). A direct relationship between these procedures and the development of SBP, however, has not yet been demonstrated. These maneuvers should be avoided whenever possible.

Hepatocellular carcinoma may result in an increase in the risk of developing SBP in cirrhotic patients by further impairing antimicrobial defense mechanisms. However, two recent studies have shown that the incidence of SBP in patients with cirrhosis and hepatocellular carcinoma is similar to that in cirrhotic patients without this tumor. These observations suggest that hepatocellular carcinoma per se does not predispose to the development of SBP (55,56). Because iron is a main factor in bacterial growth, Romero et al. (57) have evaluated the effect of free iron and transferrin concentrations on bacterial growth of *Escherichia coli* in the ascitic fluid from cirrhotic patients. These authors added iron and then transferrin to ascitic fluid samples, and observed that the growth of *Escherichia coli* was greater when high levels of free iron were present in ascitic fluid, and that this effect was inhibited by the addition of transferrin. These data suggested that cirrhotic patients with high free iron and low transferrin levels in ascitic fluid are more predisposed to develop SBP. Therefore, Kolle et al. (58) performed a clinical study to evaluate the relationship between ascitic fluid levels of iron and iron-binding proteins and the development of SBP in cirrhotic patients. In this study, there were no differences in iron, total iron binding capacity, transferrin, and ferritin levels in the ascitic fluids of patients with infected ascitic fluid and those with sterile ascites. According to these preliminary data, iron or iron-binding proteins levels in ascitic fluid do not appear to predispose to SBP in cirrhotic patients.

III. MEASURES FOR THE PREVENTION OF SPONTANEOUS BACTERIAL PERITONITIS

Several measures (59) have been proposed to be helpful in preventing bacterial infections and SBP in cirrhotic patients, such as discontinuing alcohol intake (60), reducing the time of hospitalization (1,7), avoiding unnecessary instrumentation (3), improving nutritional status (61), and preventing other complications of cirrhosis, such as ascites formation, gastrointestinal hemorrhage, and hepatic encephalopathy (59), which could favor the development of SBP.

In a recent study, Ho et al. (62) observed a high incidence of concomitant asymptomatic bacteriuria (61.4%) in cirrhotic patients with community-acquired SBP. Although a causal relationship was not demonstrated in this study, the authors hypothesized that asymptomatic bacteriuria would probably precede SBP development in these patients, and suggested that early diagnosis and treatment of asymptomatic bacteriuria could be useful for preventing SBP. Because diuresis increases the concentration of complement factors and opsonic activity of ascitic fluid in cirrhotic patients (51–53), Runyon and Van Epps proposed that diuretic therapy could prevent the development of SBP in cirrhotic patients with ascites (63). However, it is very difficult to evaluate the prophylactic effect of diuretic drugs per se, since almost all cirrhotic patients with ascites require diuretic treatment to control ascites.

In a recent retrospective study, Castells et al. (64) demonstrated that the probability of developing gastrointestinal hemorrhage, ascites, and SBP in cirrhotic patients is reduced by portacaval shunt compared to nonshunted patients treated with sclerotherapy or esophageal transection. This study confirms that not only gastrointestinal bleeding but also other major complications of cirrhosis such as ascites and SBP are prevented by decreasing portal pressure. However, the high operative mortality rate, especially in Child-Pugh C patients, the high incidence of acute and chronic encephalopathy in shunted patients, and the availability of safer alternative treatments have limited the use of surgical portacaval shunts, which are at present rarely performed to control variceal bleeding. Currently, transjugular intrahepatic portosystemic shunt (TIPS) is widely used for the treatment of variceal hemorrhage and is being evaluated in the treatment of refractory ascites (50,65). However, there are no available data as yet on the effect of TIPS on the incidence of ascites and SBP during long-term follow-up.

Bacteria arising from the patient's own intestinal flora, mainly gram-negative bacilli, are the most frequently responsible organisms for SBP (2,3,20). Moreover, bacterial translocation of enteric bacteria from the gut to mesenteric lymph nodes seems to be an important step in the pathogenesis of SBP and other infections in cirrhosis (59,66). Therefore, inhibition or eradication of intestinal gram-negative bacteria should be an effective method for preventing SBP and other infections in these patients. This is the rationale for the use of oral antibiotic agents, mainly nonabsorbable or poorly absorbable antibiotics, that have been widely evaluated to prevent SBP and other bacterial infections, both in experimental models of cirrhosis and in cirrhotic patients. This measure currently constitutes the main prophylactic treatment in cirrhotic patients at high-risk of bacterial infection (Table 13.2).

Selective intestinal decontamination (SID) consists of the inhibition of the gram-negative bacteria of the gut with preservation of the anaerobic organisms. Preservation of anaerobes seems to be extremely important in preventing intestinal colonization, overgrowth, and subsequent translocation of new po-

Table 13.2 Different Options of Antibiotic Prophylaxis of the First Episode of Spontaneous Bacterial Peritonitis in Cirrhotic Patients Reported in the Literature

I.   Short-term prophylaxis
    A. Combinations of oral nonabsorbable antibiotics
    B. Norfloxacin
            Gastrointestinal bleeding: 400 mg/12 h p.o. 7 days
            Ascites and low ascitic fluid protein levels: 400 mg/day p.o. during
               hospitalization
    C. Systemic antibiotics in gastrointestinal bleeding
            Ciprofloxacin 200 mg/12 h + amoxicillin/clavulanic acid 1g/0.2g
               first i.v. then p.o. until 3 days after control of the hemorrhage
            Ofloxacin 400 mg/day first i.v. then p.o. 10 days + amoxicillin/
               clavulanic acid 1 g/0.2 g i.v. before each emergency endoscopy
            Ofloxacin 200 mg/12 h p.o. 7–10 days
            Norfloxacin 400 mg/12 h p.o. 7 days + ceftriaxone 1 g/day i.v. 3
               days
II. Long-term prophylaxis
        Norfloxacin 400 mg/day p.o.
        Ciprofloxacin 750 mg/week p.o.
        Trimethoprim-sulfamethoxazole one double-strength (160 mg) tablet/day
           5 times a week p.o.

tentially pathogenic bacteria (67). Intestinal decontamination with combinations of nonabsorbable oral antibiotic agents has been used in the prevention of bacterial infections in neutropenic patients (68,69), in patients hospitalized in intensive care units (70), and in cirrhotic patients with gastrointestinal hemorrhage (28). However, combinations of oral nonabsorbable antibiotics have several disadvantages, such as the possible overgrowth of potentially pathogenic antibiotic-resistant bacteria, the large number of pills required, the side-effects, and the cost, especially in patients requiring long-term treatment (68,69).

Norfloxacin is an orally administered quinolone that may be an ideal drug for SID because it is incompletely absorbed by the intestine, is active against most aerobic gram-negative bacteria, and has little or no activity against gram-positive and anaerobic organisms (71). These effects have been demonstrated not only in volunteers (72), but also in neutropenic (73,74) and cirrhotic patients (75). In addition, emergence of resistance to norfloxacin appeared to be very low (75). Several studies have demonstrated that oral norfloxacin reduces the incidence of infections caused by gram-negative bacilli in neutropenic patients, without overgrowth of resistant bacteria or significant side effects (73,74).

In an experimental model of cirrhosis in rats, Runyon et al. (76) observed that norfloxacin decreases the incidence of bacterial translocation and peritonitis by gram-negative bacilli. It has also been demonstrated that norfloxacin decreases bacterial translocation in cirrhotic rats submitted to hypovolemic shock (33). In cirrhotic patients, oral norfloxacin suppresses gram-negative bacilli of the fecal flora (77,78), but total bacterial recuperation is observed one week after oral treatment is withdrawn (78). Prophylactic treatment with norfloxacin in cirrhotic patients should therefore be continued as long as the patients are at high risk of bacterial infection (78).

In addition, SID may be useful in the prophylaxis of SBP, not only because it inhibits the aerobic gram-negative intestinal flora, but also because it improves the antimicrobial capacity of the ascitic fluid in cirrhotic patients. It has been shown that the administration of oral nonabsorbable antibiotics or norfloxacin increases complement factors and protein levels in ascitic fluid in cirrhotic patients with low ascitic fluid protein concentration (79,80) and in patients with schistosomal hepatic fibrosis and low protein ascites (81).

Oral antibiotics with differential characteristics (i.e., broader antimicrobial spectra, higher systemic distribution or longer serum half-life), such as ciprofloxacin, ofloxacin, rufloxacin, and trimethoprim-sulfamethoxazole, have also been evaluated as alternatives to norfloxacin in the prevention of bacterial infections in cirrhosis (82–85) (Table 13.2).

As commented above, gastrointestinal bleeding determines an acute very high risk of bacterial infection in cirrhotic patients (28,29,34–36). In this setting, infections occur very early and are frequently due to gram-positive cocci from extraintestinal origin in addition to intestinal gram-negative bacilli, and administration of oral antibiotics may be difficult in some patients with active bleeding (34–36). These patients could, therefore, benefit from more aggressive prophylactic measures such as systemic antibiotics, which have been used in bleeding cirrhotic patients (35,36).

Several randomized clinical trials have evaluated different antibiotics and schedules of prophylactic treatment in different groups of cirrhotic patients at high risk of infection and SBP. We can group these studies into two categories: short-term prophylaxis in high-risk hospitalized patients, and long-term prophylaxis in high-risk outpatients (Table 13.2).

IV. SHORT-TERM PROPHYLAXIS OF BACTERIAL INFECTIONS IN HOSPITALIZED CIRRHOTIC PATIENTS

Several studies have demonstrated that short-term prophylactic antibiotic therapy during hospitalization dramatically reduces the incidence of nosocomial bacterial infections in cirrhotic patients admitted with gastrointestinal bleeding or with ascites with a low ascitic fluid total protein concentration.

A. Cirrhotic Patients with Gastrointestinal Bleeding

In 1985, Rimola et al. (28) published the first study on antibiotic prophylaxis of bacterial infections in cirrhotic patients. This randomized study compared the effects of prophylactic administration of nonabsorbable antibiotic agents (gentamicin, vancomycin, and nystatin or neomycin, colistin, and nystatin) in 68 bleeding cirrhotic patients treated since admission to hospital until 48 h after the hemorrhage had stopped with no prophylactic treatment in 72 control patients. The overall incidence of nosocomial bacterial infections and the incidence of severe infections (SBP or bacteremia) during the first 10 days of hospitalization was significantly lower in prophylactically treated than in nontreated patients (16% vs. 34.7% and 8.8% vs. 20.8%, respectively), but hospital mortality was not significantly different in both groups (26.5% vs. 32%, respectively). Nevertheless, as mentioned above, combinations of oral nonabsorbable antibiotic agents have several disadvantages, such as the overgrowth of potentially pathogenic antibiotic-resistant bacteria, cost, and side effects, especially in those patients requiring long-term treatment (68,69).

The efficacy of SID with norfloxacin in preventing bacterial infections in cirrhotic patients with gastrointestinal hemorrhage was evaluated by Soriano et al. (34). In this study, 109 cirrhotic patients admitted to hospital with gastrointestinal hemorrhage and free of bacterial infection were included and randomized into two groups. Sixty patients received norfloxacin 400 mg b.i.d. orally or through a nasogastric tube during the first seven days of hospitalization beginning immediately after emergency gastroscopy, and 59 patients were control subjects. The incidence of bacterial infections (10% vs. 37.2%), SBP and/or bacteremia (3.3% vs. 16.9%), and urinary infections (0% vs. 18.6%) during the hospitalization period were significantly lower in patients receiving norfloxacin than in the control group, as a consequence of a decrease in the incidence of infections caused by aerobic gram-negative bacilli. The lower hospital mortality rate observed in norfloxacin-treated patients did not reach statistical significance, however (6.6% vs. 11.8%).

Systemic antibiotics have also been used for preventing bacterial infections in cirrhotic patients with gastrointestinal hemorrhage in two different controlled studies. Blaise et al. (35) performed a prospective randomized study that included 91 noninfected cirrhotic patients with gastrointestinal hemorrhage admitted to an intensive care unit. Forty-six patients received ofloxacin 400 mg per day over a period of 10 days, first intravenously then orally, and an intravenous bolus of amoxicillin plus clavulanic acid (1 g/0.2 g) before each endoscopy performed during hemorrhage, and 45 patients received no treatment. The incidence of bacterial infections (20% vs. 66%, respectively) and respiratory infections (4% vs. 40%, respectively) during the stay in the intensive care unit was significantly lower in the treated group than in the control group. The overall incidence of infections (66%), and respiratory infections in particular (40%), in the control group were very high, probably because the study was performed in an intensive care unit; most patients had severe, Child-Pugh class C cirrhosis; more than 30% required tracheal intubation; and more than 35% needed esophageal tamponade to control hemorrhage. Mortality was higher in the control group than in the prophylactically treated group (24% vs. 35%, respectively), but this difference did not reach statistical significance.

In a second study, Pauwels et al. (36) evaluated the efficacy of prophylactic parenteral antibiotic administration in a selected subgroup of cirrhotic patients with gastrointestinal hemorrhage. These authors had previously observed that Child-Pugh class C patients or rebleeding patients constitute a subgroup with a particularly high risk of infection (37). Sixty-four patients with these characteristics were included in this randomized study. Thirty patients received ciprofloxacin (200 mg twice daily) and a combination of amoxicillin plus clavulanic acid (1 g/0.2 g three times daily) first intravenously and then orally for three days after hemorrhage and 34 patients did not receive antibiotic therapy. The incidence of bacterial infections during the first 10 days was significantly lower in treated patients than in controls (13.3% vs. 52.9%, respectively). It is of interest that the incidence of bacterial infections in non-treated patients with low risk of infection (Child-Pugh class A and B non-rebleeding patients) was higher than in patients with high risk of infection submitted to prophylaxis (18.2% vs. 13.3%, respectively). These data suggest that all cirrhotic patients with gastrointestinal hemorrhage might benefit from antibiotic prophylaxis.

Because no study has previously compared the efficacy of systemic antibiotic therapy with SID with oral norfloxacin in the prophylaxis of infections in bleeding cirrhotic patients, Sàbat et al. (86) performed a randomized study comparing oral norfloxacin alone with norfloxacin plus intravenous ceftriaxone in a group of bleeding cirrhotic patients with a high risk of infection despite norfloxacin prophylaxis (i.e., patients with shock, encephalopathy, or ascites on admission) (38). In this study, 22 patients received oral norfloxacin alone 400 mg b.i.d. for 7 days, and 24 patients received norfloxacin for 7 days plus intravenous ceftriaxone 2 g daily during the first three days of admission. The incidence of bacterial infections and the mortality rate during hospitalization were similar in both groups. Ofloxacin shows a higher activity against gram-positive cocci and higher oral absorption and systemic distribution than norfloxacin (87). Therefore, in addition to its effect on intestinal flora, ofloxacin, even when given orally, behaves as a systemic antibiotic. A multicentric randomized study recently compared oral norfloxacin with oral ofloxacin in the prevention of bacterial infections in bleeding cirrhotic patients, and the incidence of bacterial infections was similar in both groups (85).

According to these last two studies, systemic antibiotic treatment does not seem to be superior to oral norfloxacin in the prophylaxis of bacterial infections in bleeding cirrhotic patients. However, further studies are required to determine whether systemic antibiotic therapy might be useful in some subgroups of cirrhotic patients with gastrointestinal hemorrhage and high risk of infection (i.e., patients with shock, balloon tamponade, tracheal intubation, or persistent active bleeding that render the oral or nasogastric tube administration of norfloxacin difficult).

In summary, prophylactic antibiotics, preferentially norfloxacin, should be used to prevent bacterial infections in all noninfected cirrhotic patients admitted to hospital for gastrointestinal hemorrhage.

B. Cirrhotic Patients with Ascites and Low Ascitic Fluid Total Protein Levels

Hospitalized cirrhotic patients with low ascitic fluid protein concentration constitute another group at high risk of nosocomial bacterial infection, mainly SBP, as mentioned previously (25–27). Soriano et al. (88) performed a prospective randomized study to assess the efficacy of prophylactic SID with norfloxacin in 63 hospitalized noninfected patients with cirrhosis and ascitic fluid protein level <1.5 g/dL. Thirty-two patients received oral norfloxacin 400 mg daily throughout hospitalization. The incidence of bacterial infections (3.1% vs. 41.9%), SBP (0% vs. 22.5%), and extraperitoneal infections (3.1% vs. 22.5%, respectively) during hospitalization were all significantly lower in patients receiving prophylactic norfloxacin than in nontreated patients, as a consequence of a much lower incidence of gram-negative infections. The decrease in mortality observed in the group undergoing prophylactic SID did not reach statistical significance (6.2% vs. 16.1%, respectively). This study suggests that prophylactic norfloxacin should be used in hospitalized cirrhotic patients with low ascitic fluid total protein to prevent SBP and extraperitoneal infections.

In a randomized study, Henrion et al. (89) evaluated the efficacy of intestinal decontamination in the prevention of bacterial infection in 94 noninfected patients with cirrhosis admitted to an intensive care unit for various disorders, mainly gastrointestinal hemorrhage, ascites, and encephalopathy. Forty-five patients were treated with oral nonabsorbable antibiotics (neomycin 1 g, colistin 1.500.000 U, and nystatin 1.000.000 U every 6 h) or norfloxacin (400 mg b.i.d.) for at least five days. The incidence of bacteremia was significantly lower in the treated group than in the control group (8.8% vs. 24.5%, respectively), but mortality was similar in both groups. These authors recommend SID for patients with cirrhosis admitted to an intensive care unit, particularly when hepatic function is severely affected.

V. PRIMARY LONG-TERM PROPHYLAXIS OF SPONTANEOUS BACTERIAL PERITONITIS IN CIRRHOTIC OUTPATIENTS

Runyon et al. (76) evaluated long-term primary prophylaxis of SBP with norfloxacin in rats with experimental cirrhosis. Treated rats showed a lower incidence of bacterial translocation and SBP than control rats, suggesting that primary long-term antibiotic prophylaxis could be effective in the prevention of SBP in cirrhotic patients.

Ginés et al. (77) performed the first study on long-term antibiotic prophylaxis in cirrhotic patients. As mentioned elsewhere in this book, these authors demonstrated the efficacy of long-term oral norfloxacin in the prevention of SBP recurrence (i.e., secondary prophylaxis). Since then, several randomized clinical trials have been performed to assess the efficacy of different antibiotics in long-term prophylaxis in several groups of patients at risk of SBP (mainly primary prophylaxis in patients without a previous episode).

Cirrhotic patients without previous SBP and with low ascitic fluid total protein or high serum bilirubin are at increased risk of developing their first SBP episode, not only during hospitalization but also during long-term follow-up (4,5). Sixty percent of these episodes are community-acquired (4). Based on these data, it has been suggested that continuous, long-term antibiotic prophylaxis may be useful in preventing the first episode of SBP in these patients.

Grangé et al. (90) performed a multicentric, double-blind, placebo-controlled trial of primary prophylaxis of SBP in patients with cirrhosis and low ascitic fluid total protein levels (<1.5 g/dL). In this study, 54 patients were treated during six months with oral norfloxacin 400 mg daily and 53 patients received placebo. The incidence of the first episode of SBP during follow-up was significantly lower in the treated patients than in the placebo group (0% vs. 7.5%, respectively), but the incidence of other infections and mortality was similar in both groups. Only two patients exhibited nausea and hypersomnia, which are considered side effects attributable to norfloxacin.

Recently, Novella et al. (91) carried out a randomized study to evaluate long-term primary prophylaxis of SBP with norfloxacin in cirrhotic patients without previous SBP and with low ascitic fluid protein concentration and/or high serum bilirubin. In this study, 63 patients were treated continuously for a mean of 47 weeks with oral norfloxacin 400 mg daily and 59 patients were treated with norfloxacin only during periods of hospitalization. This schedule was chosen with hope of showing such patients may benefit from short-term, inpatient antibiotic prophylaxis (88), avoiding possible undesirable consequences of long-term prophylaxis, i.e., side effects, economic cost, and the development of bacterial resistance. In this study, the incidence of the first SBP episode was significantly higher in patients treated only during hospitalizations than in patients continuously treated (15.2% vs. 1.6%, respectively), due to a lower incidence of community-acquired episodes in these patients. However, no statistically significant differences were observed in the incidence of extraperitoneal infections (25.4% vs. 30.1%, respectively), other complications of cirrhosis and survival (67.8% vs. 69.8%, respectively) during follow-up. The duration of hospitalization during follow-up was longer in patients on prophylaxis only during hospitalizations than in the continuously treated group, although this did not reach statistical significance (p = 0.055). It is of interest in this study that only two episodes of nosocomial SBP were observed in more than 200 hospitalizations from high-risk patients, confirming that short-term prophylaxis is extremely effective in preventing nosocomial SBP (34,88), despite the development of bacterial resistance to norfloxacin in patients on prophylaxis (91–93).

Alternative antibiotics to norfloxacin have been evaluated for long-term prophylaxis of SBP (82–84). Rolachon et al. (82) performed a double-blind, placebo-controlled trial that demonstrated the efficacy of long-term prophylaxis with a weekly, single oral dose of 750 mg ciprofloxacin in the prevention of SBP in 60 cirrhotic patients with low ascitic fluid total protein, most of them without previous SBP (seven patients had had a previous episode). During a six-month follow-up, the incidence of SBP was significantly lower in the ciprofloxacin-treated patients than in the placebo group (3.6% vs. 22%, respectively). The duration of hospitalization during follow-up was significantly lower in the prophylactically treated group than in the placebo group. The incidence of extraperitoneal infections (11% vs. 12.5%, respectively) and mortality (14.3% vs. 18.7%, respectively) were similar in both groups. Surprisingly, in this study no acquired bacterial resistance to ciprofloxacin was observed in the bacteriological study of stools performed in 10 patients after six months of ciprofloxacin administration. In two recent studies (94,95), resistance to norfloxacin or ciprofloxacin has been observed in 40% of stool cultures of cirrhotic patients prophylactically treated with one or the other of these antibiotics. The efficacy of long-term prophylaxis of SBP with trimethoprim-sulfametoxazole has been evaluated both in experimental cirrhosis in rats and in patients with cirrhosis. Guarner et al. (96) recently observed that long-term prophylactic administration of trimethoprim-sulphamethoxazole to rats with carbon tetrachloride-induced cirrhosis delayed the development of ascites, decreased gram-negative bacterial translocation and prolonged survival. Long-term prophylactic treatment with trimethoprim-sulphamethoxazole for the prevention of SBP has been evaluated in a randomized study that included 60 patients with cirrhosis and ascites (83). Only 13 of these patients had experienced a previous SBP episode. In this study, Singh et al. (83) treated 30 patients with one double-strength tablet of trimethoprim-sulphamethoxazole (160–800 mg) orally five times a week. The incidence of SBP or spontaneous bacteremia was significantly lower in the treated group than in nontreated patients (3% vs. 27%, respectively). The incidence of other infections was similar in both groups. Mortality was lower in the treated patients than in the control group (7% vs. 20%, respectively), but the difference was not statistically significant. During a median duration of follow-up of 90 days (range 7–682 days), side effects attributed to trimethoprim-sulphamethoxazole administration, including hematological abnormalities, were not detected in any patient, demonstrating the safety of this drug for prophylaxis in cirrhotic patients.

VI. PROS AND CONS OF ANTIBIOTIC PROPHYLAXIS OF SPONTANEOUS BACTERIAL PERITONITIS

Both short-term and long-term antibiotic prophylaxis are effective in preventing in cirrhotic patients at high risk of infection. However, it is important to assess the positive and negative aspects of antibiotic prophylaxis in each clinical situation of high risk of infection before recommending the systematic use of this therapy. Therefore, the influence of antibiotic prophylaxis not only on the incidence of SBP, but also on other important parameters (Table 13.3),

Table 13.3 Pros and Cons of Primary Prophylaxis of Spontaneous Bacterial Peritonitis

I. Pros
  Efficacy in the prevention of spontaneous bacterial peritonitis
  Efficacy of short-term prophylaxis in the prevention of other infections
  Low incidence of side effects
  Improvement in survival
  Rare appearance of opportunistic infections
  Economic cost of prophylaxis is lower than treatment of SBP episodes
  Severity of SBP and other infections is similar in patients on prophylaxis than in patients without prophylaxis.
  Antibiotic sensitivity of bacteria to antibiotics more frequently used to treat SBP and other infections is similar in patients infected while on prophylaxis and in patients infected without prophylaxis
  Long-term prophylaxis reduces the length of hospitalization
II. Cons
  Long-term prophylaxis does not decrease the incidence of infections other than SBP
  Short-term prophylaxis does not reduce the length of hospitalization
  Norfloxacin prophylaxis increases intestinal bacterial overgrowth and bacterial translocation of gram-positive cocci and SBP caused by these bacteria in experimental cirrhosis
  Emergence of norfloxacin-resistant bacteria in stools and infections caused by these bacteria in patients on prophylaxis

such as the incidence of other bacterial infections, the side effects of antibiotic therapy, survival, quality of life, cost, and the development of bacterial resistance, should be taken into account in order to clarify the indications of antibiotic prophylaxis. Whereas short-term prophylaxis seems to decrease the incidence of bacterial infections other than SBP (28,34–36,88), long-term prophylaxis apparently does not prevent extraperitoneal infections (77,82, 83,90,91).

When analyzing the side effects reported in prophylactically treated patients in the randomized clinical trials, the incidence of side effects caused by antibiotic agents was very low and side effects were mild (28,34–36,77,82,83,88,90,91) (Table 13.4). Only one skin rash and one fever of unknown origin were reported among nearly 100 patients on prophylactic norfloxacin during hospitalization (34,88). Short-term prophylaxis with parenteral

Table 13.4 Side Effects of Antibiotics Used in Prophylaxis of Spontaneous Bacterial Peritonitis

I. Short-term prophylaxis

Reference	No. of patients	Side effects
Soriano et al. (88)	32	1 skin rash 1 fever of unknown origin
Soriano et al. (34)	60	No side effects
Blaise et al. (35)	46	No side effects
Pauwels et al. (36)	30	3 diarrhea

II. Long-term prophylaxis

Reference	No. of patients	Mean follow-up	Side effects
Ginés et al. (77)	40	7.6 months (1–19)	1 oral and esophageal candidiasis
Grangé et al. (90)	53	6 months	1 nausea 1 hypersomnia
Singh et al. (83)	30	90 days (7–682)	1 diarrhea
Rolachon et al. (82)	28	6 months	No side effects
Novella et al. (91)	56	47 weeks (1–139)	1 oral candidiasis

antibiotics has also been associated with infrequent mild side effects (35,36). Long-term antibiotic prophylaxis could theoretically result in a higher incidence of side effects. However, only one case each of oral and esophageal candidiasis, oral candidiasis, nausea, and hypersomnia have been reported among 149 patients on long-term prophylaxis with norfloxacin during mean periods of six, seven, and 10 months (77,90,91). Similarly, the incidence of side effects in patients who received long-term prophylaxis with ciprofloxacin or trimethoprim-sulphamethoxazole also seems to be very low as no side effects have yet been reported (82,83). However, it should be noted that the experience with these two drugs for long-term prophylaxis in cirrhotic patients is limited.

Some authors (97,98) argue against antibiotic prophylaxis because a statistically significant improvement in survival of patients on prophylaxis has not been demonstrated in any study. The previously mentioned studies that evaluate different antibiotic agents for short-term or long-term prophylaxis have consistently demonstrated a trend toward a lower mortality in patients on prophylaxis than in control patients (28,34–36,77,82,83,88,90,91), but this difference did not reach statistical significance in any study. However, Bernard et al. (99,100) recently performed two meta-analyses to assess the effect of antibiotic prophylaxis on survival in patients with high risk of infection. The first meta-analysis (99) evaluated four published trials that included 414 cirrhotic patients admitted to hospital because of gastrointestinal bleeding and treated prophylactically with oral or parenteral antibiotics. This study showed that short-term prophylaxis produces a statistically significant increase in the survival rate of patients on prophylaxis compared to control patients (87% vs. 77%, respectively). The second meta-analysis (100) assessed the effect on survival of long-term prophylactic treatment with oral antibiotic agents, including norfloxacin, ciprofloxacin, and trimethoprim-sulphamethoxazole, in cirrhotic patients with ascites with or without previous SBP. This study included 307 patients from four trials and the mean survival rate was 85% in patients prophylactically treated with antibiotics versus 76% in nontreated patients. This difference was statistically significant. According to these two meta-analysis, both short and long-term antibiotic prophylaxis seems to improve survival in cirrhotic patients with high risk of bacterial infection. Nevertheless, it should be noted that the characteristics of patients as well as the prophylactic methods used differed between the studies included in each meta-analysis, which could affect the validity of their conclusions.

It is interesting to assess the influence of antibiotic prophylaxis on the quality of life of the patients. The duration of hospitalization can be considered to be an indirect measure of the quality of life of cirrhotic patients. Although the duration of hospitalization was similar in patients receiving prophylaxis and in control patients in all the studies of short-term prophylaxis (28,34–36,88), Rolachon et al. (82) observed a statistically significant greater reduction in the duration of hospitalization during follow-up in patients on long-term prophylaxis with ciprofloxacin compared to the placebo group. Similar results were observed by Novella et al. (91) in cirrhotic patients submitted to long-term primary prophylaxis of SBP with norfloxacin, although in this study they approached but did not achieve standard levels of statistical significance (p = 0.055). Because antibiotic prophylaxis may increase the economic cost, several studies have analyzed this issue. Soriano et al. (34) observed a 62% reduction in the cost of antibiotic therapy (including prophylactic treatment) in cirrhotic patients with gastrointestinal hemorrhage on prophylaxis with norfloxacin compared to the nontreated group. Similarly, Pauwels et al. (36) observed a statistically significant decrease in the cost of antibiotic therapy in cirrhotic patients with gastrointestinal bleeding who received prophylactic systemic antibiotics. Recently, Inadomi and Sonnenberg (101) estimated the cost of long-term antibiotic prophylaxis of SBP against the cost of expected episodes over a one-year period in cirrhotic patients with ascites, based on the data reported in the literature. According to this study, prophylactic treatment with norfloxacin or trimethoprim-sulfamethoxazole significantly reduces the cost in these patients, with the patients with a higher risk of SBP (patients with low ascitic fluid total protein and especially patients with previous SBP) constituting the groups that would benefit most from prophylaxis. Younossi et al. (102) have also confirmed that prophylaxis of recurrent SBP with norfloxacin is economically cost-effective. These authors calculated that the cost of treatment of an episode of SBP exceeds the costs of prophylactic norfloxacin by $4632 per patient per year. All these data suggest that prophylaxis of SBP reduces the overall cost in cirrhotic patients, mainly in those at high risk to develop this complication.

The development of bacterial resistance is perhaps the most outstanding concern about antibiotic prophylaxis. The effectiveness of antibiotic prophylaxis might decrease with time because of the development of resistant bacterial strains that colonize the gut and might then cause SBP and other infections (93). In addition, there is the possibility that the bacteria resistant to prophylactic antibiotics could cause more severe infections in patients on prophylaxis than the infections developed by patients not on prophylaxis. Runyon et al. (76) observed bacterial overgrowth of gram-positive bacteria in gut flora and a higher incidence of gram-positive bacterial translocation and episodes of gram-positive SBP in long-term norfloxacin-treated cirrhotic rats than in untreated cirrhotic rats, suggesting that prophylaxis with norfloxacin could favor the development of SBP caused by gram-positive cocci. In cirrhotic patients, Dupeyron et al. (92) observed the emergence of bacteria resistant to quinolones in the fecal flora in more than 50% of cirrhotic patients after a mean duration of prophylaxis with norfloxacin of only 25 days. However, it has recently been suggested that the frequent development of resistant gram-negative bacteria in the fecal flora in patients on prophylaxis with quinolones is rarely associated with development of infections by these bacteria (84,94,95).

In the randomized clinical trials discussed earlier, most infections diagnosed in patients on prophylaxis were caused by gram-positive cocci, mainly streptococci (28,34–36,77,82,83,88,90,91,103), due to the antimicrobial spectrum of the antibiotic agents used, mainly norfloxacin, which is more active against gram-negative bacilli than against gram-positive cocci (71). Gram-negative bacilli were rarely isolated in these patients due to the absence of development of resistance to quinolones by these bacteria. However, recent studies have reported an increasing incidence in the resistance of gram-negative bacilli to quinolones in the general population (104), as well as in neutropenic (105) and cirrhotic patients who receive prophylaxis with quinolones (91,93,106). This is thought to be attributable to the current widespread use of quinolones in these different populations (91). Novella et al. (91) have observed that 50% of bacteria isolated in the infections diagnosed in cirrhotic patients on long-term prophylaxis with norfloxacin were gram-negative bacilli, mainly *Escherichia coli* that were resistant to norfloxacin. Also in this study, enterococci were isolated in more than 25% of the infections in these patients. It should be noted, however, that most of these infections were mild urinary infections.

Ortiz et al. (93) have observed an association between prophylaxis with norfloxacin, mainly long-term prophylaxis, and the development of infections caused by *Escherichia coli* resistant to quinolones in cirrhotic patients. In this study, most of the infections caused by *Escherichia coli* resistant to norfloxacin were urinary infections (15/19) and only two were SBP. It is of interest that the incidence of severe infections and complications, length of hospitalization, and mortality were similar in the infections caused by *Escherichia coli* resistant to norfloxacin in patients on prophylaxis and in those caused by *Escherichia coli* sensitive to norfloxacin in patients not on prophylaxis. Moreover, none of the *Escherichia coli* resistant to norfloxacin were also resistant to the antibiotics more commonly used in the empirical treatment of bacterial infections in cirrhotic patients, such as cefotaxime or amoxicillin-clavulanic acid.

Llovet et al. (107) analyzed 229 episodes of SBP and compared the clinical courses and the microbiology of SBP in cirrhotic patients with and without previous prophylactic treatment with norfloxacin. No differences were observed between the two groups in clinical features, response to treatment (cefotaxime in most cases), or short-term prognosis, suggesting that SBP episodes are not more severe in prophylactically treated patients and that cefotaxime is also effective in treating SBP in patients on prophylaxis with norfloxacin. Among the 36 episodes of ascitic fluid infection in patients on prophylaxis, there were 14 episodes in which bacteria could be identified in ascitic fluid culture. Most of these were gram-positive cocci (78.6%), mainly streptococci, although three gram-negative bacilli were also isolated. According to these data, SBP that develops in patients on prophylaxis is not more severe than that seen in patients not treated porphylactically. Moreover, in spite of the emergence of resistant bacteria in the fecal flora and the development of urinary infections by these bacteria, SBP caused by gram-negative bacilli resistant to quinolones is still rare in cirrhotic patients on prophylactic norfloxacin.

Finally, the recent studies of Das have shown that long-term prophylactic antibiotic therapy actually reduces the costs of therapy especially when the prophylaxis is limited to patients who are at high risk of developing SBP (107a).

In conclusion, after carefully considering the pros and cons of primary antibiotic prophylaxis of SBP, we recommend that antibiotic agents can be used safely and effectively in preventing SBP in cirrhotic patients at high risk of developing this complication. However, whenever antibiotic prophylaxis is performed, strict monitoring of the emergence of infections caused by resistant bacteria must be performed. Finally, nonantibiotic alternatives for preventing SBP should be investigated. Pardo et al. (108) have recently observed that cisapride, a drug that increases oral–cecal intestinal transit time, decreases intestinal gram-negative bacterial overgrowth in cirrhotic patients. Because intestinal bacterial overgrowth has been related to the pathogenesis of SBP (109), these authors have suggested that therapy with prokinetic drugs may be a useful alternative to antibiotic therapy in the prophylaxis of bacterial infections in cirrhotic patients.

REFERENCES

1. Caly WR, Strauss E. A prospective study of bacterial infections in patients with cirrhosis. J Hepatol 1993; 18:271–272.
2. Almdal TP, Skinhoj P. Spontaneous bacterial peritonitis in cirrhosis. Incidence, diagnosis and prognosis. Scand J Gastroenterol 1987; 22:295–300.
3. Carey WD, Boayke A, Leatherman J. Spontaneous bacterial peritonitis: clinical and laboratory features with reference to hospital acquired-cases. Am J Gastroenterol 1986; 81:1156–1161.

4. Andreu M, Sola R, Sitges Serra A, Alia C, Gallen M, Vila MC, Coll S, Oliver MI. Risk factors for spontaneous bacterial peritonitis in cirrhotic patients with ascites. Gastroenterology 1993; 104:1133–1138.

5. Llach J, Rimola A, Navasa M, Gines P, Salmeron JM, Gines A, Arroyo V, Rodes J. Incidence and predictive factors of first episode of spontaneous bacterial peritonitis in cirrhosis with ascites: relevance of ascitic fluid protein concentration. Hepatology 1992; 16:724–727.

6. Rimola A. Infecciones bacterianas en la cirrosis hepatica. MTA-Medicina Interna 1987; 5:161–224.

7. Wyke RJ. Problems of bacterial infection in patients with liver disease. Gut 1987; 28:623–641.

8. Runyon BA. Spontaneous bacterial peritonitis: an explosion of information. Hepatology 1988; 8:171–175.

9. Llovet JM, Planas R, Morillas R, Quer JC, Cabre E, Boix J, Humbert P, Guilera M, Domenech E, Bertran X, Gassull MA. Short-term prognosis of cirrhotic patients with spontaneous bacterial peritonitis: multivariate study. Am J Gastroenterol 1993; 88:388–392.

10. Toledo C, Salmeron JM, Rimola A, Novice M, Arroyo V, Llach J, Gines A, Gines P, Rodes J. Spontaneous bacterial peritonitis in cirrhosis: predictive factors of infection resolution and survival in patients treated with cefotaxime. Hepatology 1993; 17:251–257.

11. Rimola A, Navasa M, Arroyo V. Experience with cefotaxime in the treatment of spontaneous bacterial peritonitis in cirrhosis. Diagn Microbiol Infect Dis 1995; 22:141–145.

12. Rimola A, Salmerón JM, Clemente G, Rodrigo L, Obrador A, Miranda ML, Guarner C, Planas R, Solà R, Vargas V, Casafont F, Marco M, Navasa M, Bañares R, Arroyo V, Rodés J. Two different dosages of cefotaxime in the treatment of spontaneous bacterial peritonitis in cirrhosis. Results of a prospective, randomized, multicenter study. Hepatology 1995; 21:674–679.

13. Bernard B, Cadranel JF, Valla D, Escolano S, Jarlier V, Opolon P. Prognostic significance of bacterial infection in bleeding cirrhotic patients: a prospective study. Gastroenterology 1995; 108:1828–1834.

14. Goulis J, Armonis A, Patch D, Sabin C, Greenslade L, Burroughs AK. Infection is independently associated with failure to control hemorrhage and early rebleeding in cirrhosis (abstr). Hepatology 1997; 26:288.

15. Follo A, Llovet JM, Navasa M, Planas R, Forns X, Francitorra A, Rimola A, Gassull MA, Arroyo V and Rodes J. Renal impairment after spontaneous bacterial peritonitis in cirrhosis: incidence, clinical course, predictive factors and prognosis. Hepatology 1994; 20:1495–1501.

16. Tito L, Rimola A, Ginés P, Llach J, Arroyo V, Rodes J. Recurrence of spontaneous bacterial peritonitis in cirrhosis: frequency and predictive factors. Hepatology 1988; 8:27–31.

17. Silvain C, Besson I, Ingrand P, Mannant PR, Fort E, Beauchant M. Prognosis and long-term recurrence of spontaneous bacterial peritonitis in cirrhosis. J Hepatol 1993; 19:188–189.

18. Altman C, Grange J-D, Amiot X, Pelletier G, Lacaine F, Bodin F, Etienne JP. Survival after a first episode of spontaneous bacterial peritonitis. Prognosis of potential candidates for orthotopic liver transplantation. J Gastro Hepatol 1995; 10:47–50.

19. Hoefs JC, Canawatti HN, Sapico FL, Hopkins R, Weiner J, Montgomerie JZ. Spontaneous bacterial peritonitis. Hepatology 1982; 2:399–407.

20. Guarner C, Soriano G. Spontaneous bacterial peritonitis. Semin Liver Dis 1997; 17:203–217.

21. Rimola A, Soto R, Bory F, Arroyo V, Piera C, Rodés J. Reticuloendothelial system phagocytic activity in cirrhosis and its relation to bacterial infections and prognosis. Hepatology 1984; 4:53–58.

22. Bolognesi M, Merkel C, Bianco S, Angeli P, Sacerdoti D, Amodio P, Gatta A. Clinical significance of the evaluation of hepatic reticuloendothelial removal capacity in patients with cirrhosis. Hepatology 1994; 19:628–634.

23. Runyon BA. Patients with deficient ascitic fluid opsonic activity are predisposed to spontaneous bacterial peritonitis. Hepatology 1988; 8:632–635.

24. Runyon BA, Morrissey RL, Hoefs JC, Wyle FA. Opsonic activity of human ascitic fluid: a potentially important mechanism against spontaneous bacterial peritonitis. Hepatology 1985; 5:634–637.

25. Runyon BA. Low-protein-concentration ascitic fluid is predisposed to spontaneous bacterial peritonitis. Gastroenterology 1986; 91:1343–1346.

26. Such J, Guarner C, Enriquez J, Rodriguez JL, Seres I, Vilardell F. Low C3 in ascitic fluid predisposes to spontaneous bacterial peritonitis. J Hepatol 1988; 6:80–84.

27. Rabinovitz M, Gavaler JS, Kumar S, Kajani M, Van Thiel DH. Role of serum complement, immunoglobulins, and cell-mediated immune system in the pathogenesis of spontaneous bacterial peritonitis (SBP). Dig Dis Sci 1989; 34:1547–1552.

28. Rimola A, Bory F, Teres J, Perez-Ayuso RM, Arroyo V, Rodes J. Oral, nonabsorbable antibiotics prevent infection in cirrhotics with gastrointestinal hemorrhage. Hepatology 1985; 5:463–467.

29. Bleichner G, Boulanger R, Squara P, Sollet JP, Parent A. Frequency of infections in cirrhotic patients presenting with acute gastrointestinal haemorrhage. Br J Surg 1986; 73:724–726.

30. Deitch EA, Morrison J, Berg R, Specian RD. Effect of hemorrhagic shock on bacterial translocation, intestinal morphology, and intestinal permeability in conventional and antibiotic-decontaminated rats. Crit Care Med 1990; 18:529–536.

31. Carr F, Loegering D. Reticuloendothelial system function and humoral deficiency following acute haemorrhage. Can J Physiol 1978; 56:299–303.

32. Hamdani R, Young S, Runyon BA. Increased bacterial translocation in cirrhotic rats undergoing hemorrhagic shock (abstr). Gastroenterology 1994; 106:904.

33. Llovet JM, Bartoli R, Planas R, Viuado B, Perez J, Cabre E, Arnau J, Ojanguren I, Ausina V, Gassull MA. Selective intestinal decontamination with norfloxacin

reduces bacterial translocation in ascitic cirrhotic rats exposed to hemorrhagic shock. Hepatology 1996;23:781–787.

34. Soriano G, Guarner C, Tomas A, Villanueva C, Torras X, Gonzalez D, Sainz S, Anguera A, Cusso X, Balanzo J, Vilardell F. Norfloxacin prevents bacterial infection in cirrhotics with gastrointestinal hemorrhage. Gastroenterology 1992; 103:1267–1272.

35. Blaise M, Pateron D, Trinchet JC, Levacher S, Beaugrand M, Pourriat JL. Systemic antibiotic therapy prevents bacterial infection in cirrhotic patients with gastrointestinal hemorrhage. Hepatology 1994; 20:34–38.

36. Pauwels A, Mostefa-Kara N, Debenes B, Degoutte E, Lévy VG. Systemic antibiotic prophylaxis after gastrointestinal hemorrhage in cirrhotic patients with a high risk of infection. Hepatology 1996; 24:802–806.

37. Pauwels A, Chami N, Guivarch P, Debenes B, Florent Ch, Levy VG. Facteurs predictifs des infections survenant au decours des hemorragies digestives autes du cirrhotique (abstr). Gastroenterol Clin Biol 1990; 14:219.

38. Soriano G, Guarner C, Tomás A, et al. Predictive factors of bacterial infections in cirrhotic patients submitted to prophylactic selective intestinal decontamination (abstr). Gastroenterology 1993; 104:998.

39. Ho H, Zuckerman MJ, Wassem C. A prospective controlled study of the risk of bacteremia in emergency sclerotherapy of esophageal varices. Gastroenterology 1991; 101:1642–1648.

40. Bac DJ, de Marie S, Siersema PD, Snobl J, van Buuren HR. Post-sclerotherapy bacterial peritonitis: a complication of sclerotherapy or of variceal bleeding? Am J Gastroenterol 1994; 89:859–862.

41. Rolando N, Gimson A, Philpott-Howard J, Sahathevan M, Casewell M, Fagan E, Westaby D, Williams R. Infectious sequelae after endoscopic sclerotherapy of oesophageal varices: role of antibiotic prophylaxis. J Hepatol 1993; 18:290–294.

42. Selby WS, Norton ID, Pokorny ChS, Bernn RAV. Bacteremia and bacterascites after endoscopic sclerotherapy for bleeding esophageal varices and prevention by intravenous cefotaxime: a randomized trial. Gastrointest Endosc 1994; 40: 680–684.

43. Goff JS, Reveille RM, Stiegmann GV. Endoscopic sclerotherapy versus endoscopic variceal ligation: esophageal symptoms, complications, and motility. Am J Gastroenterol 1988; 83:1240–1244.

44. Laine L, El-Newihi HM, Migicovsky, Sloane R, Garcia F. Endoscopic ligation compared with sclerotherapy for the treatment of bleeding esophageal varices. Ann Intern Med 1993; 119:1–7.

45. Lo G-H, Lai K-H, Shen M-T, Chang Ch-F. A comparison of the incidence of transient bacteremia and infectious sequelae after sclerotherapy and rubber band ligation of bleeding esophageal varices. Gastrointest Endosc 1994; 40: 675–679.

46. Conn HO. Bacterial peritonitis: spontaneous or paracentetic? Gastroenterology 1979; 77:1145–1146.

47. Runyon BA. Paracentesis of ascitic fluid: a safe procedure. Arch Intern Med 1986; 146:2259–2261.

48. Runyon BA, Canawatti HN, Hoefs JC. Polymicrobial bacterascites: a unique entity in the spectrum of infected ascitic fluid. Arch Intern Med 1986; 146: 2173–2175.

49. Runyon BA. Care of patients with ascites. N Engl J Med 1994; 330:337–342.

50. Garcia-Tsao G. Cirrhotic ascites: pathogenesis and management. The Gastroenterologist 1995; 3:41–54.

51. Runyon BA, Antillon MR, Montano AA. Effect of diuresis versus therapeutic paracentesis on ascitic fluid opsonic activity and serum complement. Gastroenterology 1989; 97:158–162.

52. Runyon BA, Antillon MR, McHutchison JG. Diuresis increases ascitic fluid opsonic activity in patients who survive spontaneous bacterial peritonitis. J Hepatol 1992; 14:249–252.

53. Ljubicic N, Bilic A, Kopjar B. Diuretics vs. paracentesis followed by diuretics in cirrhosis: effect on ascites opsonic activity and immunoglobulin and complement concentrations. Hepatology 1994; 19:346–353.

54. Solà R, Andreu M, Coll S, Vila MC, Oliver MI, Arroyo V. Spontaneous bacterial peritonitis in cirrhotic patients treated using paracentesis or diuretics: results of a randomized study. Hepatology 1995; 21:340–344.

55. Yoshida H, Hamada T, Inuzaka S, Ueno T, Sata M, Tanikawa K. Bacterial infection in cirrhosis, with and without hepatocellular carcinoma. Am J Gastroenterol 1993; 88:2067–2071.

56. Wang SS, Tsai YT, Lee SD, Chen HT, Lu CW, Lee FY, Jeng JS, Liu YC, Lo KJ. Spontaneous bacterial peritonitis in patients with hepatitis B-related cirrhosis and hepatocellular carcinoma. Gastroenterology 1991; 101:1656–1662.

57. Romero A, Pérez-Arellano JL, González-Villarón L, Brock JH, Muñoz Bellido JL, De Castro S. Effect of transferrin concentration on bacterial growth in human ascitic fluid from cirrhotic and neoplastic patients. Eur J Clin Invest 1993; 23:699–705.

58. Kolle L, Ubeda J, Gómez C, Royo M, Sola-Vera J, Miñana J, Ricart E, Soriano G, Gimferrer E, Guarner C. Do ascitic fluid iron or iron binding proteins predispose to spontaneous bacterial peritonitis in cirrhosis? (abstr) Hepatology 1997; 26:289.

59. Guarner C, Runyon BA. Spontaneous bacterial peritonitis: pathogenesis, diagnosis and management. The Gastroenterologist 1995; 3:311–328.

60. Adams HG, Jordan C. Infections in the alcoholic. Med Clin North Am 1984; 68:179–200.

61. Cabre E, Gonzalez-Huix F, Abad-LaCruz A, Esteve M, Acero D, Fernandez Bañares F, Xiol X, Gassull MA. Effect of total enteral nutrition on the short-term outcome of severely malnourished cirrhotics. A randomised controlled trial. Gastroenterology 1990; 98:715–720.

62. Ho H, Zuckerman MJ, Ho TK, Guerra LG, Verghesse A, Casner PR. Prevalence

of associated infections in community-acquired spontaneous bacterial peritonitis. Am J Gastroenterol 1996; 91:735–742.

63. Runyon BA, Van Epps DE. Diuresis of ascites increases its opsonic activity and may prevent spontaneous bacterial peritonitis. Hepatology 1986; 6:369–399.

64. Castells A, Salo J, Planas R, Quer JC, Gines A, Boix J, Gines P, Gasull J, Teres J, Arroyo V, Rodes J. Impact of shunt surgery for variceal bleeding in the natural history of ascites in cirrhosis: a retrospective study. Hepatology 1994; 20:584–591.

65. Arroyo V, Ginès P. TIPS and refractory ascites. Lessons from the recent history of ascites therapy. J Hepatol 1996; 25:221–223.

66. Runyon BA, Squier S, Borzio M. Translocation of gut bacteria in rats with cirrhosis to mesenteric lymph nodes partially explains the pathogenesis of spontaneous bacterial peritonitis. J Hepatology 1994; 21:792–796.

67. van der Waaij D, Manson WL, Arends JP, de Vries Hospers HG. Clinical use of selective decontamination: the concept. Intensive Care Med 1990; 16(suppl. 3):S212–216.

68. Storring RA, McElwain TJ, Jameson B, Wiltshaw E, Spiers ASD, Gaya H. Oral non-absorbed antibiotics prevent infection in acute non lymphoblastic leukaemia. Lancet 1977; ii:837–840.

69. Hahn DM, Schimpff SC, Fortner CL, Smyth AC, Young VM, Wiernik PH. Infection in acute leukemia patients receiving oral nonabsorbable antibiotics. Antimicrob Agents Chemother 1978; 13:958–964.

70. Van Saene HKF, Stoutenbeek CP, Hart CA. Selective decontamination of the digestive tract in intensive care patients: a critical evaluation of the clinical, bacteriological and epidemiological benefits. J Hosp Infect 1991; 18:261–277.

71. Lee C, Ronald AR. Norfloxacin: its potential in clinical practice. Am J Med 1987; 82(suppl. 6B):27–34.

72. Nord CE. Effect of new quinolones on the human gastrointestinal microflora. Rev Infect Dis 1988; 10(suppl. 1):S193–196.

73. Karp JE, Wiliam GM, Hendricksen C, Laughon B, Redden Z, Bamberger BJ, Bartlett JG, Saral R, Burke PJ. Oral norfloxacin for prevention of Gram-negative bacterial infections in patients with acute leukemia and granulocytopenia. Ann Intern Med 1987; 106:1–7.

74. Winston DJ, Karp J, Talbot G, Levitt L, Corrado M, Ho WG, Champlin RE, Bartlett J, Finley RS, Joshi JH, Deresinski S. Norfloxacin for prevention of bacterial infections in granulocytopenic patients. Am J Med 1987; 82(suppl. 6B):40–46.

75. Ginés P, Rimola A, Marco F, Almela A, Marqués JM, Salmerón JM, Ginés A, Llach J, Jimenez de Anta MT, Arroyo V, Rodes J. Efecto de la administracion de norfloxacino sobre la flora fecal en pacientes cirroticos. Gastroenterol Hepatol 1990; 13:325–328.

76. Runyon BA, Borzio M, Young S, Squier SU, Guarner C and Runyon M. Effect of selective bowel decontamination with norfloxacin on spontaneous bacterial

peritonitis, translocation, and survival in an animal model of cirrhosis. Hepatology 1995; 21:1719–1724.

77. Ginés P, Rimola A, Planas R, Vargas V, Marco F, Almela M, Forna M, Miranda ML, Llach J, Salmeron JM, Rodes J. Norfloxacin prevents spontaneous bacterial peritonitis recurrence in cirrhosis: results of a double-blind, placebo-controlled trial. Hepatology 1990; 12:716–724.

78. Soriano G, Guarner C, Tomas A, Anguera A, Mirelis B, Fernandez C, Herrero M, Alonso C, Vilardell F. Duración del efecto de la norfloxacina sobre la fecal flora en pacientes cirróticos. Rev Esp Enferm Dig 1992; 81:322–326.

79. Soriano G, Teixido M, Guarner C, Such J, Espinos JC, Sainz S, Enriquez J, Rodriguez JL, Vilardell F. Variación del C3 en líquido ascítico de pacientes cirróticos sometidos a esterilización intestinal o a descontaminación intestinal selectiva. Ref Esp Enf Ap Digest 1989; 75:123–126.

80. Such J, Guarner C, Soriano G, Teixido M, Barrios J, Tena F, Mendez C, Enriquez J, Rodriguez JL, Vilardell F. Selective intestinal decontamination increases serum and ascitic fluid C3 levels in cirrhosis. Hepatology 1990; 12: 1175–1178.

81. el Aggan HA, el Aggan HA, Abou Seif Helmy M, Guirguis TG. Selective intestinal decontamination in patients with schistosomal hepatic fibrosis and low-protein ascites. J Egypt Soc Parasitol 1993; 23:649–657.

82. Rolachon A, Cordier L, Bacq Y, Nousbaum JB, Franza A, Paris JC, Fratte S, Bohn B, Kitmacher P, Stahl JP, Zarski JP. Ciprofloxacin and long-term prevention of spontaneous bacterial peritonitis: results of a prospective controlled trial. Hepatology 1995; 22:1171–1174.

83. Singh N, Gayowski T, Yu VL, Wagener MM. Trimethoprim-sulfamethoxazole for the prevention of spontaneous bacterial peritonitis in cirrhosis: a randomized trial. Ann Intern Med 1995; 122:595–598.

84. Navasa M y grupo colaborativo para el estudio de las infecciones en la cirrosis hepática. Norfloxacina vs. rufloxacina en la prevención de la recidiva de la peritonitis bacteriana espontánea (abstr). Gastroenterol Hepatol 1997; 20(suppl. 1):47.

85. Grupo colaborativo para el estudio de las infecciones en la cirrosis hepática. Quinolonas en la profilaxis de las infecciones bacterianas en la hemorragia digestiva de los pacientes con cirrosis hepática (abstr). Gastroenterol Hepatol 1998; 21:34.

86. Sàbat M, Kolle L, Ortiz J, Pamplona J, Novella MT, Villanueva C, Sainz S, Torras J, Soriano G, Guarner C, Balanzó J. Parenteral antibiotic prophylaxis in cirrhotic patients with gastrointestinal bleeding (abstr). Hepatology 1996; 24:448.

87. Hooper DC. Quinolones. In: Mandell GL, Bennett JE, Dolin R, eds. *Principles and Practice of Infectious Diseases*. New York: Churchill Livingstone, 1995, 364–376.

88. Soriano G, Guarner C, Teixido M, Such J, Barrios J, Enriquez J, Vilardell F. Selective intestinal decontamination prevents spontaneous bacterial peritonitis. Gastroenterology 1991; 100:477–481.

89. Henrion J, Schapira M, Derue G, Heller FR. Prevention of bacterial infection using selective intestinal decontamination in patients with cirrhosis admitted to intensive care. Controlled study in 120 patients. Acta Gastroenterol Belg 1992; 55:333–340.

90. Grangé JD, Roulot D, Pelletier G, Pariente A, Denis J, Ink O, Blanc P, Richardet JP, Vinel JP, Amiot X, Delisle F, Fischer D, Bodin F. Primary prophylaxis of bacterial infections with norfloxacin in cirrhotic patients with ascites: results of a double-blind, placebo-controlled trial (abstr). Gastroenterology 1994; 106: 901.

91. Novella M, Solà R, Soriano G, Andreu M, Gana J, Ortiz J, Coll S, Sàbat M, Vila MC, Guarner C, Vilardell F. Continuous vs inpatient prophylaxis of the first episode of spontaneous bacterial peritonitis in cirrhotic patients with norfloxacin. Hepatology 1997; 25:532–536.

92. Dupeyron C, Mangeney N, Sedrati L, Campillo B, Fouet P, Leluan G. Rapid emergence of quinolone resistance in cirrhotic patients treated with norfloxacin to prevent spontaneous bacterial peritonitis. Antimicrob Agents Chemother 1994; 38:340–344.

93. Ortiz J, Soriano G, Solà R, Gana J, Novella MT, Coll S, Sàbat M, Vila MC, Andreu M, Guarner C, Vilardell F. Characteristics of the infections caused by Escherichia coli resistant to norfloxacin in hospitalized cirrhotic patients (abstr). Hepatology 1995; 22: 166.

94. Terg R, Llano K, Cobas S, Brotto C, Barrios A, Levi D, Vasen W, Maria A. Effect of oral ciprofoxaxin on aerobic gram negative fecal flora of cirrhotic patients. Results of short and long term administration with variable dosis (abstr). Hepatology 1996; 24:455.

95. Aparicio JR, Such J, Girona E, Gutiérrez A, de Vera F, Arroyo MA, Plazas J, Palazón JM, Carnicer F, Perez-Mateo M. Increased detection of quinolone-resistant strains of Escherichia coli in rectal exudate from cirrhotic patients following selective intestinal decontamination with absence of clinical implications (abstr). Hepatology 1997; 26:289.

96. Guarner C, Runyon BA, Heck M, Young S, Sheick M. Effect of trimethoprim-sulphamethoxazole prophylactic treatment on ascites development, bacterial translocation, spontaneous bacterial peritonitis and survival in an experimental model of cirrhosis in rats (abstr). Hepatology 1996; 24:321.

97. Hoefs JC. Spontaneous bacterial peritonitis: prevention and therapy. Hepatology 1990; 12:776–781.

98. Schubert ML, Sanyal AJ, Wong ES. Antibiotic prophylaxis for prevention of spontaneous bacterial peritonitis? Gastroenterology 1991; 101:550–552.

99. Bernard B, Grange JD, Nguyen Khac E, Amiot X, Opolon P, Poynard T. Antibiotic prophylaxis for the prevention of bacterial infections in cirrhotic patients with gastrointestinal hemorrhage: A meta-analysis (abstr). Hepatology 1996; 24:1271.

100. Bernard B, Grange JD, Nguyen Khac E, Amiot X, Opolon P, Poynard T. Antibi-

otic prophylaxis for the prevention of bacterial infections in cirrhotic patients with ascites: A meta-analysis (abstr). Hepatology 1996; 24:1272.

101. Inadomi J, Sonnenberg A. Cost-analysis of prophylactic antibiotics in spontaneous bacterial peritonitis. Gastroenterology 1997; 113:1289–1294.

102. Younossi ZM, McHutchison JG, Ganiats TG. An economic analysis of norfloxacin prophylaxis against spontaneous bacterial peritonitis. J Hepatol 1997; 27:295–298.

103. Tomás A, Soriano G, Guarner C, Portorreal R, Novella MT, Vilardell F. Hospital-acquired infections in patients with cirrhosis undergoing selective intestinal decontamination. J Hepatol 1993; 18:262–263.

104. Peña C, Albareda JM, Parrarés R, Pujol M, Tubau F, Ariza J. Relationship between quinolone use and emergence of ciprofloxacin-resistant *Escherichia coli* in bloodstream infections. Antimicrob Agents Chemother 1995; 39:520–524.

105. Cometta A, Calandra T, Bille J, Glauser MP. *Escherichia coli* resistant to fluoroquinolones in patients with cancer and neutropenia. N Engl J Med 1994; 330:1240–1241.

106. Castellote J, Xiol J, Rota R, Fernández G. Spontaneous bacterial peritonitis and empyema by *Escherichia coli* resistant to norfloxacin in a patient on selective intestinal decontamination with norfloxacin. J Hepatol 1994; 20:436.

107. Llovet JM, Rodriguez-Iglesias P, Moitinho E, Planas R, Bataller R, Navasa M, Menacho M, Pardo A, Castells A, Cabré E, Arroyo V, Gassull MA, Rodés J. Spontaneous bacterial peritonitis in patients with cirrhosis undergoing selective intestinal decontamination. J Hepatol 1997; 26:88–95.

107a. Das A. A cost analysis of long term antibiotic prophylaxis for spontaneous bacterial peritonitis in cirrhosis. Am J Gastroenterol 1998; 93:1845–1900.

108. Pardo A, Viñado B, Santos J, Planas R, Cabré E, Moreno de la Vega V, Hombrados M, Ausina V, Luque T, Gassull MA. Effect of cisapride on intestinal bacterial overgrowth due to gram negative organisms in cirrhosis. A pilot, randomized, controlled study (abstr). J Hepatol 1997; 26(suppl. 1):101.

109. Guarner C, Runyon BA, Young S, Heck M, Seikh MY. Intestinal bacterial overgrowth and bacterial translocation in an experimental model of cirrhosis in rats. J Hepatol 1997; 26:1372–1378.

14

Liver Transplantation in Cirrhotic Patients with Spontaneous Bacterial Peritonitis

Antoni Rimola
Hospital Clínic i Provincial de Barcelona, University of Barcelona, Barcelona, Spain

Liver transplantation is the treatment of choice for most patients with severe, intractable, preterminal liver disease. The general indications and contraindications for liver transplantation are beyond the scope of this chapter. However, readers may consult several recent reviews dealing with these topics (1–6). In this chapter only specific issues with reference to liver transplantation in cirrhotic patients who have or have had spontaneous bacterial peritonitis (SBP) will be covered.

I. SBP AS A CRITERION FOR INDICATING LIVER TRANSPLANTATION

In general terms, liver transplantation is indicated in patients fulfilling two major criteria: (a) progressive, lethal, and otherwise untreatable liver disease; and (b) survival expectancy with conventional management clearly lower than that with liver transplantation (1–7). In this setting liver transplantation should be considered in *every* patient with SBP for the following reasons. First, SBP develops very frequently in cirrhotic patients with advanced liver disease (8–15). In a study that included a large series of consecutive, unselected patients with SBP, 76.5% of patients had Child-Pugh class C cirrhosis, 23% had class

B, and 0.5% had class A (12). Therefore, most patients with SBP satisfy the criteria for liver transplantation of severe, advanced cirrhosis with limited life expectancy.

Second, numerous authors have uniformly reported an extremely poor prognosis after SBP in patients that are treated with conventional therapy other than liver transplantation. Indeed, they have a one-year cumulative survival rate of only 30–50% and a two-year survival rate of only 25–30% (16–24). This is exemplified in Fig. 14.1 where the survival probability of a series of patients who had survived a first episode of SBP is depicted (16). Despite the generally poor prognosis, occasional patients may have prolonged survival after SBP (8,16). In one study in which a very select population was investigated (i.e., patients who survived more than 60 days after the resolution of SBP, who were younger than 66 years of age, and who were without hepatocellular carcinoma or severe extrahepatic disorders), the one-year survival probability of 11 patients with a Child-Pugh score <10 was 80%, whereas the corresponding survival rate for 26 patients with a Child-Pugh score ≥10 was only 26% (22). However, the small number of patients in this series and particularly the exclusion from the follow-up of the first 60 days after the resolution of infection, a time during which the mortality rate is the greatest in most studies, make the conclusions of this investigation not necessarily applicable to the whole population of patients who survive an episode of SBP. In contrast to

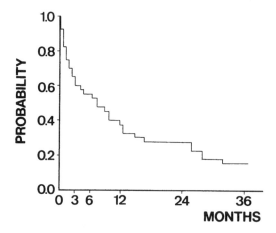

Figure 14.1 Percent survival probability of 75 cirrhotic patients who resolved their first episode of spontaneous bacterial peritonitis and who were conventionally managed without liver transplantation. (From Ref. 16.)

the poor prognosis of patients managed conventionally, survival expectancy after liver transplantion in patients with a past history of SBP is much higher, as shown in Fig. 14.2, in which a one- and two-year survival probability is 85% and 79%, respectively. Therefore, patients with SBP also satisfy the second criterion for liver transplantation. Consequently, SBP is commonly considered to be an ideal indication for liver transplantation in most centers (1,2,4–6,25,26). The only note of caution to this general opinion comes from the results of a study in which the early postoperative outcome of 25 patients with a history of SBP was worse than that of 25 age- and disease-matched control transplant recipients (mortality rate of 24% and 8%, respectively) (27). However, in that study there were several possible explanations for the conclusion that SBP patients do worse than other transplant recipients: the relatively small number of patients studied and the more severely impaired preoperative general status in the SBP group (i.e., 44% of patients were on mechanical ventilation and 36% were receiving hemodialysis, whereas the corresponding figures in the control group were 16% and 8%, respectively). Furthermore, more technical vascular and biliary complications occurred after transplantation in the SBP group than in the non-SBP group (32% versus 4%). In fact, the survival probability after liver transplantation depicted in Fig. 14.2 does not substantially differ from that reported for both liver transplant recipients as a whole and cirrhotic patients with ascites in particular (2,28–30). These

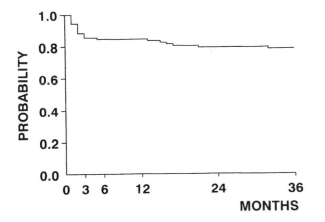

Figure 14.2 Percent survival probability after liver transplantation in 103 cirrhotic patients with past history of spontaneous bacterial peritonitis. (Results obtained in the Hospital Clínic, Barcelona, Spain.)

data further support the contention that liver transplantation should be considered in patients with SBP.

II. SBP AND SBP-RELATED COMPLICATIONS AS POSSIBLE RISK FACTORS ATTENDING LIVER TRANSPLANTATION

Assessment of possible contraindications to liver transplantation is also mandatory in patients who are potential candidates for this therapy. Patients with SBP can present with noninfectious contraindications to liver transplantation that may preclude the transplant procedure. Such contraindications include: (a) massive peritoneal adhesions; (b) complete splenic-mesenteric-portal thrombosis; (c) poor short-term prognosis because of extrahepatic malignancy or AIDS; or (d) other severe extrahepatic diseases, advanced hepatocellular carcinoma, active alcoholism or high hepatitis B virus (HBV) replicative status (1–6,25,26). In addition, several specific circumstances capable of influencing the result of liver transplantation in patients with SBP deserve adequate discussion.

A. SBP May Be a Transient Contraindication of Liver Transplantation

Due to the intraabdominal site of infection, active SBP may be considered a contraindication to liver transplantation until the infection is brought under control. However, liver transplantation can sometimes be safely performed in cirrhotic patients with SBP in whom the infection is clearly improving. In one study that specifically investigated this issue, the authors concluded that patients with SBP may be treated with liver transplantation without any increased risk of postoperative sepsis if the patient has received a minimum of four days of effective antibiotic therapy that has reduced ascitic fluid polymorphonuclear count to less than 250/mm^3 and antimicrobial treatment is prolonged for at least four more days after the transplantation procedure (31).

B. SBP-Related Complications as Risk Factors in Liver Transplant Candidates

Although survival of patients with SBP has progressively improved during the past 25 years, at present approximately 20–30% of cirrhotic patients with

SBP still die during hospitalization because of the initial infectious process, the underlying liver disease, or both (12–15,18,32–38). The impact of the development of SBP in patients on the liver transplant waiting list has recently been analyzed. In a preliminary study published in abstract form (39), 6% of patients with chronic liver disease developed SBP while awaiting transplantation, which averaged five months. More important, 62% of these patients died before receiving a liver transplant, whereas the mortality rate of patients who did not develop SBP while awaiting transplantation was only 16%. On the other hand, renal and liver function can deteriorate significantly as a consequence of SBP, and such derangements may persist after the resolution of SBP (8,14,40). Renal impairment may be related to the administration of nephrotoxic antimicrobial agents, such as aminoglycoside antibiotic agents, or to the deletereous effects of the inflammatory response itself (41–44). The existence of renal dysfunction is particularly pertinent in patients waiting for liver transplantation since renal functional impairment has almost universally been reported to be a very bad prognostic factor for postoperative survival (45–51). For example, we have recently reported that the hospital mortality rate after transplantation in cirrhotic patients with and without renal failure was 35% and 10%, respectively (51). Due to the markedly adverse effects of renal dysfunction on the results of liver transplantation, it seems reasonable to recommend the avoidance of any factor capable of impairing renal function in patients with SBP, such as the administration of aminoglycoside agents or nonsteroidal anti-inflammatory drugs, overdiuresis, or paracentesis without adequate plasma volume expansion (41–43,52–54). Conversely, the possibility of improving or preventing renal dysfunction may be of great value in these patients. In this setting, recently reported preliminary results suggest that the beneficial effects of plasma volume expansion with intravenous infusions of human albumin to patients with SBP are very promising (55).

C. SBP as a Preventable Complication

Since the development of SBP in liver transplant candidates, either at the time of transplantation or while awaiting transplantation, may seriously complicate their course, the prevention of SBP is crucial. There are three subsets of patients in whom antibiotic prophylaxis against SBP may be of benefit. These three subgroups include: (a) patients who have had a previous episode of SBP; (b) cirrhotic patients with a low ascitic fluid protein concentration (<10–15 g/L); and (c) cirrhotic patients with gastrointestinal hemorrhage (16,19,56–61). Although different strategies have been used in these patients (56,62–65), the most common form of prophylaxis consists in selective intestinal decontamination using the oral administration of norfloxacin (59–61,66). However, prophylaxis with this antimicrobial agent, particularly when it is administered for long periods of time, may be associated with the overgrowth of quinolone-resistant bacteria (67,68). However, few episodes of SBP caused by resistant organisms that occurred during norfloxacin prophylaxis have been reported (66). Nevertheless, this possibility should be taken into account for properly selecting the prophylactic administration of antibiotics in the perioperative period of liver transplantation or the therapeutic administration of antimicrobial agents in patients who develop signs of infection early after transplantation.

REFERENCES

1. Lake JR. Changing indications for liver transplantation. Gastroenterol Clin N Am 1993; 22:213–229.
2. Rimola A, Navasa M, Rodés J, Elias E, Neuberger J, Lucey MR, Shorrock C. Specific indications. Chronic parenchymal liver disease. In *Liver Transplantation: Practice and Management*, Neuberger J, Lucey MR, eds., London: BMJ Publishing Group, 1994, 34–104.
3. Rosen HR, Shackleton CR, Martin P. Indications for and timing of liver transplantation. Med Clin N Am 1996; 80:1069–1102.
4. Wiesner RH. Current indications, contraindications, and timing for liver transplantation. In: *Transplantation of the Liver*, Busuttil RW, Klintmalm GB, eds., Philadelphia: W.B. Saunders Co., 1996, 71–84.
5. Bodily K, Fitz JG. Selection of patients and timing of liver transplantation. In: *Medical Care of the Liver Transplant Patient.* Killenberg PG, Clavien P-A, eds., Malden: Blackwell Science, Inc., 1997, 3–23.
6. Yoshida EM, Lake JR. Selection of patients for liver transplantation in 1997 and beyond. Clin Liver Dis 1997; 1:247–261.
7. Kim WR, Dickson ER. The role of prognostic models in the timing of liver transplantation. Clin Liver Dis 1997; 1:263–279.
8. Hoefs JC, Canawati HN, Sapico FL, Hopkins RR, Weiner J, Montgomerie JZ. Spontaneous bacterial peritonitis. Hepatology 1982; 2:399–407.
9. Pinzello G, Simonetti RG, Craxi A, DiPiazza S, Spanò C, Pagliaro L. Spontaneous bacterial peritonitis: a prospective investigation in predominantly nonalcoholic cirrhotic patients. Hepatology 1983; 3:545–549.
10. Almdal TP, Skinhøj. Spontaneous bacterial peritonitis in cirrhosis. Incidence, diagnosis, and prognosis. Scand J Gastroenterol 1987; 22:295–300.
11. Rimland D, Hand WL. Spontaneous peritonitis: a reappraisal. Am J Med Sci 1987; 30:285–292.
12. Toledo C, Salmerón JM, Rimola A, Navasa M, Arroyo V, Llach J, Ginés A, Ginés P, Rodés J. Spontaneous bacterial peritonitis in cirrhosis: predictive factors

of infection resolution and survival in patients treated with cefotaxime. Hepatology 1993; 17:251–257.

13. Garcia-Tsao G. Spontaneous bacterial peritonitis. Gastroenterol Clin N Am 1992; 21:257–275.

14. Bac D-J, Siersema PD, Mulder PGH, DeMarie S, Wilson JHP. Spontaneous bacterial peritonitis: outcome and predictive factors. Eur J Gastroenterol Hepatol 1993; 5:635–640.

15. Rimola A, Navasa M. Infections in liver disease. In: *Oxford Textbook of Clinical Hepatology*, 2nd ed., McIntyre N, Benhamou J-P, Bircher J, Rizzetto M, Rodés J, eds., New York: Oxford University Press, 1999, 1861–1874.

16. Tító LL, Rimola A, Ginés P, Llach J, Arroyo V, Rodés J. Recurrence of spontaneous bacterial peritonitis in cirrhosis: frequency and predictive factors. Hepatology 1988; 8:27–31.

17. Ink O, Pelletier D, Salmon D, Attali P, Pessione F, Hannoun S, Buffet C, Etienne JP. Pronostic de l'infection spontanée d'ascite chez le cirrhotique. Gastroenterol Clin Biol 1989; 13:556–561.

18. Grange JD, Amiot X, Grange V, Gutmann L, Biour M, Bodin F, Poupon R. Amoxicillin-clavulanic acid therapy of spontaneous bacterial peritonitis: a prospective study of twenty-seven cases in cirrhotic patients. Hepatology 1990; 11:360–364.

19. Silvain C, Mannant P-R, Ingrand P, Fort E, Besson I, Beauchant M. Récidive de l'infection spontanée du liquide d'ascite au cours de la cirrhose. Gastroenterol Clin Biol 1991; 15:106–109.

20. Wang S-S, Tsai Y-T, Lee S-D, Chen H-T, Lu C-W, Lee F-Y, Jeng J-S, Liu Y-C, Lo K-J. Spontaneous bacterial peritonitis in patients with hepatitis B-related cirrhosis and hepatocellular carcinoma. Gastroenterology 1991; 101:1656–1662.

21. Terg R, Levi D, Lopez P, Rafaelli C, Rojter S, Abecasis R, Villamil F, Aziz H, Podesta A. Analysis of clinical course and prognosis of culture-positive spontaneous bacterial peritonitis and neutrocytic ascites. Evidence of the same disease. Dig Dis Sci 1992; 37:499–504.

22. Altman C, Grange JD, Amiot X, Pelletier G, Lacaine F, Bodin F, Etienne JP. Survival after a first episode of spontaneous bacterial peritonitis. Prognosis of potential candidates for orthotopic liver transplantation. J Gastroenterol Hepatol 1995; 10:47–50.

23. Bac DJ. Spontaneous bacterial peritonitis: an indication for liver transplantation? Scand J Gastroenterol 1996; 218(suppl.):38–42.

24. Younossi ZM, McHutchison JG, Ganiats TG. An economic analysis of norfloxacin prophylaxis against spontaneous bacterial peritonitis. J Hepatol 1997; 27:295–298.

25. Sher LS, Pan S-H, Hoffman AL, Villamil FG, Howard TK, Podesta LG, Makowka L. Liver transplantation. In: *The Handbook of Transplantation Management*, Makowka L, ed., Austin: R.G. Landes Co., 1991, 192–253.

26. Wood RP, Ozaki CF, Katz SM, Monsour HP, Dyer CH, Johnston TD. Liver transplantation. The last ten years. Surg Clin N Am 1994; 74:1133–1154.

27. Ukah FO, Merhav H, Kramer D, Eghtesad B, Samini F, Frezza E, Linden P, Mieles L, Selby R. Early outcome of liver transplantation in patients with a history of spontaneous bacterial peritonitis. Transplant Proc 1993; 25:1113–1115.

28. European Liver Transplant Registry. Data analysis 05/1969–06/1996. Hôpital Paul Brousse, Villejuif, France.

29. Kilpe VE, Krakahuer H, Wren RE. An analysis of liver transplant experience from 37 transplant centers as reported to Medicare. Transplantation 1993; 56:554–561.

30. Busuttil RW, Shaked A, Millis JM, Jurim O, Colquhoun SD, Shackleton CR, Nuesse BJ, Csete M, Goldstein LI, McDiarmid SV. One thousand liver transplants. The leasons learned. Ann Surg 1994; 219:490–499.

31. Van Thiel DH, Hassanein T, Gurakar A, Wright HI, Caraceni P, De Maria N, Nadir A. Liver transplantation after an acute episode of spontaneous bacterial peritonitis. Hepato-Gastroenterol 1996; 43:1584–1588.

32. Runyon BA, McHuntchison JG, Antillon MR, Akriviadis EA, Montano AA. Short-course versus long-course antibiotic treatment of spontaneous bacterial peritonitis. A randomized controlled study of 100 patients. Gastroenterology 1991; 100:1737–1742.

33. Kéou FXM, Bloch F, Hoi AB, Lavril M, Bélec L, Mokbat JE, Petite JP, Acar JF. Spontaneous bacterial peritonitis in cirrhotic hospital in-patients: Retrospective analysis of 101 cases. Q J Med 1992; 83:401–407.

34. Gómez-Jiménez J, Ribera E, Gasser I, Artaza MA, Del Valle O, Pahissa A, Martínez-Vázquez JM. Randomized trial comparing ceftriaxone with cefonicid for treatment of spontaneous bacterial peritonitis in cirrhotic patients. Antimicrob Agents Chemother 1993; 37:1587–1592.

35. Llovet JM, Planas R, Morillas R, Quer JC, Cabré E, Boix J, Humbert P, Guilera M, Doménech E, Bertrán X, Gassull MA. Short-term prognosis of cirrhotics with spontaneous bacterial peritonitis: multivariate analysis. Am J Gastroenterol 1993; 88:388–392.

36. Rimola A, Salmerón JM, Clemente G, Rodrigo L, Obrador A, Miranda ML, Guarner C, Planas R, Solá R, Vargas V, Casafont F, Marco F, Navasa M, Bañares R, Arroyo V, Rodés J. Two different dosages of cefotaxime in the treatment of spontaneous bacterial peritonitis in cirrhosis: results of a prospective, randomized, multicenter study. Hepatology 1995; 21:674–679.

37. Boixeda D, De Luis DA, Aller R, De Argila CM. Spontaneous bacterial peritonitis. Clinical and microbiological study of 233 episodes. J Clin Gastroenterol 1996; 23:275–279.

38. Navasa M, Follo A, Llovet JM, Clemente G, Vargas V, Rimola A, Marco F, Guarner C, Forné M, Planas R, Bañares R, Castells L, Jimenez de Anta MT, Arroyo V, Rodés J. Randomized, comparative study of oral ofloxacin versus intravenous cefotaxime in spontaneous bacterial peritonitis. Gastroenterology 1996; 111:1011–1017.

39. Chalasani N, Gitlin N. Incidence and risk factors for spontaneous bacterial peritonitis (SBP) in patients with chronic liver disease on the waiting list for orthotopic liver transplantation (OLT) (abstr). Hepatology 1997; 26:491A.

40. Follo A, Llovet JM, Navasa M, Planas R, Forns X, Francitorra A, Rimola A, Gassull MA, Arroyo V, Rodés J. Renal impairment after spontaneous bacterial peritonitis in cirrhosis: incidence, clinical course, predictive factors and prognosis. Hepatology 1994; 20:1495–1501.

41. Cabrera J, Arroyo V, Ballesta A, Rimola A, Gual J, Elena M, Rodés J. Aminoglycoside nephrotoxicity in cirrhosis: value of urinary β2-microglobulin to discriminate functional renal failure from acute tubular damage. Gastroenterology 1982; 82:97–105.

42. Felisart J, Rimola A, Arroyo V, Perez-Ayuso RM, Quintero E, Ginés P, Rodés J. Cefotaxime is more effective than is ampicillin-tobramycin in cirrhotics with severe infections. Hepatology 1985; 5:457–462.

43. Moore RD, Smith CR, Lietman PS. Increased risk of renal dysfunction due to interaction of liver disease and aminoglycosides. Am J Med 1986; 80:1093–1097.

44. Navasa M, Follo A, Filella X, Jimenez W, Francitorra A, Planas R, Rimola A, Arroyo V, Rodés J. Tumor necrosis factor and interleukin-6 in spontaneous bacterial peritonitis in cirrhosis. Relationship with the development of renal impairment and mortality. Hepatology 1988; 27:1227–1232.

45. Rimola A, Gavaler JS, Schade RR, El-Lakany S. Starzl TE, Van Thiel DH. Effects of renal impairment on liver transplantation. Gastroenterology 1987; 93: 148–156.

46. Cuervas-Mons V, Millan I, Gavaler JS, Starzl TE, Van Thiel DH. Prognostic value of preoperatively obtained clinical and laboratory data in predicting survival following orthotopic liver transplantation. Hepatology 1986; 6:922–927.

47. Shaw BW, Wood RP, Stratta RJ, Pillen TJ, Langnas An. Stratifying the causes of death in liver transplant recipients. An approach to improving survival. Arch Surg 1989; 124:895–900.

48. Baliga P, Merion RM, Turcotte JG, Ham JM, Henley KS, Lucey MR, Schork A, Shyr Y, Campbell DA. Preoperative risk assessment in liver transplantation. Surgery 1992; 112:704–711.

49. Eckhoff DE, Pirsch JD, D'Alessandro AM, Knechtle SJ, Young CJ, Geffenr SR, Belzer FO, Kalayoglu M. Pretransplant status and patient survival following liver transplantation. Transplantation 1995; 60:920–925.

50. Lafayette RA, Paré G, Schmid CH, King AJ, Rohrer RJ, Nasraway SA. Prefransplant renal dysfunction predicts poorer outcome in liver transplantation. Clin Nephrol 1997; 48:159–164.

51. González E, Rimola A, Navasa M, Andreu H, Grande L, Garcia-Valdecasas JC, Cirera I, Visa J, Rodés J. Liver transplantation in patients with non-biliary cirrhosis: prognostic value of preoperative factors. J Hepatol 1998; 28:320–328.

52. Planas R, Arroyo V, Rimola A, Pérez-Ayuso RM, Rodés J. Acetylsalicylic acid suppresses the renal hemodynamic effect and reduces the diuretic action of furosemide in cirrhosis with ascites. Gastroenterology 1983; 84:247–252.

53. Ginés P, Arroyo V, Quintero E, Planas R, Bory F, Cabrera J, Rimola A, Viver J, Camps J, Jiménez W, Mastai R, Gaya J, Rodés J. Comparison of paracentesis

and diuretics in the treatment of cirrhotics with tense ascites. Results of a randomized study. Gastroenterology 1987; 93:234–241.

54. Ginés P, Titó LL, Arroyo V, Planas R, Panés J, Viver J, Torres M, Humbert P, Rimola A, Llach J, Badalamenti S, Jimenez W, Gaya J, Rodés J. Randomized comparative study of therapeutic paracentesis with and without intravenous albumin in cirrhosis. Gastroenterology 1988; 94:1493–1502.

55. Sort P, Navasa M, and Spanish Group for the Study of Bacterial Infections in Cirrhosis. Intravenous albumin infusion prevents renal impairment (RI) and improves hospital survival in patients with spontaneous bacterial peritonitis (SBP). J Hepatol 1998; 28(suppl. 1):45.

56. Rimola A, Bory F, Terés J, Pérez-Ayuso RM, Arroyo V, Rodés J. Oral, nonasorbable antibiotics prevent infection in cirrhosis with gastrointestinal hemorrhage. Hepatology 1985; 5:463–467.

57. Llach J, Rimola A, Navasa M, Ginés P, Salmerón JM, Ginés A, Arroyo V, Rodés J. Incidence and predictive factors of first episode of spontaneous bacterial peritonitis in cirrhosis with ascites: relevance of ascitic fluid protein concentration. Hepatology 1992; 16:724–727.

58. Andreu M, Sola R, Sitges-Serra A, Alia C, Gallen M, Vila MC, Coll S, Oliver MI. Risk factors for spontaneous bacterial peritonitis in cirrhotic patients with ascites. Gastroenterology 1993; 104:1133–1138.

59. Ginés P, Rimola A, Planas R, Vargas V, Marco F, Almela M, Forné M, Miranda ML, Llach J, Salmerón JM, Esteve M, Marqués JM, Jiménez de Anta MT, Arroyo V, Rodés J. Norfloxacin prevents spontaneous bacterial peritonitis recurrence in cirrhosis: results of a double-blind, placebo-controlled trial. Hepatology 1990; 12:716–724.

60. Soriano G, Guarner C, Teixidó M, Such J, Barrios J, Enriquiez J, Vilardell F. Selective intestinal decontamination prevents spontaneous bacterial peritonitis. Gastroenterology 1991; 100:477–481.

61. Soriano G, Guarner C, Tomás A, Villanueva C, Torras X, González D, Sainz S, Anguera A, Cussó X, Balanzó J, Vilardell F. Norfloxacin prevents bacterial infection in cirrhotics with gastrointestinal hemorrhage. Gastroenterology 1992; 103:1267–1272.

62. Singh N, Gayoswski T, Yu VL, Wagener MM. Trimethoprim-sulfamethoxazole for the prevention of spontaneous bacterial peritonitis in cirrhosis: a randomized trial. Ann Intern Med 1995; 122:595–598.

63. Blaise M, Pateron D, Trinchet J-C, Levacher S, Beaugrand M, Pourriat J-L. Systemic antibiotic therapy prevents bacterial infection in cirrhotic patients with gastrointestinal hemorrhage. Hepatology 1994; 20:34–38.

64. Rolachon A, Cordier L, Bacq Y, Nousbaum JB, Franza A, Paris JC, Fratte S, Bohn B, Kitmacher P, Stahl JP, Zarski J-P. Ciprofloxacin and long-term prevention of spontaneous bacterial peritonitis: Results of a prospective, controlled trial. Hepatology 1995; 22:1171–1174.

65. Pawels A, Mostefa-Kara N, Debenes B, Lévy V-G. Systemic antibiotic prophy-

laxis after gastrointestinal hemorrhage in cirrhotic patients with a high risk of infection. Hepatology 1996; 24:802–806.

66. Llovet JM, Rodriguez-lglesias P, Moitinho E, Planas R, Bataller R, Navasa M, Menacho M, Pardo A, Castells A, Cabre E, Arroyo V, Gassull MA, Rodes J. Spontaneous bacterial peritonitis in patients with cirrhosis undergoing selective intestinal decontamination. A retrospective study of 229 spontaneous bacterial peritonitis episodes. J Hepatol 1997; 26:88–95.

67. Dupeyron C, Mangeney N, Sedrati L, Campillo B, Fouet P, Leluan G. Rapid emergence of quinolone resistance in cirrhotic patients treated with norfloxacin to prevent spontaneous bacterial peritonitis. Antimicrob Agents Chemother 1994; 38:340–244.

68. Novella M, Solá R, Soriano G, Andreu M, Gana J, Ortiz J, Coll S, Sabat M, Vila MC, Guarner C, Vilardell F. Continuous versus inpatient prophylaxis of the first episode of spontaneous bacterial peritonitis with norfloxacin. Hepatology 1997; 25:532–536.

Index

Abdominal pain, 206
Abdominal trauma and bacterial translocation, 135, 138–139
Acidosis, 207
Acinetobacter spp., 54, 221
  and selective intestinal decontamination, 157
  susceptibility to cefotaxime, 221
  susceptibility to norfloxacin, 241
Acute hemorrhagic pancreatitis and bacterial translocation, 128
Acute liver disease and SBP, 15, 65–66
Acute liver failure and bacterial translocation, 123–124
Acute necrotizing pancreatitis and bacterial translocation, 156
Acute respiratory insufficiency, 207
Adenosine deaminase in tuberculous peritonitis, 15, 93
Advanced spontaneous bacterial peritonitis, 188
Aeromonas hydrophila
  susceptibility to cefotaxime, 221
  susceptibility to quinolones, 226
Aeromonas liquifaciens, 3
Aeromonas shigelloides, susceptibility to quinolones, 226

Aeromonas sobria, susceptibility to cefotaxime, 221
Age
  as prognostic factor in SBP, 200
  and survival in SBP, 208
  and tuberculosis, 90
AIDS and tuberculosis, 89–90
Albumin
  and prevention of renal impairment, 212, 289
  and treatment of renal impairment, 212, 289
Alcoholic cirrhosis, 28
α_1-Antitrypsin-deficiency and SBP, 28
Allopurinol and bacterial translocation, 115–116, 127, 168, 175
Amphotericin B, 136
Aminoglycoside antibiotics, 13, 212
Aminoguanidine in prevention of bacterial translocation, 158, 160
Amoxicillin and clavulanic acid, 225
  and superinfections 225
Ampicillin, 222
Anaerobic bacterial peritonitis, 10, 52–54
  Bacterioides fragilis in, 52, 109–110
  Campylobacter spp., in, 54

[Anaerobic bacterial peritonitis]
  Clostridium perfringens in, 52
  Clostridium tertium in, 52
  Fusobacterium necrophorum in, 52
  Peptococcus in, 54
  Peptostreptococcus anaerobus in, 54
Analytical disturbances in SBP, 207
Antibacterial activity
  of cefotaxime, 220–221
  of quinolones, 225–226
Antibiotic therapy, 219–232
Antimicrobial mechanisms, 257
Antioxidant vitamins and prevention of bacterial translocation, 170, 175
Antipyretic substances, 31
Arizona spp., susceptibility to norfloxacin, 241
Arginine in prevention of bacterial translocation, 157–160, 168
Ascitic fluid, 51
  antimicrobial activity, 238–239, 257
  complement protein concentration, 239
    C_3 concentration, 239, 257
    C_4 concentration, 239
  culture, 13
  local defense mechanisms, 248
  opsonic activity, 238–239, 257
  total protein concentration 238–239, 248, 257
  and risk of first episode of SBP, 257–258
  and risk of nosocomial SBP, 257
Aseptic peritonitis and chronic ambulatory peritoneal dialysis (CAPD), 80
Aspergillus spp., 13
Asymptomatic bacterascites, 47, 51, 75, 77, 102
  clinical features, 47–48
  mortality, 51, 80
  prevalence, 75–76

Asymptomatic bacteriuria, 261
Atypical tuberculosis, 91
Aztreonam, 224
  and superinfections, 224

Bacillus providence and CAPD, 61
Bacterascites, 9, 76, 78
  prevalence of, 76, 80
Bacteremia, 105, 214
  in acute traumatic shock, 132
Bacterial clearance, 108–109
Bacterial endocarditis, 10, 106
Bacterial infections
  in liver cirrhosis, 206
  and risk of rebleeding, 238, 256
Bacterial overgrowth
  and bacterial translocation, 114, 127, 129, 131, 163, 178
  and SID, 136
Bacterial resistance, 227, 271, 273
  mechanisms of, 227
Bacterial translocation, 15, 102–104, 110, 113–186, 214, 258, 262
  induction of, 113- 151
    animal investigations, 116
    and bacterial overgrowth, 114, 127, 129, 131
    burns in, 125, 156
    and cirrhosis, 258
    definition of, 113
    endotoxin-induced bacterial translocation, 117, 122, 128
    gram-negative bacteria in, 245
    gram-positive bacteria in, 245
    hemorrhagic shock in, 115
    hepatectomy in, 117–118, 123, 132–133
    and hypovolemia, 258
    host immune defenses in, 114, 127
    in human disease, 119, 130–137
    inducers of, 119
    induction of, 115–116

[Bacterial resistance]
and malnutrition, 127, 130
mechanisms implicated in, 113–
115, 117
and MLN complex, 114
multiple organ failure in, 139
norfloxacin in, 245
pancreatitis in, 128
photomicrographic documentation
of, 120–123
portal hypertension in, 124–
125
and portosystemic shunting, 125
ricinoleic acid in, 115, 125–
126
shock in bacterial translocation,
102
streptozotocin in, 126
thermal injury in, 116–117, 137–
138
total parenteral nutrition (TPN)
in, 133
trauma in, 135, 138–139
"two-hit" induction in, 127
zymosan in, 127
prevention of, 118, 139–141, 153–
186
allopurinol in, 115–116, 127,
168, 175
aminoguanidine in, 158, 160
antibiotic agents in, 119–120,
154–157
antiendotoxin substances in, 169,
178–180
arginine in, 157–160, 168
bactericidal permeability-increasing protein (BPIP), 160–161
bulk-forming units in, 160–161,
171, 175, 178
cellulose in, 176, 178
kaolin in, 178
calcium in, 171–172
cholecystokinin in, 163–165
cisapride in, 165

[Bacterial resistance]
dehydroepiandrosterone in, 168–
169
dextran in, 169, 172
dietary protein in, 175–179
endotoxin in, 157
epidermal growth factor in, 179–
180
fluoroquinolones in, 156
hyperoxia in, 161, 168–169
immunoglobulins in, 169
immunostimulation in, 172
inhibition of nitric oxide synthesis in, 160
lactulose in, 161–163, 171, 178
lactobacilli in, 163
ligation of Peyer's patches in,
166–168
methotrexate in, 164
oat base, fermented in, 163–164
phosphotidylcholine in, 168–170
phosphotidylinositol in, 169, 171
protoglycan in, 179
reduction in macrophage volume
in, 165–167, 176
relief of biliary obstruction in,
172–173
selective intestinal decontamination in, 137, 139–141, 154–
157
splenectomy in, 165–167
suppression of intestinal flora in,
154–157, 162–164
Bactericidal permeability-increasing
protein (BPIP), and antiendotoxinic activity, 160
Bacterioides fragilis (*see* Anaerobic
bacterial peritonitis)
and bacterial translocation, 114
Band neutrophils
and renal impairment, 210
and resolution of infection, 208
Biliary cirrhosis, 29
Bilirubin and renal impairment, 193

Blood urea nitrogen
and renal impairment, 191, 210
and resolution of infection, 190,
208
and survival, 190, 194, 208
Bone marrow transplantation and SBP,
14
Bordetella parapertussis, susceptibility
to cefotaxime, 221
Burkholderia maltophilia, susceptibility to norfloxacin, 241
Burkholderia pseudomallei, susceptibility to norfloxacin, 241
Burn stress and bacterial translocation,
125, 156

Calcium in prevention of bacterial
translocation, 171–172
Campylobacter spp., 54–55
susceptibility to cefotaxime, 221
susceptibility to quinolones, 225
Candida albicans in CAPD, 13
Candida parapsilopsis in CAPD, 13
Candida spp. and bacterial translocation, 137
Candida tropicalis in CAPD, 61
Capnocytophaga ochraceae, 54–55
Cardiac ascites, 13, 59
Caseating granulomas and tuberculosis, 91
Causes of SBP, 29
Cefonicid, 223–224
and superinfections, 224
Cefotaxime, 220–223
antibacterial activity of, 220–221
dosage of, 223
duration of therapy, 223
pharmacokinetic properties of, 221
therapeutic efficacy of, 222–223
Ceftriaxone, 223–224
in gastrointestinal bleeding, 266
and superinfections, 224
Cellulose in prevention of bacterial
translocation, 175, 177–178

Chemotaxis, 240
Child-Pugh class
and incidence of SBP, 205
and survival, 208
Chlamydia spp., 11,13
Cholecystokinine in reduction of bacterial translocation, 164–165
Cholic acid and prevention of bacterial
translocation, 174
Chronic ambulatory peritoneal dialysis
(CAPD), 10, 12, 14, 60, 111
and aseptic peritonitis, 61
and eosinophilic peritonitis, 35
infecting organisms, 60
and tuberculous peritonitis, 41, 90,
94
and chyloperitoneum, 94
Chronic encapsulating peritonitis and
tuberculosis, 58
Chronology of SBP, 8–18
Chyluria, 58
Ciprofloxacin, 226, 263
antimicrobial activity, 241
and bacterial translocation, 130,
136
and intestinal absorption, 243
and systemic infections, 243
and tuberculosis, 95
Cisapride
in prevention of bacterial translocation, 165
in SBP prophylaxis, 275
Citrobacter spp.,
and bacterial translocation, 142
and susceptibility to cefotaxime,
220
and susceptibility to norfloxacin,
225, 241, 247
Clindamycin and bacterial translocation, 114, 126
Clinical manifestations of SBP, 25–
46, 206–207
Clinical pathogenesis of SBP, 101–
112

Clostridia and bacterial translocation, 114

Clostridial peritonitis, 54 (*see also* Anaerobic bacterial peritonitis)

Clostridium difficile colitis, 54

Clostridium perfringens, 53 (*see also* Anaerobic bacterial peritonitis)

Clostridium tertium, 53 (*see also* Anaerobic bacterial peritonitis)

Cocoon syndrome, 58

Colorectal carcinomas and bacterial translocation, 131

Community-acquired SBP, 194, 199–200

and ascitic fluid total protein concentration, 258

and hospital survival, 199, 208

and SBP resolution, 199, 208

and serum bilirubin, 258

Complement, 14, 239–240

concentrations in ascitic fluid, 110, 239–240, 248

Complications of SBP, 208–215, 256

prevalence of, 208

prophylaxis of, 208

treatment of, 208

Costs of SBP, 245

Creatinine clearance in hepatorenal syndrome, 190

Crohn's disease and bacterial translocation, 130

Cryptococcal peritonitis, 15

Culture-negative SBP (CNNA),13, 33, 47, 75, 208

clinical signs of, 49–50

history of, 13

mortality of, 198

prevalence of, 76

Culture-negative SBE, 33–34

Culture-negative SBP, 33, 47, 51, 75–76, 78, 102

prevalence of, 76, 80

prognosis of, 80

Culture-positive SBP

clinical signs of, 49–50

mortality of, 208

Curtis-Fitz-Hugh syndrome, 11, 37, 111

and chlamydial infections, 37

and pelvic inflammatory disease (PID), 37

Cyclophosphamide and bacterial translocation, 114

Cycloserine and tuberculosis, 95

Cytokines

and abdominal trauma, 139

intra-abdominal production, 197–198

prognostic value of, 197

and renal impairment, 197–198

Death

causes of, 188–189, 208

in advanced SBP, 188

in non-advanced SBP, 189

Dehydroepiandrosterone and prevention of bacterial translocation, 168

Deoxycholic acid and prevention of bacterial translocation, 174

Deoxynucleic acid (DNA) gyrase, resistance to quinolones, 227

Dexamethasone and bacterial translocation, 126

Dextran in prevention of bacterial translocation, 169, 172

Disseminated intravascular coagulopathy (DIC), 128

and peritoneovenous shunt, 56–57

in SBP, 207

Drug resistance and tuberculosis, 90

Diuretic effect, 12, 14

Ecthyma granulosum, 13 (*see also Pseudomonas aeruginosa*)

Effective plasma volume, 210–211

Empyema, 10

Encapsulating peritonitis, 15
Encephalopathy, mortality, 17
Endoscopic sclerotherapy, 16
  and antibiotic prophylaxis, 259
  and risk of bacterial infection, 63,
    258–259
Endotoxin
  and bacterial translocation, 117,
    122, 128, 160
  and gastrointestinal hemorrhage, 60
  and nitric oxide synthase, 160

Enoxacin, 226
Enteral feeding and prevention of bac-
    terial translocation, 118, 133
Enteric infections and norfloxacin, 243
Enterobacter spp.
  and susceptibility to cefotaxime,
    220
  and susceptibility to quinolones,
    225, 241, 247
  Enterococcus spp.
  and bacterial translocation, 114
  and selective intestinal decontamina-
    tion, 140–141
  and susceptibility to cefotaxime,
    221
  and susceptibility to quinolones,
    241
Eosinophilic peritonitis, 14, 35
  and hypereosinophilic syndrome, 35
Epidermal growth factor and preven-
    tion of bacterial transloca-
    tion, 179–180
Epinephrine, 108
Erythema gangrenosum, 32 (*see also
    Pseudomonas aeruginosa*)
Escherichia coli, 29
  and bacterial translocation, 114,
    122, 126–129, 142
  encapsulated, 198
    and SBP, 198–199
  nonencapsulated, 199
  and resistance to quinolones, 274

[*Escherichia coli*]
  and susceptibility to cefotaxime,
    220
  and susceptibility to quinolones,
    225, 241
  virulence, 109
Esophageal candidiasis, 247
Ethambutol, 95
Ethionamide, 95
Ethylhydroxyethyl cellulose and pre-
    vention of bacterial transloca-
    tion, 171
Experimental cirrhosis, 245

Fecal flora, 247
  and norfloxacin 245–246
Fever, 31, 206
Fibrous encapsulating peritonitis,
    58
First description of SBP, 4, 9, 25–
    26
First episode of SBP, 256–261
  ascitic fluid total protein concentra-
    tion and risk of, 257–258
  cirrhotic patients at high risk of,
    256–261
  serum bilirubin levels and risk of,
    258
Flavobacterium spp. susceptibility to
    norfloxacin, 241
Floroxacin, 226
5-Flucytosine, 155
Fluoroquinolone-resistant gram-nega-
    tive bacteria, 247
  and norfloxacin prophylaxis, 247
Fulminant hepatic failure, 65
  and galactosamine, 124
Fungal infections
  in neutropenic patients, 248
  and norfloxacin prophylaxis, 247
Functional renal failure, 191–192

Galactosamine and bacterial transloca-
    tion, 124

Gastrointestinal bleeding, 206, 208, 213–214, 13/2
and antimicrobial mechanisms, 258
and bacterial infections, 59–60
and bacterial translocation, 59, 130
as cause of death, 213
incidence of bacterial infections, 235, 258
incidence in SBP, 213
failure to control, 59
and pathogenesis of SBP, 214, 238, 258
and predictive factors of bacterial infections, 258
and prevalence of SBP, 235
as prognostic factor in SBP, 200
and risk of nosocomial infection, 258
and risk of SBP, 59, 235, 248, 258
and selective intestinal decontamination, 265
and systemic antibiotics, 264–266
Giardia muris and bacterial translocation, 126
Glutamine in prevention of bacterial translocation, 158–159, 168, 177, 179
Gonococcal perihepatitis, 11, 37
Gonococcal SBP, 55
Gram-negative aerobic bacteria
and recurrence of SBP, 243
susceptibility to cefotaxime, 220–221
susceptibility to quinolones, 225
Gram-positive aerobic bacteria
and recurrence of SBP, 243
susceptibility to cefotaxime, 221
susceptibility to quinolones, 225–226, 243, 247
Granulomas in tuberculous peritonitis, 40
Gyrase-DNA complex and quinolone resistance, 227

Haemophilus ducrei, susceptibility to cefotaxime, 221
Haemophilus influenzae
susceptibility to cefotaxime, 220
susceptibility to quinolones, 225
Halothane, 65
Hematological changes in SBP (*see also* Analytical disturbances), 207
Hematological malignancies
and bacterial translocation, 131
Hemochromatosis, 13, 28
Hepatectomy
and bacterial translocation, 117–118, 123, 132–133, 164
and cisapride, 165
Hepatic encephalopathy, 206, 208, 212–213, 256
incidence in SBP, 212
pathogenesis, 213
prognostic value, 196
and resolution of SBP, 208
severity of, 213
Hepatocellular carcinoma
prognostic factor in SBP, 200, 260
Hepatorenal syndrome, 189–190, 192, 256
type I, 190
type II, 190
History of SBP, 1–28
Hospital-acquired SBP, 17, 199
Hospital mortality of SBP, 190
and hospital-acquired SBP, 17, 199
predictive factors of, 190, 195
Hospital survival
and Child-Pugh score, 195
and liver failure, 194
Hydrothorax, 56
Hyperoxia, 161, 168
Hypertriglyceridemia and fibrous encapsulating peritonitis, 58
Hypocomplementemia, 240
Hypoglycemia, 207
Hypothermia, 11, 31–32

Hypovolemia, 258
  and bacterial translocation, 258
Hypoxemia, 207

Iatrogenic SBP, 9, 38, 63
Ileus, 206, 208, 214–215
  incidence in SBP, 214
  prognostic value, 196, 208, 214
  treatment of, 215
Imipenem, 259 (*see also* Endoscopic
    sclerotherapy)
Incidence of SBP, 255
Indian childhood SBP, 31
Infecting species, 52–54
Inflammatory response and renal im-
    pairment, 198
Ig A and bacterial translocation, 114,
    174, 179
Interleukin-1 β, 197
Interleukin-2, 127
Interleukin-6, 194, 197
  and abdominal trauma, 139
  and bacterial translocation, 118
Intestinal mucosal barrier
  and bacterial translocation, 114–
    115, 131, 137
  and hemorrhagic shock, 115
  and thermal injury, 116
Intestinal obstruction and bacterial
    translocation, 118, 130–131,
    137
Intra-uterine contraceptive devices, 62
Isoniazid, 95

Kayser-Fleischer ring, 29
Klebsiella spp., 29
  and bacterial translocation, 114,
    127, 142
  susceptibility to cefotaxime, 220
  susceptibility to quinolones, 225,
    241, 247

Lactate, 12
  prognostic value of, 196, 207

Lactitol and bacterial translocation,
    129
Lactobacillus acidophilus and bacterial
    translocation, 114, 126, 162,
    164
Lactobacillus plantarium and bacterial
    translocation, 164
Lactobacillus reuteri and bacterial
    translocation, 164
Lactulose
  and antiendotoxinic effects, 161–163
  and prevention of bacterial transloca-
    tion, 171, 178
Laennec's cirrhosis, 28
Laparoscopy in tuberculous peritonitis,
    40
Leukocyte count in SBP, 10, 12, 38
  and renal impairment, 196
Lipid peroxidation, 169–170
Liver failure, 194–195
  and hospital survival, 194
  prognostic value in SBP, 194
  and resolution of SBP, 194
  and risk of SBP, 248, 257
Liver transplantation, 66, 215, 285–
    295
  contraindications of, 288
  survival rates of, 287
Lomefloxacin, 226
Lupus erythematosus, 9, 36

Malignant SBP, 27
Malnutrition and bacterial transloca-
    tion, 127, 130, 175, 177
Management of SBP, 205–218 (*see
    also* Treatment of SBP)
Mean arterial pressure and renal im-
    pairment, 194
Meningococcal SBP, 55
Mesenteric lymph nodes (MLN), 114,
    245
Mesenteric lymphadenectomy in pre-
    vention of bacterial transloca-
    tion, 166

Metastatic hepatic malignancy, 27
Methotrexate and bacterial transloca-
        tion, 164
Metronidazol and bacterial transloca-
        tion, 126
Morganella catarrhalis
    susceptibility to cefotaxime, 220
    susceptibility to quinolones, 225
Morganella morgagnii
    susceptibility to cefotaxime, 220
    susceptibility to quinolones, 225
Multiple organ failure syndrome
        (MOFS), 116–117, 127,
        136, 154
    and bacterial translocation, 139–
        141, 157
Mycobacterium tuberculosis, 87
    bacteriological isolation of, 91
    and CAPD, 61, 90
    and polymerase chain reaction
        (PCR), 91
Mycobacterium avium intracellulare
        (MAI), 91
Myelofibrosis, 11, 27
Myeloid metaplasia, 11

Neisseria spp.
    susceptibility to cefotaxime, 220–
        221
    susceptibility to quinolones,
        225
Neomycin, 108
Neoplastic ascites, 59
Neoplastic SBP, 10, 27
Nephrogenic SBP, 16
Nephrotic syndrome, 11
Nephrotoxic drugs, 212
Neutropenic patients and quinolones,
        243
Nocardia spp., 13
    and CAPD, 61
Nonabsorbable antibiotics, 262–263
Nonadvanced SBP, 189
Noncirrhotic SBP, 59

Nonsteroidal anti-inflammatory drugs
        (NSAIDs), 212
Norfloxacin
    adverse effects of, 243, 245–248,
        263
    antibacterial spectrum of, 241–243
    and antimicrobial capacity of ascitic
        fluid, 263
    and bacterial translocation preven-
        tion, 154–157, 245, 263
    and costs of management of SBP,
        245
    duration of prophylactic treatment,
        245
    efficacy of, 243–245
    and fecal flora, 245–247
    and gram-positive cocci, 157, 247
    in neutropenic patients, 243
    pharmacokinetic properties of, 226,
        241–243
    and prevention of bacterial transloca-
        tion, 156
    and probability of recurrence of
        SBP, 243
    and renal failure, 242
    and resistant bacteria, 245–248,
        263
    and secondary prophylaxis of SBP,
        241–249
    and selective intestinal decontamina-
        tion, 245, 263
    and survival, 243–244

Obstructive jaundice-induced bacte-
        rial translocation, 172–174
Ofloxacin, 188
    in gastrointestinal bleeding, 266
    pharmacokinetic properties, 226,
        243
    in prevention of bacterial transloca-
        tion, 154
    and superinfections, 227
    and systemic infections, 243
    therapeutic efficacy of, 227

Opsonic activity of ascitic fluid, 238–239, 248, 257
Oral antibiotics, 225–229
Oral candidiasis, 247–248

Paracentesis, complications of, 67–68, 259–260
Paracetamol hepatotoxicity, 65
Parenteral nutrition
  and bacterial translocation, 130, 133, 137, 172, 177–180
Parvovirus and SBP, 15, 38–39
Pasteurella multocida, 55
  susceptibility to cefotaxime, 221
Pathogenesis of SBP, 7, 101–112, 262
  and ascites, 107
  and bacteremia, 105–107, 110
  and bacterial translocation, 103–104, 108, 110
    and arterial vasoconstriction, 109
    and bacterial overgrowth, 110
    and lymphatic system, 104, 110
    and mucosal ulceration, 109–110
  and complement, 110
  and diarrhea, 104, 107
  and mucosal barrier permeability, 104
  and portal-systemic shunting, 106–107, 110
  and reticuloendothelial system, 105–106, 110
  and spontaneous portal bacteremia, 105
Pediatric bacterial peritonitis, 8, 11
Pediatric SBP syndrome, 11, 29–30
Pefloxacin, 188, 226
  in prevention of bacterial translocation, 156
Penicillin
  and bacterial translocation, 114, 126, 130
  prevention of, 154, 172
Perforation bacterial peritonitis, 14
Perihepatitis, 11

Peritoneal pseudocyst, 62
Peritoneovenous shunt, 57
  and DIC, 57
  and peritoneal fibrosis, 57–58
  and venous thrombosis, 57
Peyer's patches and bacterial translocation, 126, 166–168
pH in SBP, 12
  prognostic value of, 196, 207
Pharmacokinetic properties
  of cefotaxime, 221
  of quinolones, 226, 241–243
Phospholipids in prevention of bacterial translocation
  phosphotidylcholine, 168, 170
  phosphotidylinositol, 171
Plasma expansion and prevention of renal impairment, 212
Plasma renin activity and renal impairment, 210
Pneumococcal infections, 29–30, 61
Pneumococcal SBP, 110
Polymixin E, 135, 155
Portal hypertension
  and bacterial translocation, 124–125
Portal-systemic shunting, 106–107, 110
  and bacterial translocation, 125
Portal vein thrombosis, 29, 288
Portosystemic encephalomyelopathy, 107
Posthepatitic cirrhosis, 28
Post-transplant SBP, 67
Practolol and sclerosing peritonitis, 58
Predictors
  of bacterial infections in bleeding cirrhotic patients, 258
  of first episode of SBP, 257
  of renal impairment, 192–194, 210
  of resolution of infection, 208
Prednisone and bacterial translocation, 114, 126
Pregnancy, 37

Prevalence of SBP, 11, 75–85, 187, 255
Prevention of SBP (*see also* Prophylaxis of SBP)
 and diuretic therapy, 261
 measures for, 261–264
 and nutritional status, 261
 and recurrence of SBP, 241–249
Primary peritonitis, 8–9, 29–30, 59, 110
Prognosis of SBP, 187–204, 255–256, 286
Prognostic factors of SBP, 189–200
Prokinetic drugs, 215
Prophylactic antibiotics in SBP prophylaxis, 16
 and sclerotherapy, 259
Prophylaxis of SBP, 241–249 (*see also* Prevention of SBP)
 bacterial resistances in, 269, 271, 273–274
 economic costs of, 273
 long-term prophylaxis of SBP, 243, 245, 256
  and bacterial translocation, 245
  and gram-positive bacteria, 228, 243, 245
 nonantibiotic alternatives, 275
 primary prophylaxis of SBP, 255–284
  alternative antibiotics, 269–270
  extraperitoneal infections, 268
  incidence of SBP, 268
  risk groups, 268
  survival, 268
 short-term prophylaxis, 264–267, 270
 side effects of, 270–272
 and survival, 272
 systemic antibiotics in, 16
Propionibacterium acnes, 172
Prosthetic devices and SBP, 11, 62

Proteus spp.
 and bacterial translocation, 114, 126–127, 142
 susceptibility to cefotaxime, 220
 susceptibility to quinolones, 225, 241, 247
Protoglycan and prevention of bacterial translocation, 179
Providencia spp. and susceptibility to quinolones, 225
Pseudomonas aeruginosa
 and ecthyma granulosum, 13
 and erythema gangrenosum, 32
 and peritoneal dialysis, 104
 susceptibility to cefotaxime, 220
 susceptibility to quinolones, 225
Pseudomonas cepacia and CAPD, 61
Pyrazinamide, 95
Pyrogenic cytokines, 31

Quinolones, 225–229
 antibacterial activity of, 225–226
 bacterial resistance to, 140, 227–228, 245–248, 263, 274–275
 pharmacokinetic properties of, 226
 therapeutic efficacy of, 227–229

Recurrence of SBP, 15, 27, 66–67
 and liver function, 235, 248
 prevention of, 241–249
 probability of, 243
 risk factors, 235
Regional enteritis and bacterial translocation, 109
Renal impairment in SBP, 16, 189–194, 209–212, 256
 categories, 191, 209–210
 hospital mortality of, 190, 193–194, 210
 incidence of, 190–191, 209
 pathogenesis of, 193, 198, 210
 prevention of, 212
Resolution of infection, 188, 205
 and Child-Pugh score, 195

Reticuloendothelial system (RES),
        105–106, 110, 132, 214
    activity of, 240, 248, 257
    and bacterial infections, 257
    and chemotaxis, 240
    and gastrointestinal hemorrhage, 59
    hepatic RES, 240
    and hypocomplementemia, 240
Rheumatoid arthritis, 9, 36
Rhodococci, 12
Ricinoleic acid and bacterial transloca-
        tion, 115, 125–126
Rifampicin, 95
Rifaximin
    and bacterial translocation, 129
    prevention of, 156
Risk factors for SBP, 233–240
Rufloxacin, 263

Salmonella enteritidis and bacterial
        translocation, 126, 171
Salmonella minnesota and bacterial
        translocation, 122
Salmonella spp., 54–55
    susceptibility to cefotaxime, 220
    susceptibility to quinolones, 225, 241
Schistosomiasis, 29
Sclerosing peritonitis, 58
Scrotal swelling in SBP, 11, 32, 35
Selective intestinal decontamination,
        16, 241–248, 262–263 (*see
        also* Prophylaxis of SBP)
    and bacterial translocation, 137
    prevention of, 139–141, 154–
        157
Septic shock, 196, 206–208
Serratia marcescens and bacterial
        translocation, 123
Serratia spp.
    susceptibility to cefotaxime, 220
    susceptibility to quinolones, 225,
        241
Serum bilirubin levels, 195, 258
Serum cholesterol and hospital mortal-
        ity, 190

Serum creatinine, 190, 193
    in hepatorenal syndrome, 190
    and hospital mortality, 190
    and resolution of SBP, 208
Serum sodium concentration
    and hospital mortality, 190
    and renal impairment, 210
Severity of infection, 195–198, 206–
        208
Shigella spp.
    susceptibility to cefotaxime, 220
    susceptibility to quinolones, 225,
        241
Shock, endotoxin-induced shock, 116
Short-chain fatty acids, 162
Silent SBP, 26, 102
Sparfloxacin, 225
Species of bacteria causing SBP, 29
Spontaneous bacterial arthritis, 58
Spontaneous bacterial cystitis, 59
Spontaneous bacterial empyema, 10,
        26, 55–57
Spontaneous portal bacteremia, 105
Splenectomy in prevention of bacterial
        translocation, 165–167
Staphylococcus aureus
    and peritoneal dialysis, 104, 111
    susceptibility to cefotaxime, 221
    susceptibility to quinolones, 225, 241
Staphylococcus enteritidis and perito-
        neal dialysis, 104, 111
Staphylococcus epidermidis
    and bacterial translocation, 126
    susceptibility to cefotaxime, 221
    susceptibility to quinolones, 226, 241
    and ventriculoperitoneal shunts, 62
Staphylococcus haemolyticus and sus-
        ceptibility to quinolones, 226
Staphylococcus saprophyticus and sus-
        ceptibility to quinolones, 226
Stenotrophomona maltophilia, suscepti-
        bility to cefotaxime, 220
Streptococcus spp.
    bovis, 131
    pneumoniae, 110

[*Streptococcus* spp.]
susceptibility to cefotaxime, 221
susceptibility to quinolones, 226,
239
Streptomycin, 95, 139–140, 154, 172
Streptozotocin nd bacterial transloca-
tion, 126
Sterile ascites, 50–51
Subacute bacterial endocarditis, 106
Superinfections, 205
Survival rate, 66, 188–189, 286
long-term survival of SBP, 248
Symptomatic bacterascites, 50–51, 79
Systemic antibiotics, 264
Systemic lupus erythematosus, 36
Systemic vasoconstrictors and treat-
ment of renal impairment in
SBP, 212

Thermal injury and bacterial translocation, 116–117, 137–138
Timolol, 58
Tobramycin, 136, 156, 222
Tosufloxacin, 226
Transjugular intrahepatic portosystemic shunt (TIPS) and SBP,
63–64, 107
Translocation (*see* Bacterial translocation)
Transmural migration of intestinal bacteria, 9
Trimethoprim-sulfamethoxazole, 139–
140, 154, 263
Tuberculosis
and AIDS, 89–90
prevalence of, 87
Tuberculous peritonitis, 9, 15, 39–40,
58, 87–100
association with other diseases, 94–
95
as cause of ascites, 90
and CAPD, 90, 94
and peritoneal fibrosis, 94
and chronic liver disease, 89–90
clinical presentation of, 87–89

[Tuberculous peritonitis]
diagnosis of, 91–94
and adenosine deaminase activity
(ADA), 15, 93
and PPD skin test, 90
differential diagnosis of, 93
and drug resistance, 90
imaging in, 94
series of cases, 88
treatment of, 95–96
immunotherapy, 95
first-line antituberculous drugs, 95
second-line antituberculous drugs, 95
Tumor necrosis factor (TNF), 197
and abdominal trauma, 139
and bacterial translocation, 118

Ulcerative colitis and bacterial trans1o-
cation, 109
Urinary tract infections, 205, 243, 247

Variations on a theme, 25–45
Vasopressin,10, 26, 38, 108
Venous thrombosis in peritoneovenous
shunt, 57
Ventriculoperitoneal shunt, 62
Vibrio spp., 33, 55
and CAPD, 60
Virulence of intestinal bacteria, 109
Vitamin C, 170
Vitamin E, 170

Widal agglutination test (*see also Yersinial* spp.), 54
Wilson's disease, 14, 28

Xanthine oxidase, 116–117, 127, 167, 175
Xanthomonas maltophilia, and norfloxacin, 140–141, 157

Yersinial spp., 13, 28, 54
and hemochromatosis, 54
susceptibility to quinolones, 225

Zymosan and bacterial translocation,
127, 154

About the Authors

Harold O. Conn is Emeritus Professor of Medicine, Yale University School of Medicine, New Haven, Connecticut, and Professor of Surgery, Division of Liver and Bowel Transplantation, University of Miami School of Medicine, Florida, where he is a consultant. Dr. Conn has published more than 300 articles in peer-reviewed medical journals and six books on various topics dealing with the liver and portal hypertension, and has presented invited lectures at more than 150 of the leading medical institutions in the United States and abroad. He has served as editor of *Hepatology* and *Gerontology* and on the editorial board of numerous journals, and is past president of American Association for the Study of Liver Disease. Dr. Conn received the B.S. and M.D. (1950) degrees from the University of Michigan, Ann Arbor, and the M.S. degree (1972) from Yale University, New Haven, Connecticut.

Juan Rodés is Professor of Medicine, University of Barcelona, Spain, and Research Director, Hospital Clinic of Barcelona, Spain. The author or coauthor of over 350 original articles, 25 books, and 80 book chapters, Dr. Rodés is editor-in-chief of the *Journal of Hepatology*. He received the M.D. degree (1967) from the University of Barcelona, Spain.

Miguel Navasa is Associate Professor of Medicine, University of Barcelona, Spain, and Senior Specialist of the Liver Unit, Hospital Clinic of Barcelona, Spain. The author or coauthor of over 135 original articles in international journals, book chapters, and reviews, Dr. Navasa is a member of the Spanish, European, and American Associations for the Study of Liver Diseases. He graduated in medicine and surgery (1979), obtained the specialty in gastroenterology (1985), and received the M.D. degree (1990) from the University of Barcelona, Spain.